DIET AND DISEASE

Other Keats Titles of Related Interest

BRAIN ALLERGIES by William H. Philpott, M.D. and Dwight K. Kalita, Ph.D.

THE HEALING NUTRIENTS WITHIN: Facts, Findings and New Research on Amino Acids by Eric R. Braverman, M.D. with Carl C. Pfeiffer, M.D., Ph.D.

MEDICAL APPLICATIONS OF CLINICAL NUTRITION edited by Jeffrey Bland, Ph.D.

MENTAL AND ELEMENTAL NUTRIENTS by Carl C. Pfeiffer, M.D., Ph.D.

THE NUTRITION DESK REFERENCE by Robert H. Garrison, Jr., M.A., R.Ph. and Elizabeth Somer, M.A.

NUTRIENTS TO AGE WITHOUT SENILITY by Abram Hoffer, M.D., Ph.D. and Morton Walker, D.P.M.

ORTHOMOLECULAR NUTRITION by Abram Hoffer, M.D., Ph.D. and Morton Walker, D.P.M.

A PHYSICIAN'S HANDBOOK ON ORTHOMOLECULAR MEDICINE edited by Roger J. Williams, Ph.D. and Dwight K. Kalita, Ph.D.

PREDICTIVE MEDICINE by E. Cheraskin, M.D., D.M.D. and W. M. Ringsdorf, D.M.D.

1984–85 YEARBOOK OF NUTRITIONAL MEDICINE edited by Jeffrey Bland, Ph.D.

1986: A YEAR IN NUTRITIONAL MEDICINE edited by Jeffrey Bland, Ph.D.

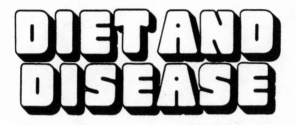

DIET AND DISEASE

E. Cheraskin, M.D., D.M.D.
W. M. Ringsdorf, Jr., D.M.D.
J. W. Clark, D.D.S.

With a New Preface to the 1987 Edition by Dr. Cheraskin

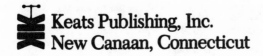
Keats Publishing, Inc.
New Canaan, Connecticut

DIET AND DISEASE

Published by arrangement with Rodale Press, Emmaus, Pennsylvania

Library of Congress Cataloging-in-Publication Data

Cheraskin, E. (Emanuel), 1916-
  Diet and disease.

  Reprint. Originally published: Emmaus, Pa. : Rodale Books, 1968.
  Includes bibliographies and index.
  1. Nutritionally induced diseases. I. Ringsdorf, W. M. II. Clark, James W., 1924- . III. Title.
[DNLM: 1. Diet Therapy—popular works. 2. Nutrition—popular works. WB 400 C521d 1968a]
RC622.C48 1987   616.3'9   87-3001
ISBN 0-87983-431-5

Printed in the United States of America

Keats Health Science Books are published by
Keats Publishing, Inc.
27 Pine Street (PO Box 876)
New Canaan, Connecticut 06840

Table of Contents

ACKNOWLEDGMENTS

WE WISH TO TAKE THIS OPPORTUNITY TO RECOGNIZE THE MANY who have shared in the creation of this book. The hundreds of experiments comprising the heart of the text are the products of scores of investigators. Citation in the bibliographic sections is admittedly an inadequate but the only feasible way of recognizing their contributions. Without the able secretarial and administrative support of Mrs. Alda McDowell, Mrs. Sybil Evans, Miss Diana Rediker, Mrs. Tonni Maddox, and Miss Virginia Chybowski, this monograph could not have come to completion. Skillful artistic and photographic assistance was provided by Doctor A. T. S. H. Setyaadmadja and Doctor R. A. Barrett. Our own research efforts would not have been possible without the technologic assistance of Mrs. Dorothy Ginn and Mrs. Frances Medford. A great indebtedness is owed to Mrs. Sarah Brown and her patient staff for their library research contributions. We are especially grateful to the University of Alabama Medical Center Administration, particularly Doctor J. F. Volker and Doctor C. A. McCallum, for providing an academic atmosphere conducive to research and scientific writing. Finally, a great debt is owed many others for many reasons. However, the synthesis of the material and its interpretation is all our own, for which we must accept full responsibility.

E. Cheraskin, M.D., D.M.D.
W. M. Ringsdorf, Jr., D.M.D., M.S.
J. W. Clark, D.D.S.

PREFACE TO THE 1987 EDITION:

Happy Anniversary!

MY COLLEAGUES, THAT IS DR. JAMES W. CLARK AND DR. WARREN MARSHALL Ringsdorf, Jr., are excited to be here with me to share in the twentieth birthday of DIET AND DISEASE. After all, what are birthdays for if not to celebrate and reminisce?

This is a good time to recall that DIET AND DISEASE was conceived in 1966, more than twenty years ago. All three of us had been trained in classical medicine and dentistry—there were not then nor are there now groovy medical or dental schools—and our traditional orientation should have convinced us of the relative unimportance of diet as a factor in disease. But all three of us, for reasons we shall never know, happily sought out each, other convinced that man is a food-dependent creature (if you stop feeding him, he will die) and that when man dies, all parts of man die. Then, and regretfully even now in some cases, that was strange talk from fringe groups (meaning outside of conventional medical/dental circles).

But the evidence was there—true, largely ignored but right smack in the publications of the American Medical Association and the American Dental Association, the *Journal of the American Dietetic Association*, the *American Journal of Clinical Nutrition*, the *New England Journal of Medicine* and scores of other standard texts and conventional periodicals. And really, all that has changed is that there is more information today than in 1968 . . . and nothing that contradicts what we reported then in DIET AND DISEASE.

And what we learned (as have others) is what we knew already. Those who do not read history must repeat it, and this is precisely what has been happening during the past twenty years.

For example, the revered RDA took a big tumble last year. The National Academy of Sciences/National Research Council (the famous quasigovernmental agency that has been providing the nation with the "gold standard" for our eating habits from 1943 through nine editions of its publication) just last year turned down its own subcommittee's recommendation. It argued that some of the suggestions from its Committee on Recommended Dietary Allowances were preposterous. For its unpublished tenth revised edition, it has left us, to some extent, for the first time in forty years with a non-RDA!

The prestigious American Heart Association and the world-renowned National Heart Institute, along with many other cardiology and cardiovascular bodies during most of the past two decades, have started to suggest that diet may well be the single most important ingredient in the causation of overall heart disease. The business of cholesterol in the food and in the diet, the role of fiber, for example, sound almost like the food faddists in the thirties and forties. *In the interest of accuracy, I have to point out that this was reported in* DIET AND DISEASE *twenty years ago!*

The famous National Cancer Institute and the prominent American Cancer Society, as well as other oncologic agencies, are now claiming that a significant amount of cancer may be directly related to what we eat—*just as we described in* DIET AND DISEASE *twenty years ago!*

A more humorous, though not necessarily less serious or significant, note is stuck by a poll recently conducted of the eating habits of registered dietitians in the State of Washington. Parenthetic mention should be made that the American Dietetic Association has as one of its principal tenets that a good diet meets all nutritional needs—supplementation is not necessary. Interestingly enough, the recent poll suggests that approximately sixty percent of registered dietitians in the State of Washington consume on a more or less regular basis multivitamin/trace mineral supplements. *Let the record show that we talked about the need for supplementation in* DIET AND DISEASE *twenty years ago!*

We knew then and know now that all disease is not due to diet. However, with the burgeoning interest in tobacco, alcohol, physical activity and pollution, we may well be approaching a realistic mosaic of lifestyle and disease and putting into proper focus the great significance of the relationship between diet and disease.

Emanuel Cheraskin, M.D., D.M.D.
March 1987

DIET AND DISEASE

You would be surprised at the number of years it took me to see clearly what some of the problems were which had to be solved.... Looking back, I think it was more difficult to see what the problems were than to solve them.

Charles Darwin

PREFACE

ONE OF THE MOST PERPLEXING PROBLEMS FACING A CONSCIENTIOUS
student in any field of endeavour is how to winnow the wheat
from the chaff in the twentieth-century publication explosion.

In most fields, the *number* of available texts seems adequate. One more manuscript adds not so much to man's store
of knowledge as to the task of winnowing. Hence a new book,
to justify its publication--be it about nature, nurture, or navi-
gation--should make a distinctive contribution. What then,
one may reasonably ask, is the justification for this book? As
simple as it may appear, the rightful place of diet in the
ecology of health and disease as witnessed in the United
States, has seemingly not been accorded just consideration.

Therefore, DIET AND DISEASE opens with a description of
what the average American eats. This story, to our knowledge,
has not been attempted in book form. It continues with a
survey of the most killing and crippling diseases which plague
him. This is followed with a discussion of the ingredients,
including diet, which make for health and disease. Insight
into the amazingly intricate interdependency of the major
nutrients is provided in the closing chapter of Part One.

Part Two attempts to tell the story of the role of diet but
not in the rare classical deficiency diseases. Rather, it describes the more common and seemingly diverse ailments and
problems in man's womb-to-tomb journey. Thus, it begins
with infertility, the commencement of life, and concludes
with ischemic heart disease and cancer in the autumnal days.
The material covered in this section has been culled from
many sources. This is attested to by the considerable, if not
complete, appended references. The *real* contribution of this
section is the focusing of attention upon the role of diet in

common afflictions not usually regarded as "nutritional" in nature.

In the final section (Part Three), the common dietary threads observed in the syndromes reported in Part Two are examined. Lastly, the diets characteristic of health and disease are delineated.

Considered collectively, the information within these pages suggests that the role of diet as a factor in the development of diseases afflicting the nation may have been grossly underestimated. To quote Charles Darwin: "Looking back, I think it was more difficult to see what the problems were than to solve them."

DIET AND DISEASE is a beginning. We shall look for counsel from our readers for subsequent revisions. More importantly, it is hoped that these words will catalyze more and better understanding of the relationship between diet and disease.

E. Cheraskin, M.D., D.M.D.
W. M. Ringsdorf, Jr., D.M.D., M.S.
J. W. Clark, D.D.S.

PART ONE

INTRODUCTION

DIET AND DISEASE SUGGESTS POSSIBLE PARALLELISMS BETWEEN dietary derangement and disease. To set the stage for such an analysis, it is first imperative to examine independently the dietary patterns of the public and the scope, both qualitatively and quantitatively, of disease.

It is well established that the food supplies in this country are warranty against starvation. Despite this incontrovertible fact, the adequacy of the American diet remains the subject of debate. Surprisingly, a systematic analysis of the many links in the garden-to-gullet chain has seldom been reported in a clinically-oriented nutrition text. For this reason, this section opens with a study of the American diet based upon governmental and other institutional reports.

The prevailing climate of both morbidity and mortality attests to the rising importance of the chronic diseases. In addition to the obviously ill, silent sickness of increasing magnitude is being uncovered during the routine screening examination of apparently well people. It is noteworthy that the health and sickness patterns of the nation, and particularly those of the common killing and crippling disorders, are not a principal feature in nutrition books although most authors allude to dietary relationships. It is fitting, therefore, that Chapter Two is dedicated to a study of the incidence and prevalence of some of the more commonplace diseases.

Ecologic observations have provided two essential conclusions regarding the nature of disease; namely, disease is the result of a constellation of factors and, second, it occurs in an endless series of gradations. The interplay of host factors and environmental challenges constitutes the only tenable basis for the etiology of health and disease. This book departs from traditional practice by weaving diet into the very fabric of the ecology of all disease. Consequently, the third chapter describes the factors which contribute to health and disease with particular emphasis placed upon diet.

The customary description of a nutritional disorder leaves the reader with the conclusion that dietary afflictions can be neatly catalogued on the basis of single nutrients. To a degree, this obtains in classical nutritional syndromes where it may be related to a prominent clinical characteristic (e.g. bleeding in scurvy) the result of an obvious and severe deficit. However, in the more common instances of allegedly non-nutritional disorders (e.g. mental retardation), the dietary effect is based upon a disruption of nutritional balance rather than simply a deficit or excess of a single nutrient. Thus, the last chapter in Part One explores the interdependency of putatively independent nutrients.

1. THE AMERICAN DIET

THE RAISON D'ETRE OF THIS TEXT IS TO ILLUMINATE KNOWN relationships between *diet* and *disease*. Accordingly, it is appropriate in this introductory chapter to consider the first of the ingredients, namely the diet of the American public.

The late Doctor Tom D. Spies (Professor of Nutrition and Metabolism, Northwestern University Medical School and Director of the Nutrition Clinic, Hillman Hospital, Birmingham, Alabama) epitomized the place of diet in health and disease *(32):*

> Today germs are not our principal enemy. Our chief medical adversary is what I consider a disturbance of the inner balance of the constituents of our tissues, which are built from and maintained by necessary chemicals in the air we breathe, the water we drink and the food we eat. For a generation we have worked on the concept that our cells are never static and that in time must be replaced in varying degrees by the nutrients obtained from food. More specifically, our working hypothesis has been that all disease is chemical and, when we know enough, chemically correctable.

Doctor Willard A. Krehl (Research Professor of Medicine at the Clinical Research Center, University Hospitals, Iowa City) delivered a notable prognostication before the *Symposium on Recent Advances in the Appraisal of the Nutrient Intake and the Nutritional Status of Man* at the Massachusetts Institute of Technology on 6-7 March 1962 *(23):*

> Greater realization is needed in medicine and in public health that good nutrition along with good hygiene are the best weapons available in the prevention of disease. If one were bold enough to make a prediction, it would be that *the most important measure* (italics added) that could be taken to prevent the development of many chronic diseases would be the provision

of consistently good individual nutrition, supervised by physicians with a strong assistance from the housewife, from conception to the grave.

TRENDS IN THE AMERICAN DIET

In 1962, Doctor Margaret A. Ohlson (formerly Director of Nutrition Services and Professor, Department of Internal Medicine, State University of Iowa) presented arresting data on available retail foods *(28)*:

Estimates of food available in retail channels per capita of population can be found in the reports of the U.S. Department of Commerce and, for recent years, the U.S. Department of Agriculture (for the period from 1889 to the present). Certain well marked trends can be identified.

The consumer supplies of two basic sources of starch, i.e. cereals and potatoes, have decreased sharply. At the same time, the form of market cereals has changed from bread flour to highly processed bakery products and the prepared type of breakfast cereal. The per capita supply of refined sugar has increased from 50 pounds per man per year to about 100 pounds.

Even more recently, Doctor Ohlson and her associates published an exhaustive account of changes in retail market food supplies in the United States. An analysis of trends in the American diet over the last seventy years revealed the following alterations *(2)*:

The data presented indicate clearly that the major changes in the American diet over the last seventy years are a slight decrease in supply of total calories per man per day; a considerable decrease in the consumption of total carbohydrates with a greater progressive decline in the intake of complex carbohydrate from flours, cereals and potatoes and a concurrent dramatic increase of simple sugars, especially in the first part of this century; a slight increase in total fat consumption contributed mainly by the increase of unsaturated fatty acids and due to the lesser supplies of cereal and milk proteins, total protein consumption has decreased.

The dramatic major change in carbohydrate supplies is vividly portrayed in Figure 1.1 *(2)*. The most obvious shift is a *reduction* of approximately 54 per cent in complex carbohydrates in parallel with a 50 per cent *increase* in simple sugars netting a reversal from a dominantly complex to a simple carbohydrate diet. Parenthetic mention should be made that, during the same time interval, sugars and syrups collectively more than doubled. Fluctuations in the retail total fat (an increase of 12 per cent) and protein (a decrease of 6 per cent) supplies have been surprisingly small. Actually a 37 per cent increase in the ratio of polyunsaturated to saturated fatty acids is thought to be a favorable trend (2).

In the light of the striking trends in carbohydrate consumption during the twentieth century, Doctor Samuel Soskin and Doctor Rachmiel Levine, in their contribution to the classical text, *Modern Nutrition in Health and Disease,* postulate (31):

> It is known that the vitamin B complex plays an integral part in carbohydrate metabolism and that the need for this group of vitamins depends upon the amount of carbohydrate eaten. Why was knowledge of its existence not acquired much earlier in human experience and why did the race not suffer from lack of that knowledge? The answer to these questions is that it was only in comparatively recent times that the natural union between the vitamin B complex and carbohydrate, a union existing in whole grain and plants, was broken by the industrial processing of foods. Before this occurred, the supply of B vitamins was automatically adjusted to the amount of carbohydrate eaten; the occurrence of vitamin B deficiency with its consequent disturbance in nutrition is, therefore, a comparatively recent development in the Western World.

Thus, not only has there been a considerable change in available quantities of carbohydrate, but a critical qualitative mutation has also transpired. In addition to the relatively diminished nutritional value of some of the carbohydrate consumed today, its replacement of high quality foods, in the diets of children (20) and adults (Table 1.1) (27, 35), may invite nutritional disturbances (27, 35). From this chart, it is evident that the consumed sweets and desserts exceed by two to threefold the recommended amounts. In the case of animal protein, the average intake is approximately one-half to one-fifth the suggested consumption.

Considerable changes in the nutrient content of the retail food supply have taken place during the past few decades. Table 1.2 (18) highlights the magnitude of change for the period 1944 to 1958 for eleven nutrients. The American dietary paradox, according to the author, is spelled out (18):

The United States has the greatest food production capability in the world, the widest varieties of food products and the largest surpluses of food. Yet there is widespread nutritional starvation or malnutrition which is often shown by clinical or subclinical signs and symptoms.

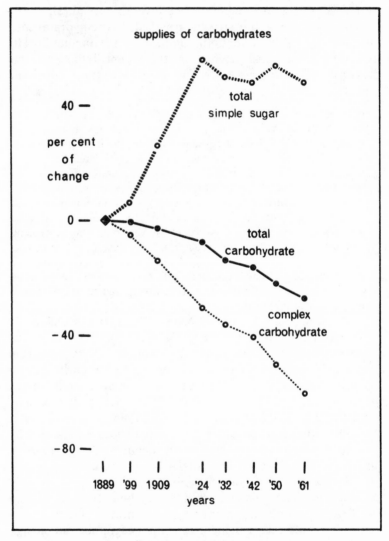

Figure 1.1. Percentage changes in supplies of carbohydrates available to retail markets from 1889 to 1961.

Table 1.1
average amounts of foods eaten by adults (27)*
and those recommended (35)** in pounds per week

region	age and sex	meat, poultry, fish		cereal products		sweets and desserts	
		*	**	*	**	*	**
North Central	30-39F	1.71	4.25	2.16	2.25	1.52	0.75
	40-49F	1.60	4.25	2.21	2.25	1.50	0.75
	50-59F	1.63	4.25	2.04	2.25	1.49	0.75
California	50-59F	1.80	4.25	1.62	2.25	2.09	0.75
North Central	60-69F	1.32	4.25	2.22	2.25	1.31	0.75
California	60-69F	1.78	4.25	1.69	2.25	1.95	0.75
North Central	70+F	0.93	4.25	2.10	2.25	1.10	0.75
California	70+F	1.48	4.25	1.60	2.25	1.75	0.75
California	50-59M	2.75	5.25	2.41	3.50	3.13	1.25
	60-69M	2.51	5.25	2.36	3.50	2.87	1.25
	70+M	2.05	5.25	1.80	3.50	2.32	1.25

Table 1.2
differences in nutrients
available for consumption per
capita between 1944 and 1958

nutrient	per cent difference between 1944 and 1958
ascorbic acid	−23
vitamin A	−22
thiamine	−16
folic acid	−14
iron	−13
niacin	−8
calories	−7
riboflavin	−6
protein	−5
calcium	−3
fat	+1

RELATED DIETARY TRENDS

In their text, *Nutrition and Atherosclerosis*, Doctors Louis N. Katz, Jeremiah Stamler, and Ruth Pick *(22)* (Michael Reese Hospital, Medical Research Institute) have noted the association of economic prosperity with a "rich" diet throughout history:

...contemporary American patterns of diet represent relatively recent innovations in nutrition. They are diets markedly different in composition, qualitatively and quantitatively from any ever consumed by wild animals or most pre-literate peoples. These nutritional patterns are relatively recent products of a long and complex development. In terms of the time scale of human evolution, their origins go back only about 8,000 years. Prior to that time, man had been exclusively a food gatherer. He had not yet learned to be a food producer. Inevitably, therefore his eating habits differed markedly from ours. Composed of a variety of natural unprocessed foods, yielding a high ratio of essential nutrients to calories, his diets were invariably well nourishing and well balanced (as long as nature's bounty was adequate). In the Fertile Crescent of the Middle East, man made the decisive historic leap from food gathering to food producing, and became a farmer and herder. This Neolithic transition created the economic pre-conditions for urban life. It also made available for the first time many of the foods commonly consumed by most Americans today, e.g. dairy products, eggs, cereals, breads and other foods. In the economically developed countries a marked change in nutritional patterns has occurred during the last century. In conjunction with industrialization, urbanization and increase in per capita national income, 'richer' diets have become commonplace — diets containing sizable quantities of the more expensive high-lipid foods of animal origin plus 'elegant' white bread and refined sugar. These foods are now consumed en masse in countries like the United States.

An increase in protein consumption has accompanied the increase in fat and sugar in some of the wealthier countries. However, the protein increases have not been of equal magnitude and have been evident largely in the lower classes. For example, in the United Kingdom, this is well illustrated by observing these changes when grouped according to annual income *(38)*. It can be noted (Table 1.3) that the only rise (10 per cent) in meat consumption since 1936 occurred in the lower income group despite the relative stability of the distribution of the economic groups.

In summarizing the basic flaws in the dietary of economically developed countries, Doctor Katz and his associates *(22)* have emphasized that bad nutrition (malnutrition) is more descriptive of the prevailing situation than undernutrition. The nature of the aberration is (1) an excess of total calories, empty calories, total fat, saturated fat, cholesterol, refined sugar, salt, and (2) an inadequacy (relative and/or absolute) of essential nutrients (vitamins, minerals, essential amino acids and essential fatty acids) and bulk. Thus malnutrition of a different type is actually widespread in the economically developed countries — malnutrition in the literal meaning of the word, bad nutrition.

Table 1.3
United Kingdom meat consumption
per capita related to income and
percentage of population in each income class

income class	consumption ounces/ week 1936	1960	per cent change	percentage of population 1936	1960
lower	32	35	+10	50	52
middle	43	36	−16	40	38
upper	49	38	−22	10	10

There has been an increasing anxiety among nutritionists concerning the competition between sugar-containing foods and the much needed protein-rich foodstuffs in poorer countries. In the rapid growth areas of some of these countries, there is a tendency for the poorest people to buy sweet foods and drinks for their children in lieu of milk *(38)*.

It has been reported that the quarter of the world's population with the lowest food consumption had even less to eat in 1954 than prior to World War II. The deficit was greatest for milk and meat. During the same period, sugar consumption had increased by more than 50 per cent *(38)*.

Calculations (1958) for nine low-income countries (Brazil, Ceylon, Chile, Egypt, Greece, India, Pakistan, Philippines, and Yugoslavia) with a collective population of some 650 million people, revealed that caloric intake compared with the prewar period had increased by 9 per cent. During this same interval, however, meat consumption declined 9 per cent, animal protein decreased 7 per cent, and sugar consumption increased 105 per cent *(38)*. The drastic increase in dietary sugar in various regions of the world may be noted in Table 1.4 *(38)*.

It is obvious that North America has set the pace for sugar consumption. The per capita intake that the United States had achieved before World War II is now being approached by Western Europe and South America. The remainder of the world is rapidly closing the gap. In Britain, sugar in all its forms, excluding that used in brewing and distilling, now provides 18 per cent of the total calories consumed and 37 per cent of the total carbohydrate — twice as much as at the turn of the century *(14)*. As a result of the demand for sugar and sugar products, its production increase has outstripped that of all other food items (Figure 1.2) *(38)*. Summarily, the yearly world per capita sugar consumption increased 282 per cent from 1899 to 1957 *(38)*.

Thus, a change in the pattern of carbohydrate intake appears to be the most obvious alteration in the world's dietary during the twentieth century. This pattern essentially involves a reduction in complex carbohydrates and an increase in simple ones *(1, 2, 9, 14, 33, 38)*.

Table 1.4
regional per capita increase in
yearly sugar consumption (kilograms)

region	prewar	1957	per cent increase
Near East	4.9	12.4	145
Africa	5.0	10.0	100
Eastern Europe + USSR	12.9	25.8	100
South America	16.8	29.1	73
Central America	16.6	28.3	70
Far East (excluding China)	4.7	6.6	40
Western Europe	25.2	32.4	27
Oceania	43.3	45.4	5
North America	46.5	46.1	−1

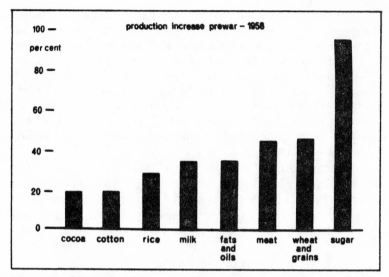

Figure 1.2. Percentage increase in 1958 over prewar production of some agricultural commodities.

According to Doctor John Yudkin (Professor of Nutrition and Dietetics, Queen Elizabeth College, University of London) the separation of nutrition and palatability has been partially responsible for the changes in carbohydrate consumption (37). He points out that the ability of the food technologist to effect this change means that taste is no longer a guide to the ingestion of nutritious foods.

One may note from the discussion thus far that American dietary habits are influencing food consumption around the world. If United States plant breeders are equally influential in the underdeveloped nations in substituting plant varieties for native ones, the nutrient content of the foods of these nations may be further reduced. This is vividly demonstrated by comparing the nutritional quality of food varieties grown in this country and in Mexico and Central America. Doctor Robert S. Harris (15) (Professor of Biochemistry of Nutrition, Massachusetts Institute of Technology) pointed out that foods grown in the United States do not always favorably compare with those of other countries.

A detailed examination of data on Mexican foods revealed that in a number of instances the variety of a food plant produced in Mexico or Central America was higher in nutritional value than the same food grown in the United States. The Latin American varieties were generally more nutritious. In his eagerness to produce more kernels per row, more rows per ear, and more ears per stalk, the plant breeder has sacrificed nutrient content. In his desire to produce lovelier apples, sweeter oranges, blander vegetables, ship-resistant foods, he has often produced varieties which are less nutritious per pound. It is usually possible to obtain all these desirable effects without impairing the nutritional quality, if the plant breeder adds the nutritional factor to his working equation.

A comparison of middle American (Central American and Mexican) versus United States varieties of foods may be noted in Table 1.5 *(15)*. Considering each nutrient analyzed, there are Central American food varieties which exceed the maximal United States value in every case except nicotinic acid.

ADEQUACY OF THE AMERICAN DIET

A marked difference of opinion prevails as to what constitutes an adequate diet. To some, a sufficient caloric intake and the absence of classical deficiency diseases is proof that the prevailing American diet is adequate. On the other hand, there are those who hold that dietary inadequacies are common in the United States even though an abundance of food exists. Doctor Robert S. Goodhart, President and Scientific Director of the National Vitamin Foundation, in two interesting reports, *How Well Nourished Are Americans?*, I and II *(12, 13)*, has carefully researched the findings fundamental to this controversy.

The papers summarized in this report indicate that variable but substantial proportions of subgroups of our population consume diets which fall short of the Recommended Dietary Allowances for Vitamin A, thiamin, riboflavin and ascorbic acid, the vitamins routinely studied in nutrition survey work. Wherever body fluid levels were determined, like proportions of the population were found to have levels of these vitamins below accepted normal values.

For different groups of persons and for the different vitamins, the proportion consuming less than two-thirds of the Recommended Dietary Allowances ranges from less than five to more than 70 per cent....

While the studies discussed here do not represent a valid cross

Table 1.5

comparison of the number of plant foods
(as listed in food tables) in Middle
America versus United States which exceed
a specified minimal nutrient value

		number of foods which exceed standard	
nutrient	standard	Middle America	United States
nitrogen	2,500.0	20 (1)*	8
calcium	100.0	39 (6)	12
iron	3.0	51 (10)	19
carotene	2.0	32 (3)	14
thiamine	0.2	42 (5)	16
riboflavin	0.2	34 (1)	13
nicotinic acid	2.0	31 (0)	13
ascorbic acid	75.0	48 (20)	7

*number of Middle American plant foods with nutrient values exceeding the highest found in the United States noted in parenthesis

section of the population of the United States, we believe that they, in conjunction with those in our first report on How Well Nourished Are Americans? (National Vitamin Foundation, 1960 Annual Report) provide incontrovertible proof that a great many Americans of all ages and socio-economic brackets are subsisting on diets which fall substantially short of the Recommended Dietary Allowances in respect to one or more essential nutrients.

Doctor R. S. Harris *(15)* noted in a comparison of United States and Middle American foods that the Latin American varieties were generally more nutritious. A comparable situation exists within the United States. Not only are inter- and intravariety differences in food nutrient content present within a particular state in this country, but they are no less evident in interstate comparisons *(18)*. For instance, Table 1.6 shows a difference of 12 grams of vitamin C per 100 grams of juice for two varieties of California oranges and between Valencia oranges from two different geographic locales.

The urbanization of America, with all of its advantages, has been fraught with many problems not the least of which is the diet. For example, the unrivaled transportation network has brought a variety of foods, previously not attainable, to the city dweller throughout the year. Yet, it is quite rare today for one to purchase locally grown foods within 24 hours of their harvest time. Most fresh produce must be shipped for long distances and stored for varying periods of time. Additionally, because of the time lapse between harvest and consumption, processors have extended the shelf life of many foods. This, plus food preparation, invites nutrient loss. Illustrative of this problem are the effects of these factors upon the nutrient content of the Irish potato (Table 1.7) *(4)*. An analysis of the ascorbic acid content of potatoes revealed a 91.4 per cent loss from the raw potato after harvest (October 1960) to the reconstituted flakes (May 1961). In a repeat of this study the College of Agriculture of the University of Idaho has substantiated these findings *(5)*.

Table 1.6

variation in vitamin C content
of oranges within the United States*

type of orange	average amount of ascorbic acid per 100 grams of juice
California Navel	61
California Valencia	49
Florida Valencia	37

*In a review of data from several thousand samples of oranges, ascorbic acid content ranged from a minimum of 20 mg. per 100 grams of juice in one orange to more than 80 mg. per cent maximum in another.

Regardless of the availability of nutrients in the market place, obviously only the food eaten is beneficial. The consumption of less than two-thirds of the R.D.A. (Recommended Dietary Allowance) established by the Food and Nutrition Board, National Research Council, National Academy of Sciences, for any nutrient is considered suboptimal. Doctor Agnes Fay Morgan *(27)* (Emeritus Professor of Nutrition and Biochemistry in the California Agricultural Experiment Station, University of California) recently pointed out the ubiquity of such suboptimal consumption (Table 1.8). Analyses of the intake of eight nutrients revealed that the per cent of persons consuming less than two-thirds of the R.D.A. for all nutrients ranged from five (for protein) to sixty per cent (for calcium). Even where the family as a whole reports an adequate nutrient consumption, the children frequently exhibit poor eating habits (Table 1.9) (27).

Table 1.7
mean total ascorbic acid content in potatoes
harvested in autumn 1960 and sampled
periodically (estimated on a fresh
weight basis in mg. per 100 gm. of potato)

	raw	fresh, peeled, cooked and mashed	reconsti- tuted flakes
October 1960	29.3	18.8	8.0
February 1961	11.7	8.2	3.1
May 1961	10.6	6.8	2.8

Table 1.8
percentage of men and women 30-60
years of age from all sections of the
United States who ate less than two-thirds
R.D.A. of various nutrients

	per cent eating less than 2/3 R.D.A.	
	women	men
protein	10	5
iron	18	12
thiamine	20	15
riboflavin	30	10
niacin	20	9
vitamin A	45	20
ascorbic acid	35	35
calcium	60	30

Table 1.9
per cent of 9-11 year old Kansas children
with nutrient intake less than two-thirds
of the Recommended Dietary Allowance
from families consuming adequate diets

	boys	girls
thiamine	8	5
iron	10	7
riboflavin	10	11
niacin	18	14

The authoritative text, *Nutritional Evaluation of Food Processing*, by Doctor R. S. Harris and Mr. H. V. Loesecke, provides a panoramic view of the effect of culture on man's diet *(17)*. A glance at topics discussed (e.g. agricultural practices, commercial processing, packaging and storage, and home preparation) indicates the breadth of possible links in the chain of nutrient loss. In the home, the choice of food is limited by many factors. These include not only what food is purchased, but all the steps from washing to cooking.

Nutrient loss during food preparation may occur not only as a result of peeling or trimming foods, but through such seemingly harmless procedures as cleansing with a water rinse. Table 1.10 *(26)* points out the magnitude of nutrient loss by simply washing rice in three changes of water. The fact that as much as one-fourth of the content of a nutrient (available iron) may be lost is quite alarming when one considers how diligently the housewife washes many foods.

An innovation of food preparation in the home, of rather recent introduction, is the popular use of frozen foods. The possibility of nutrient loss during thawing is usually overlooked. The potential loss is exemplified in Table 1.11 *(29)*. Although the vitamin and amino acid loss from this study of defrosting frozen pork averages only about 8 per cent, the magnitude of the problem becomes apparent when it is realized that the modern family prepares a large proportion of its meat and other foods in such a fashion.

The most severe loss of nutrients may result during the cooking of foods. According to the United States Department of Agriculture *(19)*, preparation and cooking can effect as much as a 40 to 55 per cent loss of B complex fractions or ascorbic acid in certain foods (Table 1.12). Not only is there a significant nutrient loss from food as it is being cooked, but the lapse of time between cooking and eating is still another hazard *(24)*. Table 1.13 *(21)* points out this source of ascorbic acid loss for potatoes prepared in a variety of ways.

Table 1.10
per cent loss of nutrients from rice
during three equal volume water
washings

nutrient	mean of five varieties of rice
available iron	24.7
iron	21.3
riboflavin	16.9
calcium	10.1
niacin	9.1
ash	8.0
phosphorus	4.7
thiamine	4.6
phytin phosphorus	3.8
nitrogen	2.3
total solid	0.5

Table 1.11
the vitamin and amino acid content
of the drip obtained while defrosting
frozen pork

nutrient	per cent loss
isoleucine	11.08
niacin	10.69
leucine	9.71
thiamine	9.02
vitamin B6	8.71
lysine	8.60
methionine	7.58
tryptophan	7.15
pantothenic acid	6.95
vitamin B12	5.06
riboflavin	4.15

Although not usually recognized, considerable protein destruction takes place as foods are heated *(6, 8, 10)*. This has been underscored by an editorial in Nutrition Reviews *(30)*.

It has been postulated the dry heat processing of proteins produces a new lysine linkage which is either not digestible by enzymes or is so slowly digested that lysine enters the blood stream too late to participate with the rest of the assimilated amino acids in tissue formation.

More severe heat damage to proteins results when moist heat is used. When reducing sugars (e.g. glucose) are present true destruction of amino acids has been repeatedly corroborated. This destruction may account for a loss of 50 per cent of the lysine, arginine, tryptophane and histidine content *(30)*.

A startling example of protein destruction during the cooking of food was reported at the Mead Johnson Research Center in Evansville, Indiana. It was discovered that the stockpile of survival biscuits and crackers developed by the Office of Civil Defense for use in catastrophic emergencies was significantly deficient in essential amino acid content *(25)*. Actually two-thirds of the lysine was destroyed presumably during the baking of these foods (Table 1.14). As one may note in Table 1.14, there was a great discrepancy between the lysine content of the survival rations as calculated from food tables and the actual amount based on chemical analysis.

Table 1.12
per cent of vitamin loss during
the preparation and cooking of food

food groups	B1	B2	niacin	C
fats, oils, bacon, salt pork	55	0	0	0
eggs	15	5	0	0
meat, poultry, fish	25	5	10	0
potatoes, sweet potatoes	25	20	20	35
leafy green, yellow vegetables	45	40	40	50
other vegetables, fruits	20	20	20	25
flour and uncooked cereals	10	0	10	0

Table 1.13
percentage loss of ascorbic acid during
the preparation of potatoes for eating

method of preparation	minutes allowed to stand after preparation (steam table)			
	30	45	60	75
potatoes steamed in skins	0	0		
potatoes baked in skins	34	59		
potatoes, peeled, cut and baked	48			
French-fried potatoes	34	30		
potatoes, peeled, cut in halves, steamed, mashed or creamed	63	64		95
potatoes, peeled, cut, soaked in water 2 hours, baked	76		89	

Table 1.14
the essential amino acid composition
of survival biscuits and crackers
stockpiled by the Office of Civil Defense

amino acid	survival biscuits		survival crackers	
	calculated gm./ 100 gm.	analysis gm./ 100 gm.	calculated gm. 100 gm.	analysis gm./ 100 gm.
lysine	3.1	1.0	2.7	0.8
methionine	1.4	1.5	1.5	1.6
methionine + cystine	3.4	2.5	3.4	2.4
isoleucine	4.3	3.6	4.2	3.4
leucine	6.8	7.5	8.0	7.4
phenylalanine	4.7	5.1	4.6	—
threonine	2.8	2.9	3.0	2.7
valine	4.5	4.2	4.4	4.0

Investigators who have compared the calculated and analyzed nutrient content of foods almost invariably have found that the table values are too high (16, 34). In a 1962 *Symposium on Recent Advances in the Appraisal of the Nutrient Intake and the Nutritional Status of Man* at the Massachusetts Institute of Technology (16), Doctor Robert S.

Harris, when asked how dietary calculations agree with dietary values in respect to nutrient content, replied:

> They seldom agree closely. Some years ago we studied the vitamin content of meals already prepared to eat in homes. We weighed and calculated the nutrient contents in each meal item using food tables, and compared the calculated amounts with the analysis amounts. In most cases the calculated value exceeded the analyzed value by 5 to 30 per cent.... More recently we conducted a study of dinner meals with the same results. The ascorbic acid content of the prepared meals by analysis was about 60 per cent of the calculated value, the fat content was about 70 per cent of the calculated value, etc.... Thus food tables tend to give values that are too high....

This discrepancy is of great significance in view of the fact that most nutrition surveys base the nutrient content of consumed foods on such food tables. Thus, this makes even more significant the findings by Doctor Robert S. Goodhart in his *How Well Nourished Are Americans? I and II (12, 13).* Doctor Goodhart pointed out that for different groups of people and for different vitamins, the proportion consuming less than two-thirds of the Recommended Dietary Allowances ranges from less than 5 to more than 70 per cent.

Two recent and interesting reports emphasize the frequent recognition of hypovitaminemia in both dental *(7)* and hospital *(36)* patients. From a survey of 861 routine care patients at the University of Alabama School of Dentistry by the Department of Oral Medicine, it was noted that 6.6 per cent showed zero plasma ascorbic acid levels and approximately one-half had concentrations indicative of a possible vitamin C deficiency state *(7).* A survey of 120 randomly selected patients admitted to ward service at the Jersey City, New Jersey, Medical Center revealed that 88 per cent had a significant deficit in the circulating level of at least one vitamin and 63 per cent in two or more vitamins *(36).*

SUMMARY

The American dietary pattern of a decreased consumption of complex carbohydrates (starches) and an increase in simple ones (sugar) is rapidly spreading around the world. These eating habits tend to reduce the intake of protein, vitamins, and minerals since many of the simple carbohydrate foods are relatively low in these nutrients. The substitution of sugar-rich foods by the individual for more nutritious ones further invites a nutrient-deficit. The dramatic progress in food handling has assured a constant supply notwithstanding population explosion and distribution. Actually, these advances have made larger urban complexes possible. Such consumer demands have led to the creation of many environmental hazards that reduce the biologic value of many nutrient-rich foods. Such factors as transportation, storage, processing, preparation, cooking, and time lapse before eating can contribute to nutrient depletion.

The evidence thus far suggests serious flaws in the American diet. The profound public health implications of the present-day diet have been underscored by Doctor Frank G. Boudreau in *Food, the Yearbook of Agriculture 1959* (a publication of the United States Department of Agriculture).

If all that we know about nutrition were applied to modern society, the result would be an enormous improvement in public health, at least equal to that which resulted when the germ theory of infectious disease was made the basis of public health and medical work.

REFERENCES

1. Albrink, M. J. *Diet and cardiovascular disease.* J. Am. Dietet. Assn. 46: #1, 26-29, January 1965.
2. Antar, M. A., Ohlson, M. A., and Hodges, R. E. *Changes in retail market food supplies in the United States in the last seventy years in relation to the incidence of coronary heart disease, with special reference to dietary carbohydrate and essential fatty acids.* Am. J. Clin. Nutrit. 14: #3, 169-178, March 1964.
3. Boudreau, F. G. in U. S. Department of Agriculture. *Food, the yearbook of agriculture 1959.* 1959. Washington, D.C., U.S. Government Printing Office.
4. Bring, S. V., Grassl, C., Hofstrand, J. T., and Willard, M. J. *Total ascorbic acid in potatoes.* J. Am. Dietet. Assn. 42 #4, 320-324, April 1963.
5. Bring, S. V. and Raab, F. P. *Total ascorbic acid in potatoes.* J. Am. Dietet. Assn. 45: #2, 149-152, August 1964.
6. Butterworth, M. H. and Fox, H. C. *The effects of heat treatment on the nutritive value of coconut meal, and the prediction of nutritive value by chemical methods.* Brit. J. Nutrit. 17: #4, 445-452, 1963.
7. Cheraskin, E. and Ringsdorf, W. M., Jr. *Vitamin C state in a dental school patient population.* J. South. California State Dent. Assn. 32: #10, 375-378, October 1964.
8. Clarke, J. A. K. and Kennedy, B. M. *Availability of lysine in wholewheat bread and in selected breakfast cereals.* J. Food Sc. 27: #6, 609-616, November-December 1962.
9. Cohen, A. M. *Fats and carbohydrates as factors in atherosclerosis and diabetes in Yemenite Jews.* Am. Heart J. 65: #3, 291-293, March 1963.
10. Gates, J. C. and Kennedy, B. M. *Protein quality of bread and bread ingredients.* J. Am. Dietet. Assn. 44: #5, 374-377, May 1964.
11. Goodhart, R. S. *Some comments on the American diet and household consumption data.* Am. J. Clin. Nutrit. 7: #5, 508-513, September-October 1959.
12. Goodhart, R. S. *How well nourished are Americans?* National Vitamin Foundation Report for 1960. New York, New York. July 1961.
13. Goodhart, R. S. *How well nourished are Americans? II.* National Vitamin Foundation Report for 1961-1963. New York, New York.

14. Greaves, J. P. and Hollingsworth, D. F. *Changes in the pattern of carbohydrate consumption in Britain.* Proc. Nutrit. Soc. 23: #2, 136-143, 1964.

15. Harris, R. S. *Influence of culture on man's diet.* Arch. Environ. Health 5: #2, 144-152, August 1962.

16. Harris, R. S. (Moderator) *Panel discussion: food composition and availability of nutrients in foods.* Am. J. Clin. Nutrit. 11: #5, 400-405, November 1962.

17. Harris, R. S. and Loesecke, H. V. *Nutritional evaluation of food processing.* 1960. New York, John Wiley and Sons.

18. Hubbard, A. W. *The American diet paradox.* Modern Med. Topics 23: #12, December 1962.

19. Information Bulletin 112, Human Nutrition Research Branch, United States Department of Agriculture, 1954.

20. Jackson, R. L., Hanna, F. M., and Flynn, M. A. *Nutritional requirements of children.* Pediat. Clin. North America 9: #4, 879-910, November 1962.

21. Kahn, R. M. and Halliday, E. G. *Ascorbic acid content of white potatoes as affected by cooking and standing on steam table.* J. Am. Dietet. Assn. 20: #4, 220-222, April 1944.

22. Katz, L. N., Stamler, J., and Pick, R. *Nutrition and atherosclerosis.* 1958. Philadelphia, Lea and Febiger. pp. 16-20.

23. Krehl, W. A. *Factors affecting utilization and requirements; vitamins and minerals.* Am. J. Clin. Nutrit. 11: #5, 389-399, November 1962.

24. Leichsenring, J. M., Pilcher, H. L., and Norris, L. M. II. *Effect of baking and of pressure-cooking on the ascorbic, dehydroascorbic, and diketogulonic acid contents of potatoes.* Food Research 22: #1, 44-50, January-February 1957.

25. Longenecker, J. B. and Sarett, H. P. *Nutritional quality of survival biscuits and crackers.* Am. J. Clin. Nutrit. 13: #5, 291-296, November 1963.

26. Malakar, M. C. and Banerjee, S. N. *Effect of cooking rice with different volumes of water on the loss of nutrients and on digestibility of rice in vitro.* Food Research 24: #6, 751-756, November-December 1959.

27. Morgan, A. F. *Nutritional status U.S.A.* 1959. Berkeley, California Agricultural Experiment Station, Bulletin 769.

28. Ohlson, M. A. *Dietary patterns and effect on nutrient intake.* Illinois M. J. 122: #5, 461-466, November 1962.

29. Pearson, A. M., West, R. G., and Luecke, R. W. *The vitamin and*

amino acid content of drip obtained upon defrosting frozen pork. Food Research 24: #5, 515-519, September-October 1959.

30. Present status of heat-processing damage to protein foods. Nutrit. Rev. 8: #7, 193-196, July 1950.

31. Soskin, S. and Levine, R. The role of carbohydrates in the diet. In Wohl, M. G. and Goodhart, R. S. Modern nutrition in health and disease. 1960. Philadelphia, Lea and Febiger.

32. Spies, T. D. Some recent advances in nutrition. J. A. M. A. 167: #6, 675-690, June 7, 1958.

33. Takahashi, E. An epidemiological approach to the relation between diet and cerebrovascular lesions and arteriosclerotic heart disease. Tohoku J. Exper. Med. 77: #3, 239-257, August 25, 1962.

34. Tucker, R. E., Brown, P. T., and Hedrick, D. I. Ascorbic acid content of fruits and vegetables served college students. Rhode Island Agricultural Experiment Station, Bulletin 331, 1955.

35. United States Department of Agriculture. Nutrition, up to date, up to you. 1960, Washington, D.C., U.S. Government Printing Office.

36. Vitamin defects found in many hospitalized. Med. Tribune and Med. News 6: #35, 1, 26, March 22, 1965.

37. Yudkin, J. Nutrition and palatability, with special reference to obesity, myocardial infarction, and other diseases of civilization. Lancet 1: #7295, 1335-1338, June 22, 1963.

38. Yudkin, J. Patterns and trends in carbohydrate consumption and their relation to disease. Proc. Nutrit. Soc. 23: #2, 149-162, 1964.

2. NATIONAL DISEASE STATUS

IN THE FIRST CHAPTER, ATTENTION WAS DIRECTED TO ONE OF THE factors, diet, in the title of this text. Consideration will now be given to the other ingredient, namely disease. This will be undertaken through an analysis of mortality and morbidity in the general population.

MORTALITY FINDINGS

Doctor Iwao M. Moriyama (Chief of the Office of Health Statistics Analysis), in a recent report (15) released by the United States Department of Health, Education, and Welfare, pointed out that, in the period 1939-1960, the crude death rate dropped from 17.2 to 9.5 per 1000 population (Figure 2.1). However, current figures indicate that the trend now appears to have levelled off during the last recorded decade (1950-1960). Doctor Moriyama expressed concern about the stationary 1950-1960 trend:

> The failure to experience a decline in mortality during this period is unexpected in view of the intensified attack on medical problems in the postwar years....In this setting it would seem reasonable to expect further reductions in mortality. On the other hand, the possible adverse effects on mortality of radioactive fallout, air pollution, and other manmade hazards cannot be completely ignored....If the levelling off of the death rate has resulted from failure to prevent deaths that are preventable, this is of public health significance.

It is noteworthy that the *quantitative* mortality pattern is paralleled by significant *qualitative* differences since 1900 (Figure 2.2). According to Doctor William H. Stewart (formerly of the Division of Public Health Methods, United States Public Health Service), there has been a dramatic curtailment of acute infectious diseases leading to death and a gradual rise in mortality due to chronic disorders *(23)*. For the most part, the overall downward trend has been checked (Figure 2.1) by the current trends among the chronic disorders. Despite intensified research, heart disease, cancer and stroke continue to rate overwhelmingly as the leading causes of death in the United States at the present time. In 1963, these three groups of disorders, collectively, accounted for 71 per cent of all deaths in the nation *(19)*.

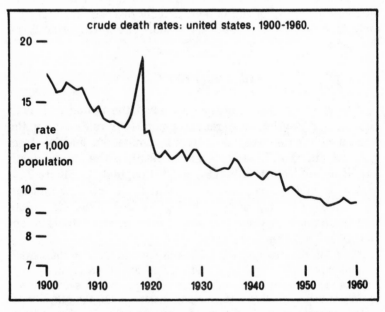

Figure 2.1. Crude death rate per 1000 population in the United States from 1900 to 1960.

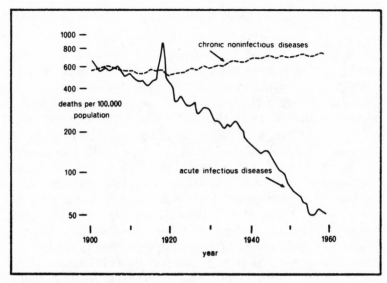

Figure 2.2. Incidence of deaths from acute and chronic diseases in the United States from 1900 to 1960.

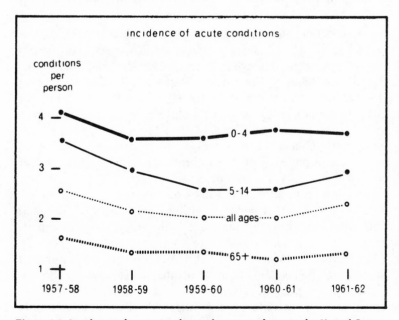

Figure 2.3. Incidence of acute conditions by years of age in the United States from 1957 to 1962.

MORBIDITY PATTERNS

While the risk of death from acute diseases has been steadily declining since 1900, the incidence of these conditions in the general population is still a considerable problem among the youngest age groups. The acute disorders most often reported by the National Health Survey are respiratory disorders, infective and parasitic diseases, and digestive problems. The incidence of acute diseases in all age groups has been relatively stable since 1958. The number of acute conditions per person in the United States in 1961-1962 was 2.2. For the age groups 0-4, the value was 3.7 but for persons over 65 years, the incidence was only 1.3. Thus, the youngest age groups had approximately three times as much acute disease as elderly persons (Figure 2.3) according to the United States Department of Health, Education, and Welfare *(26)*. Public Health Service statistics recently revealed an incidence of 2.1 acute illnesses per person in the civilian non-institutionalized population for the period July 1963 to June 1965 *(17)*

In contrast, the frequency of chronic disorders during the last three decades has been increasing. This has been particularly evident in the aging groups. The National Center for Health Statistics of the United States Public Health Service *(16)* noted that in the four-year period from July 1957 to June 1961 an annual average of 72 million persons was reported to have one or more well-established chronic diseases or impairments. Almost 20 per cent of this population under 15 years of age had one or more chronic disorders while 80 per cent of those over 65 were affected (Figure 2.4). Not only are death rates from chronic diseases on the increase, but an additional 38,000,000 Americans suffer specifically (Figure 2.5) with arthritis, rheumatism, mental illness, and other impairments which do not enter into mortality statistics *(21)*. In 1960, physicians attending the Association of American Medical Colleges Teaching Institute in Hollywood Beach, Florida, were presented with a startling estimate *(21)* of the prevalence of specific chronic diseases (Figure 2.5). Public Health Service statistics for the period July 1961-June 1963 indicate that 80.3 million persons or 44.1 per cent of the civilian, noninstitutionalized population reported one or more chronic problems *(18)*. For July 1963-June 1964 the incidence had increased to 45.2 per cent *(17)* and for the period July 1964 to June 1965 an estimated 87.3 million persons or 46.3 per cent of the civilian, noninstitutionalized population reported one or more chronic conditions or impairments *(17)*. Thus, within a span of four years, there has been a 2.2 per cent rise in the frequency of reported chronic disease.

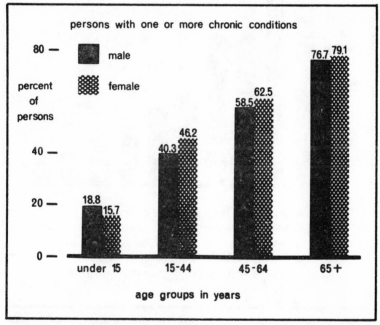

Figure 2.4. Percentage of persons with one or more chronic conditions in the United States from 1957 to 1961.

Although not usually reported in the epidemiology of chronic disease, most health authorities readily concur that oral pathosis is a major chronic problem in the United States. Doctor Wesley O. Young, in his contribution to the Commission on the Survey of Dentistry in the United States, summarized its enormity *(29)*:

The most obvious measure of the dental health problem is its sheer magnitude. It is estimated, for example, that the 180,000,000

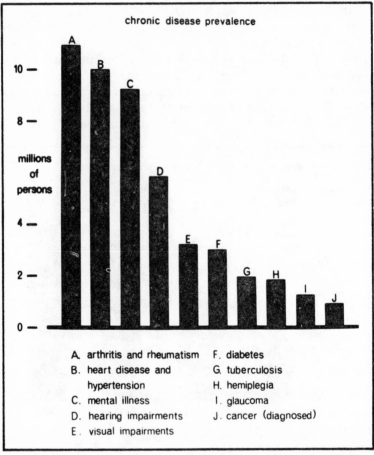

Figure 2.5. Estimated prevalence of specified chronic diseases and physical impairments in the United States.

people in the United States in the year 1960 have accumulated at least 700,000,000 unfilled cavities....

Diseases of the supporting bone and gingival tissues affect at least half of the population by the age of 50 and almost every one by age 65.

The eventual outcome of dental caries and periodontal disease is tooth loss. Statistics from the National Health Survey from 1960 through 1962 (25) reveal that by 60 years of age, 35 per cent of the American public is edentulous (Figure 2.6).

An important economic aspect of illness is the loss of manpower. According to figures cited by the United States Department of Health, Education, and Welfare, the number of employed civilians absent from work on an average day in 1962 was 1,300,000. This amounted to 1.94 per cent of the working civilian population *(26)*. These values become even more significant when one realizes that not only is absenteeism greater today than in the fifties but that it prevails in spite of the continuing exponential rise in public and private expenditures for health and medical care. For example *(26)*, total dollar outlay has swelled threefold in the past fifteen years (Figure 2.7).

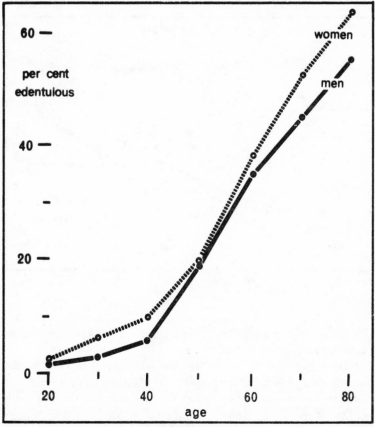

Figure 2.6. Percentage of edentulous men and women of different ages in the United States from 1960 to 1962.

Not only are there millions of obviously ill people, but the morbidity figures from examinations of apparently healthy individuals present shocking evidence of what may be called silent sickness. Table 2.1 presents a representative summary from a number of multiphasic examinations conducted on *presumably healthy* persons *(1-4, 6-10, 12, 20, 24, 27, 28)*. It is significant to note that the percentage with newly discovered disease ranges from 8.3 to 59.9. This, it should be underlined, excludes previously known illness. When these two groups are combined, those designated as healthy are in the minority (7.7 to 36.3 per cent). Needless to say, the more refined the testing procedures, the greater is the disease yield. For example, replacing urinalysis by blood sugar studies

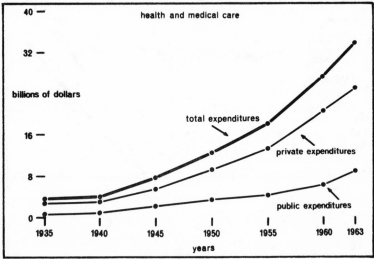

Figure 2.7. Private and public expenditures for health and medical care in the United States from 1935 to 1963.

(20) enhances the detection of abnormal carbohydrate metabolism by 61 per cent (Table 2.2).

Doctor Henrietta Herbolsheimer (Director, Student Health Service and Associate Professor of Medicine, University of Chicago), in a screening survey of entering college and university students in 1956, discovered a total of 589 abnormalities per 1000 students *(11)*. Doctor Harold Jacobziner (Assistant Commissioner of Health, New York City), in a paper presented before the Joint Session of the American School Health Association, the Food and Nutrition, Maternal and Child Health and School Health Sections of the American Public Health Association at the Ninetieth Annual Meeting in Miami Beach, Florida (17 October 1962), introduced data from 20,000 children examined during well-child conferences in 78 child health stations. It was concluded that 39 per cent had one or more adverse conditions *(13)*.

Table 2.1
per cent healthy and with newly discovered
disease from health-maintenance examinations
of presumably healthy people

sample number	per cent healthy	per cent with significant newly discovered disease	investigators
500	48.0	40.6	Bolt et al (1)
500	10.6	32.6	Huth et al (12)
500	15.0	39.0	Elsom (7)
14,965	13.6	37.5	Roberts (20)
957	28.0	25.3	Borhani (2)
3,994		19.4	Weinerman et al (28)
*14,132	36.3	29.7	Culbert and Jacobziner (6)
707	50.5	35.3	Franco (9)
600	7.7	59.9	Thompson and Staack (24)
352	10.5		Wade (27)
1,000	22.3	36.2	Collen and Linden (4)
5,711		8.3	Carroll et al (3)
717	41.3	52.6	Franco et al (10)
1,513	28.0	40.0	Elsom et al (8)

*public school children

Table 2.2
refinement of testing in the
diagnosis of abnormal
carbohydrate metabolism

number tested	method used	per cent abnormal
396,800	urine sugar	2.56
507,383	blood sugar	4.11

SHORTCOMINGS OF MORBIDITY STUDIES

Although the practice of multiphasic screening of presumably healthy people is a forward step and has altered the concepts of health and sickness, it suffers two glaring omissions. In general, these health maintenance examinations have not included an evaluation of the oral cavity nor an estimate of nutritional status.

As previously noted, caries and periodontal diseases are the most prevalent chronic conditions today (p. #33). Therefore, an estimate of their extent should also be included in the morbidity index. The oral cavity has been recognized as a barometer of general health and particularly reflects the nutritional status.

The failure to include nutritional appraisal in multiple testing programs has evoked much concern. Doctor Willard A. Krehl (Research Professor of Medicine and Director of the Clinical Research Center, State University of Iowa School of Medicine) discussed some of the reasons for this apathy toward nutrition in a recent article (14):

> The nutritional evaluation of the patient is as important as any other aspect of the total evaluation. All too often one finds the nutritional status dismissed with the cursory statement that the patient is well-nourished and well-developed or that the patient seems to be getting a satisfactory diet. Alertness to the importance of nutritional well-being may have been dulled somewhat by the fact that frank deficiency diseases such as scurvy, pellagra, beriberi and rickets have largely disappeared....

> It is reasonable to assume, however, that nutritional deficiencies of all grades exist and do not necessarily appear as the florid evidence of the classical deficiency diseases. Just as atherogenesis and atherosclerosis commonly have a long silent course before coronary heart disease is clinically evident, so too one may have inadequate or less than optimal nutritional status without overt evidence of nutritional disease; the deficits may begin early in life and continue for long periods of time. They may contribute ultimately to an illness without themselves becoming identified as the cause of or even related to the illness.

The Council on Foods and Nutrition of the American Medical Association is also aware of the dilemma and voiced one solution (5):

> Undergraduate teaching of nutrition often is centered around

nutritional deficiency diseases. This is too-limited a focus for present-day problems. It is necessary to think more in terms of disturbances of the metabolic and biochemical reactions of the body. Nutritional diagnosis implies evaluation of biochemical changes within and outside the cell, as well as abnormalities of function and structure of the organs and tissues of the body. The basic scientists and the clinicians, especially the biochemists, pediatricians, and internists, must integrate their knowledge so that the student may better appreciate the practical application of biochemistry to prevention and treatment of disease.

While disease is obviously multifactorial (see Chapter Three), there are those who hold that there may be dietary denominators.

SUMMARY

An examination of mortality trends during this century has shown a gratifying progressive decline in crude death rate. However, the evidence suggests that, for the last decade, there is no further decline. A more detailed analysis reveals a significant decrease in the acute infectious diseases. On the other hand, there appears to be a true rise in chronic disorders. The innovation of multiple testing has unearthed much previously unrecognized disease among so-called healthy people. There has been a glaring failure to utilize nutritional testing procedures, not only in the ill but in examinations of presumably well individuals.

Doctor T. D. Spies *(22)*, formerly Professor of Nutrition and Metabolism, Northwestern Medical School, Chicago, and Director, Nutrition Clinic, Hillman Hospital, Birmingham, Alabama, suggests the possibility of a nutritional factor in *all* disease:

Today germs are not our principal enemy. Our chief medical adversary is what I consider a disturbance of the inner balance of the constituents of our tissues, which are built from and maintained by necessary chemicals in the air we breathe, the water we drink and the food we eat. For a generation we have worked on the concept that our cells are never static and that in time they must be replaced in varying degrees by the nutrients obtained from food. More specifically, our working hypothesis has been that all disease is chemical and, when we know enough, chemically correctable.

REFERENCES

1. Bolt, R. J., Tupper, C. J., and Mallery, O. T., Jr. *An appraisal of periodic health examinations.* Arch. Indust. Health 12: #4, 420-434, October 1955.
2. Borhani, N. O. *Screening tests find longshoremen with organized medical follow-up.* Amer. J. Pub. Health 42: #12, 1552-1567, December 1952.
3. Carroll, B. E., Kurlander, A. B., and Nester, H. G. *Multiple screening pilot study. Report of the Indianapolis, Indiana project.* Pub. Health Rep. 6: #12, 1180-1184, December 1956.
4. Collen, M. F. and Linden, C. *Screening in a group practice prepaid medical care plan.* J. Chron. Dis. 2: #4, 400-408, October 1955.
5. Council on Foods and Nutrition. *Nutrition teaching in medical schools.* J. A. M. A. 183: #11, 955-957, March 16, 1963.
6. Culbert, R. W. and Jacobziner, H. *What does the school physician see?* Amer. J. Pub. Health 40: #5, 567-574, May 1950.
7. Elsom, K. A. *Personal communications of September 14, 1954, and February 16, 1955. Cited by Roberts, N. J. Periodic health-maintenance examinations. In The early detection and prevention of disease* edited by J. P. Hubbard. 1957. New York, Blakiston Division, McGraw-Hill Book Company. p. 30.
8. Elsom, K. A., Schor, S., Clark, T. W., Elsom, I. O., and Hubbard, J. P. *Periodic health examination: nature and distribution of newly discovered diseases in executives.* J. A. M. A. 172: #1, 55-60, January 2, 1960.
9. Franco, S. C. *The early detection of disease by periodic examination.* Indust. Med. and Surg. 25: #6, 251-257, June 1956.
10. Franco, S. C., Gerl, A. J., and Murphy, G. T. *Periodic health examinations, a long term study, 1949-1959.* J. Occupat. Med. 3: #1, 13-20, January 1961.
11. Herbolsheimer, H. and Ballard, B. L. *Multiple screening in evaluation of entering college and university students.* J. A. M. A. 166: #5, 444-453, February 1, 1958.
12. Huth, E., Meidt, C., Vernon, W., Spoont, S., and Dohan, F. C. *Periodic health status examination program.* Unpublished report, June 29, 1954. Cited by Roberts, N. J. *Periodic health-maintenance examinations. In The early detection and prevention of disease* edited by J. P. Hubbard. 1957. New York, Blakiston Division, McGraw-Hill Book Company. p. 30.
13. Jacobziner, H., Rich, H., Bleiberg, N., and Merchant, R. *How well are well children?* Amer. J. Pub. Health 53: #12, 1937-1952, December 1963.

14. Krehl, W. A. *The evaluation of nutritional status.* Med. Clin. North America 48: #5, 1129-1140, September 1964.
15. Moriyama, I. M. *The change in mortality trend in the United States.* National Center for Health Statistics, United States Department of Health, Education, and Welfare. Public Health Service Publication 1000, Series 3, #1, March 1964.
16. National Center for Health Statistics. *Bed disability among the chronically limited, United States July 1957-June 1961.* Series 10, #12, September 1964. Washington, D. C., Superintendent of Documents, United States Government Printing Office.
17. National Center for Health Statistics. *Current estimates from the health interview survey, United States July 1964-June 1965.* Series 10, #25, November 1965. Washington, D. C., Superintendent of Documents, United States Government Printing Office.
18. National Center for Health Statistics. *Chronic conditions and activity limitation, United States July 1961-June 1963.* Series 10: #17, May 1965. Washington, D. C., Superintendent of Documents, United States Government Printing Office.
19. The President's Commission on Heart Disease, Cancer and Stroke. *Report to the president; a national program to conquer heart disease, cancer and stroke.* Vol. 1, December 1964. Washington, D. C., Superintendent of Documents, United States Government Printing Office. 1965.
20. Roberts, N. J. *Periodic health-maintenance examination.* In *The early detection and prevention of disease* edited by J. P. Hubbard. 1957. New York, Blakiston Division, McGraw-Hill Book Company. pp. 27-57.
21. Sheps, C. G. *The dynamics of medical care.* 1960. Evanston, Illinois, Association of American Medical Colleges.
22. Spies, T. D. *Some recent advances in nutrition.* J. A. M. A. 167: #6, 675-690, June 7, 1958.
23. Stewart, W. H. *Who gets what care and how?* In *The health care issues of the 1960's.* 1963. Group Health Insurance, Inc., 221 Park Avenue South, New York, New York.
24. Thompson, C. E. and Staack, H. F. *Executive health--diagnostic study of 600 executives.* Indust. Med. and Surg. 25: #4, 175-176, April 1956.
25. United States Department of Health, Education and Welfare, Public Health Service, Health Statistics from the United States National Health Survey. *Selected dental findings in adults by age, race and sex, United States, 1960-1962.* Series 11: #7, February 1965. Washington, D. C., Superintendent of Documents, United States Government Printing Office.
26. United States Department of Health, Education and Welfare.

Health, education and welfare trends. 1963. Washington, D. C., Superintendent of Documents, United States Government Printing Office.

27. Wade, L. *Physical examinations for executives.* Arch. Indust. Health 17: #3, 175-179, March 1958.

28. Weinerman, E. R., Breslow, L., Belloc, N. B., Waybur, A., and Milmore, B. K. *Multiphasic screening of longshoremen with organized medical follow-up.* Amer. J. Pub. Health 42: #12, 1552-1567, December 1952.

29. Young, W. O. *Dental health.* In Hollinshead, B. S. *The survey of dentistry.* 1961. Washington, D. C., American Council on Education. pp. 5-16.

3. DIET AND THE NATURE OF HEALTH AND DISEASE

EVIDENCE HAS BEEN PRESENTED (CHAPTER ONE) TO SUGGEST THAT a significant number of Americans consume a suboptimal diet. From Chapter Two it is apparent that the health of the American public leaves room for improvement. It is the purpose of this chapter to study the role of diet in the genesis of disease.

There are many and diverse definitions of health and illness. However, there are two points upon which there is general agreement. First, the extent to which health or disease prevails is, in part, a function of the absence or presence of one or more environmental challenges (e.g. physical insult, microbial invasion, chemical stressor). But, to complete the story, one must recognize that health or disease is the end-result of the capacity of the organism to cope with the many and constant environmental threats. This capacity is identified as host resistance and susceptibility. Second, while there are undoubtedly classical expressions of disease states, sickness more commonly is marginal and can be clinically categorized in a graduated series.

MULTICAUSAL CONCEPT OF DISEASE

The evidence is truly overwhelming that disease is pluricausal *(1, 2, 6, 7, 10, 12, 15, 16, 18, 21, 22, 27-33)*. Doctor Rene J. Dubos, of the Rockefeller Institute, in his superb text, *Mirage of Health (10)*, points out the past contributions of the doctrine of specific etiology but warns of the futility of basing future research on this hypothesis:

> Unquestionably the doctrine of specific etiology has been the most constructive force in medical research for almost a century and the theoretical and practical achievements to which it has led constitute the bulk of medical practice. Yet few are the cases

in which it has provided a complete account of the causation of disease. Despite frantic efforts, the causes of cancer, of arteriosclerosis, of mental disorders, and of other great medical problems of our times remain undiscovered. It is generally assumed that these failures are due to technical difficulties and that the cause of all disease can and will be found in due time by bringing the big guns of science to bear on the problems. In reality, however, search for the cause may be a hopeless pursuit because most disease states are the indirect outcome of a constellation of circumstances rather than the direct result of single determinant factors.

The view just expressed is enlarged upon by Doctor E. S. Rogers *(27)*, Professor of Public Health and Medical Administration at the University of California, in his textbook, *Human Ecology and Health*:

There is a growing suspicion that many a form of pathology heretofore considered as the specific consequence of a specific cause may not be so at all....Thus, we are led to the concept of multiple causation of illness. This concept maintains that illness is rarely the result of the impact of a single, discrete, disease-causing agent (such as the tubercle bacillus) upon an otherwise normal and healthy man. Rather, it holds that most, if not all, illness is an expression of a basic unbalance in man's physiologic adaptation to multiple physical and emotional stresses that are initiated, for the most part, in the condition of his external environment.

Doctor Jacques M. May, Director of the Medical Geography Department of the American Geographical Society, viewing the problem from a third vantage point, echoes the views of the other authorities and prognosticates *(21)*:

I think that we have been very near to committing the major sin in disease etiology, that is, to consider that what we call disease may have a single cause. There is no such thing. A multiplicity of causes are always needed to produce that alteration of tissues creating maladjustment....I stress that I think this subject (the host) is the field of the future. Our forefathers had a good awareness of the importance of the individual, which they called the 'terrain,' in shaping the clinical forms of disease. Following the enlightening Pasteurian discoveries we have been mesmerized by the action of a single stimulus to produce disease, and have forgotten completely to explore the reasons that make the host respond in the way he does.

It is as though I had on a table three dolls, one of glass, another of celluloid, and a third of steel, and I chose to hit the three dolls with a hammer, using equal strength. The first doll would break, the second would scar, and the third would emit a pleasant sound.

It is clearly impossible to cite all of the evidence for a multicausal thesis of disease. Authorities representing many disciplines are concerned with this concept. Doctor B. Bronte-Stewart and Doctor L. H. Krut *(1)*, in a report entitled *The Interdependence of Prospective and Retrospective Studies in Research on Ischaemic Heart Disease,* published in the Journal of Atherosclerotic Research, indicated that the only rational approach to the etiology of ischemic heart disease must be founded on a multifactorial basis. Doctor Robert J. Hagerty *(14),* Professor and Chairman of the Department of Pediatrics at the University of Rochester School of Medicine, in an article *Host and Environmental Factors in Infection,* presented before the Eighty-Fourth Annual Meeting of the Louisiana State Medical Society (5 May 1964), discusses quite lucidly the relationship among the host, the infecting organisms, and other environmental determinants which make for disease. The point being made by all of these authorities, and others cited at the end of the chapter, is that disease is multifactorial and that disease is a sequela to an environmental change in a host incapable of tolerating the hostile environment.

All carefully studied natural phenomena seem to follow mathematical laws and may, therefore, be depicted in equation form. Thus, arithmetic expressions of renal clearance and cardiac output have been derived. It is reasonable to assume that health and disease may also be described in a simple arithmetic or algebraic system.

GRADATIONS OF HEALTH AND DISEASE

The present teaching methods in professional schools are such that the student is early introduced to disease in its *classical* form. Hence, the future doctor learns early to recognize *clearcut* acromegaly with its pronounced prognathism, excruciating chest pain in *obvious* ischemic heart disease, and *classical* scurvy because of a bleeding diathesis. It is quite comprehensible that this should be the technique in the early training years since these are convincing expressions of disease states. Regretfully, the student leaves the medical center still wedded to the binomial concept that man is either essentially healthy or obviously sick.

The fact that health and disease are not clearcut entities has been well described by many authorities (2, 6, 9, 17, 20, 25, 27, 28, 34, 35).

Doctor G. R. Wadsworth (35), of the Sir John Atkins Laboratories, Queen Elizabeth College, University of London, makes a plea for quantitation of health and disease:

Ill-health, whether through inadequate nutrition or some other cause, should ultimately be measurable and that although there is no sharp contrast between optimal health and various degrees of departure from it, grades of health status are evident. An individual's health status may be: optimal health, undefined ill-health, disease, or death.

Doctor E. S. Rogers (27, 28), in his text Human Ecology and Health (pages 158-160) graphically supports the concept:

One has little difficulty in distinguishing between life and death, but the distinction between illness and health is not an easy one to make. Except for certain acute illnesses the transition from health to ill health is often almost imperceptible. A useful approach is to view health as a spectrum. This spectrum ranges from perfect health to the complete absence of health, or death. Between these two extremes there is little agreement on criteria for differentiating the various degrees of ill health. Nevertheless, the need to make these distinctions has been growing in recent years....(Figure 3.1) presents a schematic classification dividing man's status into four stages: a state of optimum health....a state of suboptimum health or incipient illness; a state of overt illness or disability; and finally a state of very serious illness or of approaching death....The point of major importance is the concept of a spectrum or range at some point along which every individual has a place at any given time even though it may not be possible to determine it. Also, individuals move up and down on this scale as their health improves or deteriorates.

Parenthetic mention should be made that Doctor Rogers believes that the medical profession has been primarily concerned with overt illness (c) and approaching death (d) as shown in Figure 3.1. Only secondary and tertiary effort and interest has been accorded marginal illness (b) and optimal health (a), respectively.

Doctor T. S. Danowski, Chairman of the Section of Endocrinology and Metabolism in the School of Medicine at the University of Pittsburgh, was quoted in an interview

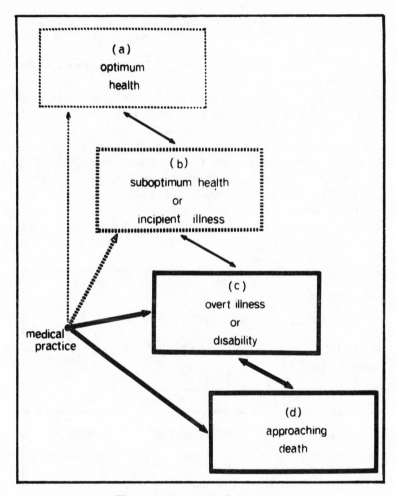

Figure 3.1. Spectrum of disease.

released in the Journal of the American Medical Association in which he elaborated on the possibility of even more precise quantitation *(9)*:

> The researchers took as their hypothesis the concept that health and disease are not absolutes, but occur in a spectrum ranging from perfect health to death....'We have been thinking that the time has come to speak in terms of percentage of disease,' Danowski said. 'For example, some people have difficulty holding down their weight. Some of these people may have 14 per cent Cushing's

disease. Yet, by present techniques, they might not be detected.'
...Aging itself might be a progression of disease along a scale from
zero to 100 per cent....

From these and like comments, it seems reasonable to
characterize health and disease in a simple equation
(Figure 3.2). For illustrative purposes only, numbers are
assigned to the two variables on the left side of the formula
(Figure 3.3). Here is the situation where host susceptibility
is zero in a subject under no (zero) environmental stress. It
would follow that the end result would be perfect health or
zero per cent disease. On the other hand, the value 10 may
be assigned to each of the two factors on the left side of the
equation (Figure 3.4). Now the subject with maximal host
susceptibility (scored as 10) is being challenged maximally
by the environment (graded as 10). The end result is 100 per
cent disease or death.

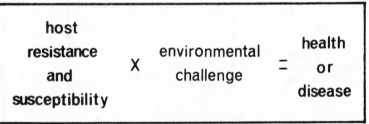

$$\text{host resistance and susceptibility} \times \text{environmental challenge} = \text{health or disease}$$

Figure 3.2. An ecologic formula for health and disease.

$$\text{host susceptibility} \times \text{environmental challenge} = \text{health (no disease)}$$
$$0 \times 0 = 0$$

Figure 3.3. The formula for perfect health.

$$\text{host susceptibility} \times \text{environmental challenge} = \text{death}$$
$$10 \times 10 = 100$$

Figure 3.4. The formula for the ultimate in disease (death).

The two extremes, 0 x 0 = 0 and 10 x 10 = 100, are simple to comprehend. The gradations or intermediate stages are obviously more difficult to discriminate one from the other. A color analogy can be used with white representing health (0 x 0 = 0), black signifying total disease or death (10 x 10 = 100), and an infinite number of shades of gray between these two limiting poles of black and white *(2)*. It is in this transitional gray zone where the common clinical problems exist. For example, disease as typically encountered may be expressed by the formula 5 x 5 = 25 (Figure 3.5). Here one observes an individual with a suboptimal metabolic state (which is the case for many if not most people, as shown in Chapter Two) being minimally challenged by the environment. Thus, most disease is certainly not a function of only the environment or the host, but of both these variables on the left side of the equation.

DIET AND HOST STATE

The mechanisms of host resistance and susceptibility are still incompletely understood. It is clear, nonetheless, that the capacity of the organism to survive the many and diverse environmental threats can be improved or worsened in a number of different ways.

Doctor Howard A. Schneider, of the Laboratories of the Rockefeller Institute for Medical Research, participating in a symposium *Nutrition in Relation to Tropical Medicine* discussed the separateness of resistance and susceptibility *(30)*:

> Resistance and susceptibility, in the minds of many, are relative terms applying to the same over-all phenomenon, infection, and merely point to different ends of the same scale of events as they occur in the infected host. In this view, for example, "more resistant" and "less susceptible" are equivalent, interchangeable, and of equal usefulness. Indeed, as long as we are content to use these terms in making *descriptive* statements in comparing, say, one host with another, we are in no particular difficulties. For simplicity let us say Host A has survived and Host B has died. It matters little whether we say "Host A is less susceptible than Host B," or "Host A is more resistant than Host B."

But Doctor Schneider is not content to view host resistance and susceptibility in just a *descriptive* fashion. His *analytic approach* is particularly pertinent to this discussion:

host susceptibility	X	environmental challenge	=	minimal disease
5	X	5	=	25

Figure 3.5. The formula for the common man.

It is now a necessity, for purposes of unambiguous interpretation of results and the improved design of experiments, that susceptibility and resistance be regarded as separate and distinct biological attributes, each capable of separate manipulations, be it enhancement or diminution.

When experiment shows us that withholding a nutrient decreases the effect of an infection and supplying the nutrient increases the effect, then we can say that the given nutrient is a susceptibility factor, and what we have thereby affected is the character "susceptibility." When experiment shows us that withholding a nutrient increases the effect of an infection, and supplying the nutrient decreases the effect, then we can say that the given nutrient is a resistance factor, and what we have thereby affected is the character "resistance."

While Doctor Schneider utilizes the infectious states to illustrate his point, the cardinal items being stressed are twofold. First, host resistance and susceptibility are not just antonyms. Second, host response may be nutritionally altered in four ways: (1) by supplying a nutrient which enhances or, (2) diminishes the host potential, and (3) by depriving the organism of a nutrient which enhances, or (4) diminishes host capacity. For the present, it is well to illustrate these relationships.

The following findings demonstrate a susceptibility factor (5). Seventy-six presumably healthy dental students shared in this program. Forty of the group were instructed to consume a relatively low-sugar diet for four days. Of the remaining 36, 22 students were supplied with sucrose drinks and 14 served as the control group. Gingival state was graded before and after the four-day experimental period. It will be noted (Figure 3.6) that the overwhelming percentage (82.5 per cent) of the group with sugar deprivation improved. The majority of the group given sucrose supplementation worsened (77.3

per cent). Finally, the control group was relatively unchanged. Thus, on the basis of this study and within the limits of the definition, sugar foods may be regarded as a susceptibility factor.

Conversely, to illustrate a *resistance* variable, a study *(3)* is presented in which 22 subjects were supplied with a wafer prepared from the essential amino acids while another 22 individuals were given an indistinguishable placebo wafer. The experimental design was exactly that utilized in the sugar study *(5)*. Gingival state was graded on Monday and Friday of the same week. Figure 3.7 shows that 19 of the 22 subjects (87 per cent) demonstrated gingival improvement with the protein supplement; 20 of the 22 participants (91 per cent) in the placebo group showed no improvement. Thus, here is a simple demonstration of a nutrient which, when supplied, adds to the *resistance* factor.

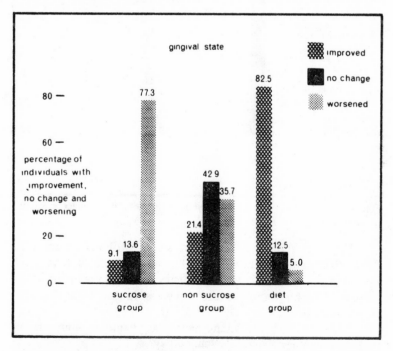

Figure 3.6. The effect upon gingival state of the elimination and addition of refined carbohydrate foodstuffs.

HOMEOSTASIS: THE CRUX OF THE PROBLEM

In the final analysis, life or death is a function of homeostasis (the ability of the body to maintain metabolic equilibrium). The cells collectively as a total organism survive when the host can cope successfully with the many and diverse environmental threats. When the homeostatic machinery collapses, the same hostile environment now overwhelms the system, and disease and then death ensue.

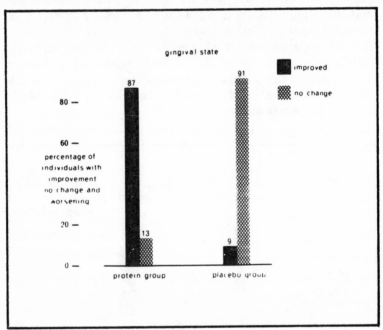

Figure 3.7. The effect upon gingival state of protein versus placebo supplementation.

While much about homeostasis is still unknown, it is clear that metabolism echoes the steady state. One such measure is carbohydrate metabolism. Its relationship to homeostasis may be found in the answers to the following five questions (4):

1. What is the carbohydrate metabolic picture of a presumably healthy person during a routine day?
2. How does carbohydrate metabolism relate to the sugar equivalent of carbohydrate foods in a regular diet?

3. What changes in carbohydrate metabolism follow a decrease in refined carbohydrates (sugar and white flour) ingestion?
4. Is there any relationship between carbohydrate metabolism and the physiologic state (e.g. blood pressure)?
5. Can physiologic state (e.g. blood pressure) be significantly altered by reducing refined carbohydrate intake?

Seven dental practitioners participated in a program during a two-week period *(4)*. On Monday through Thursday of the first week, the seven subjects carried out their usual activities while consuming their regular diets. On Thursday, each participant reported to the clinic at 8:00 A.M. fasting (immediately before an 8:15 A.M. breakfast), 10:00 A.M. (about 30 minutes after the usual 9:30 A.M. break), 12:00 Noon (about 30 minutes prior to the 12:30 P.M. lunch), 2:00 P.M. (about one hour before the customary 3:00 P.M. coffee break), and at 4:00 P.M. At each visit, the blood glucose (Somogyi-Nelson method) was determined. Also, at each of the sessions, blood pressure was recorded.

The following Monday through Thursday, the subjects carried out their usual duties. However, as far as possible, refined carbohydrates (sugar and white flour products) were eliminated from the diet. On Thursday, the subjects reported to the clinic for blood glucose and blood pressure measurements as earlier reported for the initial visit.

Figure 3.8 pictorially portrays the mean blood glucose values for the seven subjects at the five different intervals during the initial visit (interrupted line). The overall individual spread is 115 mg. per cent (from a low of 60 to a high of 175). The mean spread for the entire group is approximately 46 mg. per cent (73.4 to 119.0 mg. per cent). Within the limits of these observations (and supported by the reported literature), carbohydrate metabolism, as measured by blood glucose, fluctuates significantly during the day.

There are undoubtedly many factors which govern the metabolism of carbohydrates. Certainly, one of the important variables is the diet. The sugar equivalent for total carbohydrate intake at any one temporal point varied from 0 to 28.9 teaspoonsful. Figure 3.9 graphically shows the mean sugar equivalent intake for the experimental days (hatched columns). The range for the group is approximately 29 teaspoonsful

(0 to 29). It is reasonable to conclude, from these data, that the carbohydrate intake fluctuates widely and significantly during the day.

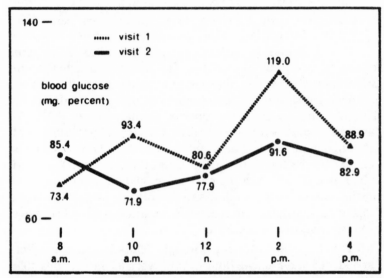

Figure 3.8. Daily fluctuations in mean blood glucose following a three-day regular diet (visit 1, interrupted line) and after a three-day decrease in refined-carbohydrate foods (visit 2, continuous line).

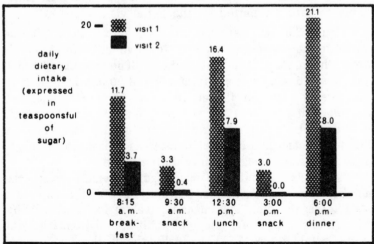

Figure 3.9. Mean sugar equivalent intake (expressed in teaspoonsful) after a three-day regular diet (visit 1, hatched columns) and following a three-day reduction in refined-carbohydrate foods (visit 2, dark columns).

An analysis of Figure 3.10 shows the relationship between the ingestion of carbohydrate foods (as expressed in sugar equivalents) and the blood glucose levels. It appears from the available data that orderly relationships prevail between the dietary sugar equivalent for total carbohydrate intake and carbohydrate metabolism. In brief, after carbohydrate intake, the blood glucose rises. Parenthetic mention should be made of published data showing that the glycemic responses are more severe following sucrose ingestion than after isoglucogenic quantities of other carbohydrates or protein (8). While the observations thus far are of interest, no cause-and-effect relationships of carbohydrate intake to blood glucose can be drawn.

Earlier mention was made of the fact that, on Monday through Thursday of the second week, the subjects were instructed to reduce sugar and white flour intake to a minimum. The mean sugar equivalent intake for subjects at the initial (hatched columns) and the final (black columns) visit is summarized in Figure 3.9. It is abundantly clear from this chart that the sugar equivalent intake at every temporal point has been sharply curtailed. With this background information, it is now possible to reiterate the question as to what effect this dietary change exerted upon the blood glucose pattern.

Figure 3.8 shows the mean glucose values initially with a regular diet (interrupted line) versus the scores following a reduction in sugar equivalent intake (continuous line). On a regular diet, the mean spread of values is about 46 mg. per cent. At the second visit, the range is 20 mg. per cent. Hence, the mean spread has been halved.

It is now possible to answer the third question: what changes in carbohydrate metabolism occur with dietary alteration? Within the limits of these observations, it appears that significant blood glucose changes follow the elimination of refined carbohydrate foods from the diet. Thus, the relative omission of sugars and white flour products seems to yield a more homeostatic picture of carbohydrate metabolism as evidenced by fewer and less abrupt fluctuations in the diurnal blood glucose concentration. This is consistent with published reports (8,23).

The point now at hand is to determine whether the

demonstrated changes in carbohydrate metabolism are of physiologic import. In other words, is the organism biologically better when there is a steadier (more homeostatic) carbohydrate metabolic state?

Figure 3.11 pictorially portrays the mean systolic pressure at the initial visit. It can be seen (interrupted line) that the pressure fluctuates during the day. Figure 3.12 provides the opportunity of comparing the daily mean blood glucose and blood pressure changes while subsisting on a regular diet. It is interesting (Figure 3.12) that the systolic pressure at the various temporal points (interrupted line) parallels almost precisely the fluctuations in blood glucose (continuous line).

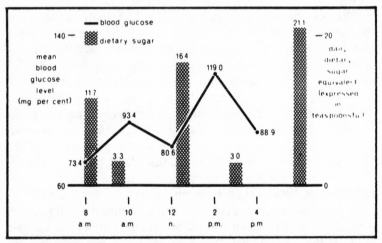

Figure 3.10. Relationship of the daily fluctuations in mean blood glucose (continuous line) to the mean sugar equivalent intake (expressed in teaspoonsful) of a regular diet (stippled columns).

It is now possible to answer the fourth question: is there any relationship between carbohydrate metabolism and the physiologic state (e.g. blood pressure)? It would appear, from these data and an earlier study *(26)*, that parallelisms do indeed exist. Certainly, in the case of the systolic blood pressure, when the blood glucose rises, the systolic pressure increases; when the glucose decreases, the pressure drops.

Now we may return to the all-important point. Is the organism biologically improved when the carbohydrate meta-

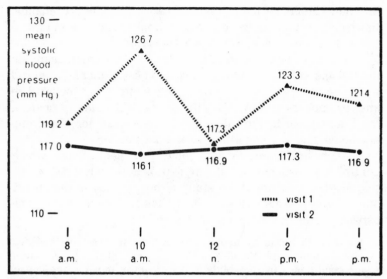

Figure 3.11. Daily fluctuations in mean systolic blood pressure following a three-day regular diet (visit 1, interrupted line) and after a three-day relatively low-refined-carbohydrate intake (visit 2, continuous line).

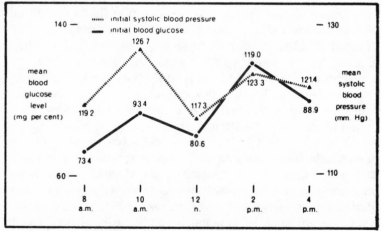

Figure 3.12. Comparison of the daily variations in the mean blood glucose (continuous line) and the mean systolic blood pressure (interrupted line) after a three-day regular dietary regimen.

bolic pattern is more steady? Figure 3.11 provides the opportunity of comparing the initial mean blood pressure values (interrupted line) and the mean final scores (continuous line).

Mention should be made that, following the dietary change, the mean systolic range decreased from 9 mm. Hg (117.3 to 126.7) to about 1 mm. Hg (116.1 to 117.3).

It is now possible to answer the fifth question: can the physiologic state (e.g. blood pressure) be significantly altered by reducing the intake of sugar and white flour foods? The answer appears to be in the affirmative. With dietary change, the fluctuations in the individual subjects and for the group are fewer and the amplitude variations smaller.

Much has been written about the mechanisms which control homeostasis (the steady state). Relatively little attention has been accorded the study of how steady is the steady state. Dubos, in his writings about Claude Bernard and homeostasis, made the following statement *(10)*:

> He (Claude Bernard) emphasized that at all levels of biological organization, in plants as well as in animals, survival and fitness are conditioned by the ability of the organism to resist the impact of the outside world and maintain constant *within narrow limits* (italics added) the physicochemical characteristics of its internal environment.

Surely, during health, body temperature fluctuates during the day. Any sudden rise or abrupt fall is immediately reflected in the clinical state (e.g. sweating and chilling). Ordinarily, the average man during the usual day has his moments of pleasure and displeasure. When these fluctuations are exaggerated, so that the subject is at once manic and moments later catatonic, disease is obvious (Figure 3.13). It would seem that health and disease could be plotted on the basis of the extent of the amplitudes of a constellation of physiologic, biochemical, and clinical parameters. For example, it would follow that carbohydrate metabolism (as reflected in blood glucose) also possesses its physiologic limits. Thus, during the normal day of a healthy man, blood glucose should vary. The question is, how much amplitude is physiologically acceptable?

The simple study reported here shows that a daily blood glucose variation exists. This experiment demonstrates that the blood glucose concentration parallels dietary habits. In this report, there is evidence to indicate that the ups and downs in blood glucose can be muted by decreasing the sugar and white flour intake. Thus, as far as carbohydrate metabolism is concerned, the end result is a more steady state, a more homeostatic pattern.

That this biochemical phenomenon is not without physiologic benefits is demonstrated by a study of the cardiovascular system as reflected in blood pressure. Daily fluctuations are evident in the average man. The blood pressure changes correlate with the blood glucose levels. The restriction of sugar and white flour products seems to parallel a more steady state in the cardiovascular system as reflected by the systolic blood pressure.

The point of this story is that small fluctuations in homeostatic mechanisms may be more significant than heretofore recognized. The experiment just cited (4) in no way implies that these minor blood glucose fluctuations cause physiologic changes (e.g. in blood pressure). What is exciting about these feedback systems is that small variations in one area can presage widespread physiologic changes in another region. Evidence of one such servosystem has been recently pub-

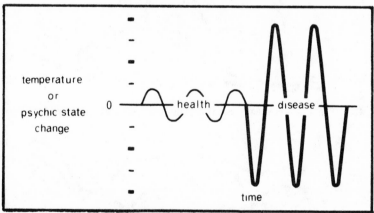

Figure 3.13. Apparently health and disease may be expressed in terms of amplitudes; the smaller ones appear more consonant with health.

lished by investigators from the Karolinska Hospital in Stockholm, Sweden, and Southwestern Medical School in Dallas, Texas (19). It is apparent from Figure 3.14 that a minor decrease in blood glucose, of a magnitude which occurs daily in the average person, produces a significant increase in plasma growth hormone. On the basis of these findings, the authors suggest that growth hormone is one of the most sensitive regulators of blood glucose homeostasis.

SUMMARY

The relationship of diet and disease is predicated on the principle that health and sickness are the result of the inter-

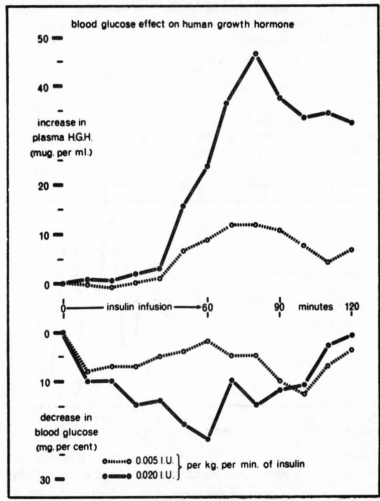

Figure 3.14. Small changes in blood glucose are paralleled by significant alterations in the release of hypophyseal growth hormone.

play of host factors and environmental challenges. When the host can successfully cope with the environment, high resistance or low susceptibility prevails. If the host succumbs to the many and diverse environmental bombardments, low resistance or high susceptibility is operative. Diet can serve in four different ways to modify the host state. Nutrients, when added, may increase resistance or susceptibility; conversely, withholding nutrients can enhance resistance or exaggerate susceptibility.

REFERENCES

1. Bronte-Stewart, B. and Krut, L. H. *The interdependence of prospective and retrospective studies in research on ischaemic heart disease.* J. Atheroscl. Res. 2: 317-331, 1962.

2. Cheraskin, E. *The arithmetic of disease.* J. Dent. Med. 14: #2, 71-82, April 1959.

3. Cheraskin, E. and Ringsdorf, W. M., Jr. *Periodontal pathosis in man: IX. Effect of combined versus animal protein supplementation upon gingival state.* J. Dent. Med. 19: #2, 82-85, April 1964.

4. Cheraskin, E. and Ringsdorf, W. M., Jr. *Homeostasis: a study in carbohydrate metabolism.* J. Med. Assn. State of Alabama 35: #3, 173-182, September 1965.

5. Cheraskin, E., Ringsdorf, W. M., Jr. and Setyaadmadja, A. T. S. H. *Periodontal pathosis in man: XII. Effect of sucrose drinks upon gingival state.* Pakistan Dent. Rev. 15: #4, 143-147, October 1965.

6. Clark, K. G. *Preventive medicine in medical schools: report of Colorado Springs Conference, November 1952.* 1953. Baltimore, Waverly Press.

7. Coburn, A. F. *The pathogenesis of rheumatic fever–a concept.* Perspec. Bio. and Med. 6: #4, 493-511, Summer 1963.

8. Conn, J. W. and Newburgh, L. H. *The glycemic response to isoglucogenic quantities of protein and carbohydrate.* J. Clin. Invest. 15: #5, 665-671, November 1936.

9. Danowski, T. S. and Moses, C., Jr. *Cholesterol levels reduced by hormone 'replacement doses,'* J. A. M. A. 181: #9, 27-28, 1 September 1962.

10. Dubos, R. J. *Mirage of health.* 1959. New York, Harper and Brothers. p. 86.

11. Dubos, R. J. *Pasteur and modern science.* 1960. New York, Anchor Books, Doubleday and Company. p. 136.

12. Engel, G. L. *A unified concept of health and disease.* Perspec. Bio. and Med. 3: #4, 459-485, Summer 1960.

13. Grunberg, E. *Aspects of cancer research.* Trans. New York Acad. Sc. 25: #4, 433-443, February 1963.

14. Haggerty, R. J. *Host and environmental factors in infections.* J. Louisiana State Med. Soc. 116: #9, 309-317, September 1964.

15. Keys, A. *The role of the diet in human artherosclerosis and its complications.* In Sandler, M. and Bourne, G. H. *Atherosclerosis and its origin.* 1963. New York, Academic Press.

16. King, S. H. *Perceptions of illness and medical practice*. 1962. Philadelphia, William F. Fell Company. pp. 14-15.

17. Krehl, W. A. *The evaluation of nutritional status*. Med. Clin. North America 48: #5, 1129-1140, September 1964.

18. Kruse, H. D. *The interplay of noxious agents, stress, and deprivation in the etiology of disease*. In Galdston, I. *Beyond the germ theory*. 1954. New York Health Education Council. p. 17.

19. Luft, R., Cerasi, E., Madison, L. L., von Euler, U. S., Casa, L. D. and Roovete, A. *Effect of a small decrease in blood-glucose on plasma-growth-hormone and urinary excretion of catecholamines in man*. Lancet 2: #7457, 254-256, 30 July 1966.

20. May, J. M. *The ecology of human disease*. 1958. New York, MD Publications, Inc.

21. May, J. M. *The ecology of human disease*. Ann. New York Acad. Sc. 84: #17, 789-794, December 8, 1960.

22. Meerloo, J. A. M. *Illness and cure*. 1964. New York, Grune and Stratton.

23. Page, M. E., Ringsdorf, W. M., Jr. and Cheraskin, E. *The effect of a low-refined-carbohydrate high-protein diet upon nonfasting blood sugar*. Odont. Revy 12: #1, 1-24, 1961.

24. Payne, A. M. *Teaching preventive medicine*. Arch. Environ. Health 4: #6, 625-629, June 1962.

25. Piersol, G. M. *Foreword: the mechanisms of disease*. In Stambul, J. *The mechanisms of disease*. 1952. New York, Froben Press.

26. Ringsdorf, W. M., Jr., Cheraskin, E. and Hollis, C. F. *Effect of a low-refined-carbohydrate diet upon nonfasting blood pressure*. Alabama Dent. Rev. 9: #3, 18-30, Spring 1962.

27. Rogers, E. S. *Human ecology and health*. 1960. New York, The Macmillan Company. pp. 167, 170.

28. Rogers, E. S. *Human ecology and health*. 1960. New York, The Macmillan Company. p. 174.

29. Ryan, E. J. *The editor's page*. Dent. Dig. 68: #10, 479, October 1962.

30. Schneider, H. A. *Nutrition and resistance—susceptibility to infection*. Am. J. Trop. Med. 31: #2, 174-182, March 1951.

31. Scrimshaw, N. S. *Ecological factors in nutritional disease*. Am. J. Clin. Nutrit. 14: #2, 112-122, February 1964.

32. Selye, E. H. *The pluricausal cardiopathies*. 1961. Springfield, Charles C. Thomas. p. xiii.

33. Spain, D. M. *The failure to extend the horizons of preventive medicine*. Arch. Environ. Health 7: #3, 263-265, September 1963.

34. Spies, T. D. *Some recent advances in nutrition.* J. A. M. A. 167: #6, 675-690, 7 June 1958.

35. Wadsworth, G. R. *Nutrition surveys--clinical signs and biochemical measurements.* Proc. Nutrit. Soc. 22: #1, 72-78, 20 July 1962.

36. Wolf, S. *A new view of disease.* J. A. M. A. 184: #2, 143-144, 13 April 1963.

4. DIETARY INTERRELATIONSHIPS

THE ECOLOGIC FACTORS WHICH ENTER INTO THE GENESIS OF HEALTH and disease have been evolved in the preceding chapter. The point was underlined that diet plays a role in host defense mechanisms. This becomes particularly relevant in the light of what the average American consumes (Chapter One) as it relates to the disease pattern of the nation in terms of mortality and morbidity. (Chapter Two).

In the next section *specific* nutrients will be analyzed for their contribution to various disease syndromes. Actually, this is an artificial situation. Realistically, the biologic effects of a single nutrient will vary with the other nutrients consumed at the same time. Hence, there is need for an understanding of the dynamics of nutrient interdependency.

The vast number and complexity of nutrient interactions have been graphically described by Robert A. Harte (American Society of Biological Chemists, Washington, D. C.) and Doctor Bacon Chow *(19)* of the Johns Hopkins University School of Public Health and Hygiene:

> In the first edition of this book a comprehensive, critical review of relevant literature to 1953 included well over 200 references on the various facets of the problem of dietary interrelationships. Since then additional reports have appeared to further elucidate such dietary interrelationships. Perhaps the most striking impression received from evaluation of the literature is that hardly any study undertaken with any pair of nutrients has failed to show a significant interaction in terms of some nutritional or biochemical criterion. This is not surprising, though, since each step of the chain of reactions through which a nutrient goes as it follows an appropriate metabolic pathway is mediated by at least one enzyme system, and the functioning of every enzyme system calls for the combined action of an apoenzyme (made up for the most part of

amino acids) and a coenzyme (which usually includes a vitamin and/or a mineral element). However, the breadth of the experimental interrelationships brought out by these various studies underlines the statement that 'the recognition of the large number of them re-emphasizes the basic soundness of the principle of maintaining variety in food in order to provide the most nutritious diet.'

This insight into nutrient interplay is the basis for a changing concept of deficiency disease. For example, the late Doctor Richard H. Follis (14) of the Nutritional and Metabolic Disease Section, Veterans Administration Control Laboratory for Anatomical Pathology and Research, Armed Forces Institute of Pathology, has noted that perhaps the most important point to realize in a consideration of the naturally occurring deficiency diseases in man is that:

...These diseases result from a lack of multiple nutrients rather than the deficit of a single essential....More and more attention is being given to the multiple nature concept of most deficiency disease syndromes; this should help to clarify our understanding of them and allow us to investigate them more intelligently.

Because of the interaction of nutrients, it is possible that much of nutritional knowledge, derived from experimental situations where only one nutrient is deficient, is incomplete. Robert A. Harte and Doctor Bacon Chow (19) have also commented on this neglected aspect of nutrition research.

The usual experimental situation in which a vitamin deficiency state is studied involves the feeding of an otherwise adequate diet containing all the known nutrients except the one being tested. It is generally assumed, implicitly, that such a diet will create a deficiency only of the essential nutrient; but there are important fallacies in this assumption. First, the administration of a diet deficient in a nutrient is very frequently followed by a marked reduction of food intake. As a result the intake of all of the other nutrients is reduced....Second, in many instances the deficiency of a certain vitamin may adversely affect the absorption of one or more other vitamins, thus giving rise to secondary deficiencies. Third, an effect of a dietary deficiency in a single vitamin may be an increase in requirement for one or more other nutrients, so that relative secondary deficiencies may arise.

Because the number of nutrient interrelationships is quite large, the selection of examples must of necessity be very incomplete. The following data will attempt to summarize some of the interclass activity and provide, where possible, both lower animal and human evidence. Since the major change in the American diet during the last century has been in carbohydrate consumption (Chapter One, The American Diet) and since abnormal carbohydrate metabolism is so prevalent and is evident in many of the current major health problems (Chapter Twelve, Disease State Interrelationships), the association of carbohydrates with the other nutrient groups will be especially emphasized.

MAJOR FOODSTUFFS INTERRELATIONSHIPS

The intricate associations among carbohydrates, fat, and proteins have been summarized by Doctor Rachmiel Levine, Professor and Chairman of the Department of Medicine at the New York Medical College *(24)*:

> The tricarboxylic acid cycle assumes a significance far beyond its function in carbohydrate breakdown. The catabolisms of carbohydrate, protein and fat, respectively, pursue more or less independent courses until they reach the stage of the alpha or beta keto acids....From this point on, the lower intermediates of all three foodstuffs are indistinguishable from one another; and from this "pool" of 2-carbon and 3-carbon intermediates, any of the three foodstuffs can be built up again. Hence, the cycle is probably the final common pathway for carbohydrate, protein and fat, as well as the locus for interconversions between the three foodstuffs.

It must be borne in mind that, in the utilization of carbohydrates, fats, and proteins for energy, calories from any one of these sources may be regarded as completely replaceable by calories from any other of these sources. However, this is dependent upon the integrity of a variety of enzyme systems which, in turn, depend upon exogenous supplies of vitamins, minerals, and amino acids *(19)*.

CARBOHYDRATE-FAT INTERRELATIONSHIPS

Because of the prominent role played by the dietary lipids and their metabolism in the cardiovascular diseases, the relationships between carbohydrate intake and fat metabolism are worthy of further elaboration.

Doctor Robert E. Olson of Washington University in Saint Louis, in a presentation to the Council on Foods and Nutrition and the Council on Scientific Assembly at the 109th Annual Meeting of the American Medical Association (13 June 1960) in Miami Beach, Florida, described the importance of the 2-carbon chain as a common pathway for the metabolism of carbohydrates and fats (33) and especially the synthesis of ketone bodies, fatty acids and cholesterol.

In an excellent review article entitled *Inter-relationships of Glucose and Lipid Metabolism,* Doctor Marvin D. Siperstein (Department of Internal Medicine, The University of Texas Southwestern Medical School, Dallas, Texas) discussed the mounting evidence for the influence of glucose on various phases of lipid metabolism. He concludes that (37):

> ...it is becoming increasingly apparent that fatty acid synthesis and oxidation, cholesterol synthesis, and ketone body accumulation all are in part controlled by the rate at which glucose is broken down within the cell....In particular, it has been emphasized that glucose, in addition to serving the vital function of supplying substrate for the operation of Krebs cycle, acts as a generating system for the reduced pyridine nucleotides, and that it is through these coenzymes and in particular TPNH, that glycolysis may be able to exert its regulatory influence on lipid metabolism.

Thus, one may conclude that glucose, in addition to being utilized for energy, affects the synthesis of lipids through the active 2-carbon metabolite, acetyl coenzyme A, and the reduced pyridine nucleotide coenzymes (di- and triphosphopyridine nucleotide).

Less well known is the importance of the type of dietary carbohydrate in lipid metabolism. Reviews of animal studies (4,27,35) challenge the commonly held belief that simple sugars and more complex forms of carbohydrate are alike in their effect upon lipid metabolism. The evidence indicates that simple sugars such as sucrose are more lipogenic. In fact, human studies enlarge the view (1,5,6,25,26) that, while sucrose does indeed elevate serum lipid levels, dietary starch actually lowers these fractions (6,15,25,26).

Typical findings are those of Doctor I. McDonald (25) of the Physiology Department, Guy's Hospital Medical School, London, England, who studied the effects of dietary starch and sucrose upon blood lipids in adult males (Table 4.1). As indicated in the starch diet column, none of the lipid parameters rose; however, with the sucrose diet, total serum lipids and serum glycerides increased. Doctor Margaret A. Ohlson *(6)*, formerly Director of Nutrition Services and Professor, Department of Internal Medicine, State University of Iowa, and her associate, Mohamed A. Antar, recently conducted a similar investigation using four healthy 20 to 25 year old men and a like group of women as subjects. Each person served as his own control by consuming on two different occasions both the high simple carbohydrate and high complex carbohydrate diets in a crossover fashion. Total serum lipids, phospholipids, and nonphospholipids were found to be significantly reduced with the high cereal diet and increased with the high sugar diet when the total calories and fats were held constant for both men and women (Table 4.2) *(5)*.

Table 4.1
changes in the concentration of serum
lipid and its fractions found in
adult males on a diet low in fat
and high in starch or sucrose

	starch diet	sucrose diet
total serum lipids	decreased	**increased**
serum sterol esters	decreased	unchanged
serum glycerides	unchanged	**increased**
serum phospholipid	decreased	unchanged
total serum cholesterol	decreased	unchanged

CARBOHYDRATE-VITAMIN INTERRELATIONSHIPS

It is known that vitamin B fractions are an integral part of carbohydrate metabolism and that the need for this group of vitamins depends upon the amount of carbohydrate consumed. Doctor Samuel Soskin (Consultant in Medicine, Cedars of Lebanon Hospital, Los Angeles; Consulting Editor, "Metabolism, Clinical and Experimental Medicine") and Doctor R. Levine (Professor and Chairman, Department of Medicine, New York Medical College, New York City) have explained why there was not an earlier awareness of this interdependency *(38)*.

Why was knowledge of its existence not acquired much earlier in human experience and why did the race not suffer from lack of that knowledge? The answer to these questions is that it was only in comparatively recent times that the natural union between the vitamin B complex and carbohydrate, a union existing in whole grain and plants, was broken by the industrial processing of foods. Before this occurred, the supply of B vitamins was automatically adjusted to the amount of carbohydrate eaten; the occurrence of B deficiency with its consequent disturbance in nutrition is, therefore, a comparatively recent development in the Western World....

Since the breakdown of carbohydrate is essentially similar in all tissues and organs, it follows that a vitamin B deficiency will impair carbohydrate metabolism in every structure of the body.

Table 4.2
mean serum lipid levels during
self selected, high simple carbohydrate
and high complex carbohydrate diet periods

number of subjects	pre-experimental diet	Period 1 high simple carbohydrate diet	Period 2 high complex carbohydrate diet	Period 3 high simple carbohydrate diet	Period 4 high complex carbohydrate diet
total lipids, mg/100 ml.					
men (4)	563	616	545	691	470
women (2)	467	545	478	589	446
women (2)*	563	532	450	512	431
nonphospholipids (neutral), mg/100 ml.					
men (4)	364	393	350	454	292
women (2)	336	345	301	364	266
women (2)*	347	346	275	319	260
phospholipids, mg/100 ml.					
men (4)	196	212	192	226	173
women (2)	156**	189	174	209	170
women (2)*	200	179	171	185	174
phospholipids, % of total lipids					
men (4)	35.4	35.1	35.7	33.2	37.4
women (2)	37.1**	35.3	37.4	36.3	39.2
women (2)	37.3	34.0	38.4	37.0	40.1

*pregnancy occurred during period 3
**one case

Consideration of Figure 4.1 (illustration added) also shows the fallacy of regarding any single factor of the B complex as more important than another, for the normal chain of events can be broken by a lack of any one of them.

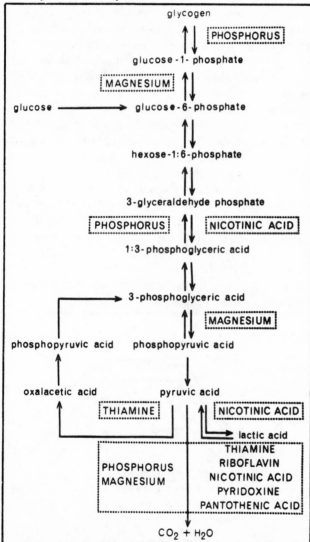

Figure 4.1. Points of action of vitamins and minerals in carbohydrate metabolism (substances required for a particular reaction are necessary in both directions).

Relatively recent reviews of the literature on carbohydrate-vitamin interaction cite both lower animal and human studies of the role of B complex fractions in the maintenance of optimal carbohydrate metabolism *(30,41)*. On the other hand, it has been noted that the type of dietary carbohydrates may also influence vitamin requirements. For example, dextrin and cornstarch appear to be less demanding on the common B complex fractions *(30)*. Recently, even B_{12} has been shown to enhance significantly glucose utilization in a group over 70 years of age *(17)*.

Evidence has accumulated from lower animal and human studies that there is a significant relationship between ascorbic acid and the metabolism of carbohydrates. As representative of this relationship, one may observe in Figure 4.2 *(36)* that a progressive and significant decrease in glucose tolerance parallels the successive stages of vitamin C depletion in guinea pigs. Doctor Emanuel Cheraskin (Professor and Chairman, Department of Oral Medicine, University of Alabama Medical Center) and co-workers, from human experimental data *(36)*, concluded that the commonly noted progressive decrease in glucose tolerance with age in the human does not occur in the presence of a relatively physiologic vitamin C state (Table 4.3).

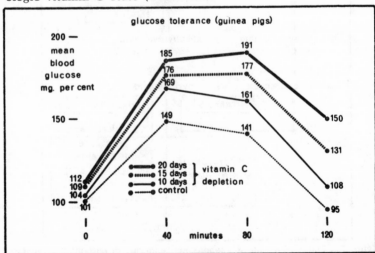

Figure 4.2. The glucose tolerance of control and vitamin C depleted guinea pigs.

Table 4.3
glucose tolerance in two age groups
(≤ 35 versus ≥ 36) with a relatively poor*
(≤ 0.5 mg. %) and good** (≥ 0.6 mg. %) plasma
ascorbic acid level

*relatively poor plasma ascorbic acid level

cortisone glucose tolerance test	age ≤ 35 years		age ≥ 36 years		P
	mean	S.D.	mean	S.D.	
fasting	76.6	12.8	87.7	16.0	≤ 0.005
30 minutes	134.2	27.4	148.1	42.9	> 0.050
1 hour	129.4	40.0	157.9	54.9	≤ 0.005
2 hours	96.6	32.2	120.8	51.4	≤ 0.010
3 hours	73.6	29.6	91.8	46.2	≤ 0.025

**relatively good plasma ascorbic acid level

fasting	81.7	11.9	79.8	15.5	> 0.500
30 minutes	128.9	29.9	129.7	23.4	> 0.500
1 hour	123.0	31.7	138.9	35.2	> 0.050
2 hours	94.0	23.3	107.0	31.9	> 0.050
3 hours	76.5	21.1	84.1	28.8	> 0.200

CARBOHYDRATE-PROTEIN INTERRELATIONSHIPS

Although the protein-sparing action of carbohydrate has been recognized for nearly a century, the underlying mechanism still remains obscure. Fructose induces a greater nitrogen retention than sucrose, glucose, or a maltose-dextrin mixture. This finding in studies of children and convalescent adults *(3)* underscores the different sparing action of different carbohydrates.

Possibly more important than the protein-sparing effect of carbohydrates is the relationship between dietary protein and carbohydrate as reflected in the organism's ability to maintain a steady state. It will be recalled that this concept has been previously discussed (Chapter Three). Doctor Stewart Wolf (Department of Medicine, University of Oklahoma, and the Oklahoma Medical Research Foundation) emphasized the importance of metabolic homeostasis in the following comments before the Seventy-Fifth Annual Meeting of the American Clinical and Climatological Association at French Lick, Indiana, in November 1962 *(42):*

There is some reason to believe that organ disturbances are more likely to occur when the alternation of positive and negative forces is poorly damped, that is when a system is labile or vacillates relatively a great deal. Harold Wolff showed several years ago that if a daily record of temporal-artery pulsations is obtained, those persons subject to migraine can be recognized at times when no headache is present, by the fact that there is considerable variability in the amplitude of temporal-artery pulsations from day to day. It is a common experience that patients in whom diabetes ultimately develops may in earlier life have had troublesome episodes of hypoglycemia. Hypertensive patients often give a history of hypotensive episodes in youth.

My thesis, not really new, therefore, would hold that (1) many diseases represent simply too much or too little of essentially normal adaptive reactions, (2) regulation of these reactions is often achieved thru [sic] cyclic variations in the homeostatic systems, (3) wide swings in a cycle may constitute the evidences of disease, and thus (4) modifications in these wide swings to a point of equilibrium between health and disease may be achieved through influences on the regulatory processes from the higher centers of the central nervous system.

The glycemic response to isoglucogenic quantities of protein and carbohydrate was effectively demonstrated by Doctor Jerome W. Conn and Doctor L. H. Newburgh *(21)* of the Department of Internal Medicine, University of Michigan Medical School in 1936 (Figure 4.3) *(9),* (Figure 4.4) *(10).* A comparison was made between the glycemic and glycosuric responses after ingestion of equivalent amounts of glucose derived from glucose per se, protein and carbohydrate foods in normo-, hyper-, and hypoglycemic individuals. Within the limits of these studies one may note a decided contribution to homeostasis in deriving glucose from protein. The slow rate of liberation of glucose, in the liver, from the glycogenic amino acids produced no glycosuria and very little change in the blood sugar concentration. This is consistent with the experiment described earlier (Chapter Three).

Not only are blood sugar levels more homeostatic when protein replaces dietary glucose, but the simultaneous ingestion of both yields a more steady level than glucose consumption alone. Doctor M. Srinivasan (Assistant Director, Division of Biochemistry and Nutrition, Central Food Technological Research Institute, Mysore, India) has demonstrated that proteins ingested before or with glucose produce a much more physiologic glucose tolerance pattern in hyperglycemic subjects than when only glucose is taken (Figure 4.5) *(39)*.

Elsa Orent-Keiles and Lois F. Hallman, of the United States Department of Agriculture, Circular 827 *(34)*, provide an excellent review of the literature on the glycemic response to protein and carbohydrate ingestion. They noted that sustained blood sugar levels and a sense of well-being were more closely related to the quantity and quality of protein than to the carbohydrate or fat content of the breakfast meal. They concluded that the favorable effect may be due to the relatively slower digestion, absorption, and metabolism of protein and consequently to a steadier supply of glucose to the blood.

CARBOHYDRATE-MINERAL INTERRELATIONSHIPS

From Figure 4.1 it is apparent that both phosphorus and magnesium are essential for the anaerobic metabolism of glucose or glycogen to carbon dioxide and water and for the synthesis of glycogen. Magnesium, in addition, plays a prominent role in the metabolism of galactose, fructose, and mannose (Figure 4.6) *(2)*.

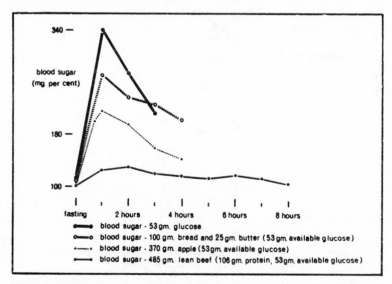

Figure 4.3. Glycemic response to isoglucogenic quantities of protein and several carbohydrate foods.

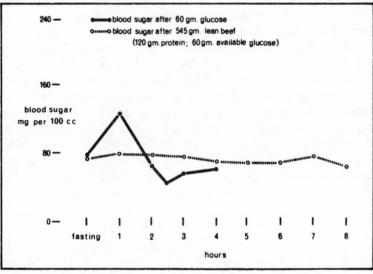

Figure 4.4. Glycemic response to isoglucogenic quantities of glucose and protein.

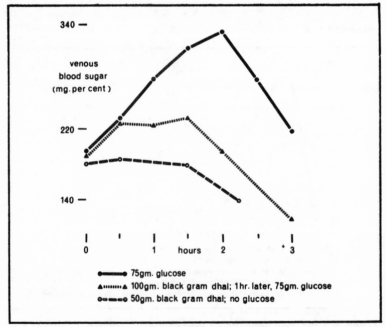

Figure 4.5. Dietary protein and glucose tolerance patterns.

Aerobic metabolism also utilizes magnesium at many levels. The specific areas are described by Doctor Jerry K. Aikawa, Associate Professor of Medicine, University of Colorado School of Medicine *(2)*:

The initial oxidation of pyruvic acid requires magnesium. In the tricarboxylic acid cycle, magnesium is necessary for the conversion of alpha-ketoglutaric acid to succinic acid. In the assimilation of carbon dioxide, the reaction, pyruvate $\longleftrightarrow$ oxaloacetate, requires magnesium. In the pentose monophosphate shunt, the conversion of xylulose-5-phosphate to glyceraldehyde-3-phosphate is magnesium-dependent.

OTHER DIETARY INTERRELATIONSHIPS

As was mentioned earlier in this chapter, dependency exists not only between classes of nutrients but in addition intra- and interclass associations of individual nutrients are common. In fact, from the existing evidence in this field, it is not speculative to state that *every nutrient has interrelationships with every other nutrient (14,19,40)*.

There are countless other correlations between foods and chemicals that are ingested and nutritional status. Several examples will be briefly considered in order to demonstrate the magnitude of the problem.

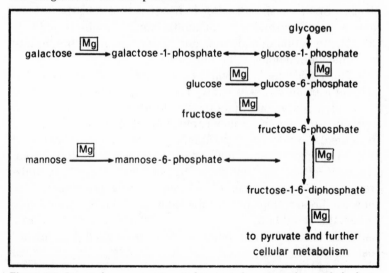

Figure 4.6. Steps where magnesium is known to be essential in carbohydrate metabolism.

Chemicals are available which will reverse or block the effects of related substances in biologic systems. The compounds responsible for these blocking effects are termed *antimetabolites* because they are concerned with preventing the utilization by living tissues of normally-occurring nutritional substances. Actually, antimetabolites now exist, from foods or by synthesis, for practically all known nutrients *(20)*. Since most of the nutrient antimetabolites are not found in the human diet, they are not of primary concern. Of those which occur in the American dietary, avidin and the goitrogens are among the most widely publicized examples *(8)*. Avidin is a biotin antagonist found in raw egg white; goitrogens prevent iodine uptake by the thyroid. These are found in the cabbage family and soy bean group.

Metabolic interrelationships have been demonstrated between nutrients and drugs *(11,43)*. Recently, the teratogenic effect of thalidomide upon the human fetus has received much publicity. As a result, animal experimentation has revealed that most species demonstrate the embryotoxic effects of this drug. Thalidomide has been reported to act as an antagonist of several nutrients in experimental animals: folic acid *(21, 22)*, vitamin B_6 *(21,22)*, glutamic acid *(7,12,23)*, and vitamin B_2 *(23)*. Since these and other nutrient deficiencies have been shown to induce multiple congenital abnormalities in animals *(31,32)*, the thalidomide-nutrient reactions may precipitate maternal deficiencies (Chapter Seven).

The Department of Pharmacology of the Geigy Research Laboratories in Ardsley, New York, has released *(15)* some interesting data on thalidomide teratogenicity in vitamin deficient and control rats (Table 4.4). It may be noted that in animals rendered hypovitaminotic by diets deficient in riboflavin, pantothenic acid, and alpha-tocopherol, the embryotoxic effect was enhanced by the daily peroral administration of 150 mg./kg. of thalidomide during pregnancy. The increased resorptions or malformations induced by thalidomide under the condition of certain hypovitaminic states in rats may, according to the authors, provide a lead for further testing of the assumption that thalidomide may act as an antimetabolite.

Doctor Edmund B. Flink *(29)* (Professor and Chairman,

Department of Medicine, West Virginia University School of Medicine) and others (13) have demonstrated in both normal and alcoholic individuals that the ingestion of ethanol leads to significant body losses of magnesium.

Dietary interrelationships have been demonstrated between protein foods and nutrient utilization. Amino acid imbalances may produce not only an increase in the requirements for specific amino acids but also a depression in food intake (18). An important form of the malabsorption syndrome is that due to an inability to handle wheat or rye gluten. The reason for improvement of this enteropathy on a gluten-free regime is not understood and still under investigation (16).

In this atomic age everyone is concerned about the effects of radiation upon the human body. There may even be indirect effects as well that could alter the nutritional status. The recent idea of preserving foods for human consumption by irradiation is being carefully investigated. A current report from the College of Veterinary Medicine, University of Illinois, and the Illinois Agriculture Experimental Station indicated that such practices might be harmful. They stated that the primary cause of hemorrhage in rats fed an irradiated beef ration appears to be due to a vitamin K deficiency (28).

Many other examples of dietary interrelationships have been reported, but the illustrations cited in this chapter are sufficient to underline the complexity and interdependence of nutrient activity. It would appear that the evidence cited in this chapter suggests the fallacy of therapeutic dietary regimes which do not cover all aspects of the diet and which attempt to administer only one or several vitamins and minerals.

Table 4.4
significant effect of thalidomide on
embryonic development in hypovitaminic rats

vitamin deficiency	per cent fetal resorption	
	control	thalidomide
E	0.0	27.3
riboflavin	32.9	77.9
pantothenic acid (12-15 days)	17.2	44.7

SUMMARY

The biologic activity of carbohydrates, proteins, fats, vitamins, and minerals is so interdependent that an imbalance of any one will likely affect one or more of the others.

The relationships between carbohydrates and other nutrients were given more detailed citation for the following reasons:

1. The major dietary change during the past century has been the caloric substitution of nutrient-free sugar for starch (Chapter One, The American Diet).
2. Abnormal carbohydrate metabolism is increasingly being recognized as a very prevalent problem.
3. A decreased tolerance for glucose has been cited as a prominent feature of many pathologic states.

Additional examples of the changes in nutritional status initiated by the ingestion of antimetabolites, drugs, and irradiated foods are provided in an attempt to emphasize further the complexity of dietary interrelationships.

REFERENCES

1. Ahrens, E. H., Jr., Hirsch, J., Oette, K., Farquhar, J. W., and Stein, Y. *Carbohydrate-induced and fat-induced lipemia.* Trans. Assn. Am. Physicians 74: 134-146, 1961.
2. Aikawa, J. K. *The role of magnesium in biologic processes.* 1963. Springfield, Illinois, Charles C. Thomas. pp. 49-52.
3. Albanese, A. A., Orto, L., Rossy, J., DiLallo, R., and Belmont, A. *Effect of carbohydrate on blood amino nitrogen.* Metabolism 4: #2, 160-165, March 1955.
4. Al-Nagdy, S., Miller, D. S., Qureshi, R. U., and Yudkin, J. *Metabolic differences between starch and sucrose.* Nature 209: #5018, 81-82, January 1, 1966.
5. Anderson, J. T., Grande, F., Matsumoto, Y., and Keys, A. *Glucose, sucrose and lactose in the diet and blood lipids in man.* J. Nutrit. 79: #3, 349-359, March 1963.
6. Antar, M. A. and Ohlson, M. A. *Effect of simple and complex carbohydrates upon total lipids, nonphospholipids and different fractions of phospholipids of serum in young men and women.* J. Nutrit. 85: #4, 329-337, April 1965.
7. Boylen, J. B., Horne, H. H., and Johnson, W. J. *Teratogenic effects of thalidomide and related substances.* Lancet 1: #7280, 552, March 9, 1963.
8. Broquist, H. P. and Jukes, T. H. *Antimetabolites, effect on nutrition.* In Wohl, M. G. and Goodhart, R. S. *Modern Nutrition in health and disease.* Third Edition. 1964. Philadelphia, Lea and Febiger. pp. 486-521.
9. Conn, J. W. and Newburgh, L. H. *The glycemic response to isoglucogenic quantities of protein and carbohydrate.* J. Clin. Invest. 15: #6, 665-671, November 1936.
10. Conn, J. W. *The advantage of high protein diet in the treatment of spontaneous hypoglycemia.* J. Clin. Invest. 15: #6, 673-678, November 1936.
11. Conney, A. H., Bray, G. A., Evans, C., and Burns, J. J. *Metabolic interactions between L-ascorbic acid and drugs.* Ann. New York Acad. Sc. 92: #1, 115-127, April 21, 1961.
12. Faigle, J. W., Keberle, A., Riess, W., and Schmid, K. *The metabolic fate of thalidomide.* Experientia 18: #9, 389-397, 1962.
13. Fankushen, D., Raskin, D., Dimick, A., and Wallach, S. *The significance of hypomagnesemia in alcoholic patients.* Am. J. Med. 37: #5, 802-812, November 1964.
14. Follis, R. H., Jr. *Deficiency disease.* 1958. Springfield, Illinois, Charles C. Thomas.

15. Fratta, I. D., Sigg, E. B., and Maiorana, K. *Teratogenic effects of thalidomide in rabbits, rats, hamsters, and mice.* Toxicol. and Appl. Pharmacol. 7: #2, 268-286, March 1965.

16. Frazer, A. C. *Deleterious effects due to wheat gluten.* Food and Cosmetics Toxicol. 2: #6, 670-672, December 1964.

17. Hadnagy, C., Horvath, E., Elekes, I., Puia, A., and Nicoara, E. *Effect of vitamin B12 and cortisone on the glucose tolerance of aged persons.* Gerontologia 9: #2, 71-77, 1964.

18. Harper, A. E. *Amino acid toxicities and imbalances.* In Munro, H. N. and Allison, J. B. *Mammalian protein metabolism.* Vol. II. 1964. New York, Academic Press. pp. 87-134.

19. Harte, R. A. and Chow, B. *Dietary interrelationships.* pp. 534-544. In Wohl, M. G. and Goodhart, R. S. *Modern nutrition in health and disease.* Third Edition. 1964. Philadelphia, Lea and Febiger.

20. Hockster, R. M. and Ouastel, H. J. *Metabolic inhibitors.* 1963. New York, Academic Press.

21. Kemper, F. *Effect of thalidomide on growth and sexual development of cockerels.* Ztschr. ges. exp. Med. 135: 454-459, 1962. Abstract in Nutrit. Abst. and Rev. 33: #2, 396, April 1963.

22. Kemper, F. and Berger, H. *Changes produced by thalidomide in the blood of chickens.* Ztschr. ges. exp. Med. 136: 86-96, 1962. Abstract in Nutrit. Abst. and Rev. 33: #2, 396, April 1963.

23. Leck, J. M. and Millar, E. L. *Incidence of malformations since the introduction of thalidomide.* Brit. Med. J. 2: #5296, 16-20, July 7, 1962.

24. Levine, R. *Carbohydrate metabolism.* In Duncan, G. G. *Diseases of metabolism.* Fifth Edition. 1964. Philadelphia. W. B. Saunders Company. p. 131.

25. Macdonald, I. *Dietary carbohydrates and lipid metabolism.* Proc. Nutrit. Soc. 23: #2, 119-123, 1964.

26. Macdonald, I. and Braithwaite, D. M. *The influence of dietary carbohydrates on the lipid pattern in serum and in adipose tissue.* Clin. Sc. 27: #1, 23-30, August 1964.

27. Macdonald, I. *Dietary carbohydrates and lipid metabolism.* Nutrit. Rev. 22: #9, 257-259, September 1964.

28. Malhotra, O. P., Reber, E. F., and Norton, H. W. *Effect of methionine and vitamin K3 on hemorrhages induced by feeding a ration containing irradiated beef.* Toxicol. and Appl. Pharmacol. 7: #3, 402-408, May 1965.

29. McCollister, R. J., Flink, E. B., and Lewis, M. D. *Urinary excre-*

tion of magnesium in man following the ingestion of ethanol. Am. J. Clin. Nutrit. 12: #6, 415-420, June 1963.

30. Miller, S. Dietary interrelationships and antimetabolites. In Nizel, A. E. Nutrition in clinical dentistry. 1960. Philadelphia, W. B. Saunders Company. pp. 232-233.

31. Nelson, M. M., Baird, C. D., Wright, H. V., and Evans, H. M. Multiple congenital abnormalities in the rat resulting from riboflavin deficiency induced by the antimetabolite galactoflavin. J. Nutrit. 58: #1, 125-134, January 1956.

32. Nelson, M. M. Production of congenital anomalies in mammals by maternal dietary deficiencies. Pediatrics 19: #4, 764-776, April 1957.

33. Olson, R. E. The two-carbon chain in metabolism. J. A. M. A. 183: #6, 471-474, February 9, 1963.

34. Orent-Keiles, E. and Hallman, L. F. The breakfast meal in relation to blood sugar values, December 1949. U. S. Department of Agriculture, Circular #827. Washington, D. C., U. S. Government Printing Office.

35. Ringsdorf, W. M., Jr. and Cheraskin, E. Effect of a relatively high-protein low-refined-carbohydrate diet upon serum cholesterol concentration. J. Amer. Geriat. Soc. 11: #2, 156-165, February 1963.

36. Setyaadmadja, A. T. S. H., Cheraskin, E., and Ringsdorf, W. M., Jr. Ascorbic acid and carbohydrate metabolism: I. The cortisone glucose tolerance test. J. Amer. Geriat. Soc. 13: #10, 924-934, 1965.

37. Siperstein, M. D. Inter-relationships of glucose and lipid metabolism. Amer. J. Med. 26: #5, 685-702, May 1959.

38. Soskin, S. and Levine, R. The role of carbohydrates in the diet. In Wohl, M. G. and Goodhart, R. S. Modern nutrition in health and disease. Third Edition. 1964. Philadelphia, Lea and Febiger. pp. 208-210.

39. Srinivasan, M. Effects of certain protein foods on blood-sugar levels and glucose tolerance. Lancet 2: #6990, 317-320, August 17, 1957.

40. Sure, B. Dietary interrelationships. In Wohl, M. G. and Goodhart, R. S. Modern nutrition in health and disease. 1955. Philadelphia, Lea and Febiger. pp. 404-428.

41. Sure, B. Dietary interrelationships. In Wohl, M. G. and Goodhart, R. S. Modern nutrition in health and disease. 1955. Philadelphia, Lea and Febiger. pp. 416-417.

42. Wolf, S. *A new view of disease.* J. A. M. A. 184: #2, 143-144, April 13, 1963.

43. Yeh, S. D. J., Chow, B. F., and Goodhart, R. F. *Marginal deficiencies of vitamins. I. In animals.* J. New Drugs 1: #1, 10-17, January-February 1961.

PART TWO

DISEASE STATES

THE SUCCEEDING PAGES ARE A DISTILLATION OF THE RESEARCH efforts of many and varied experts. The singularity of this section lies in its design. It is felt that the reviews of the literature should be comprehensive, yet not overwhelming. Hence, typical findings are described with a more complete tabular review of the pertinent literature. Each table is planned to insure maximum convenience, clarity, and conciseness. Thus, none exceeds a page. The order in which the various nutrients are listed is consistent throughout the tables and irrelevant data have been avoided. It is recognized that simplification invites distortion. It is hoped that the tabular technique will minimize this hazard. Additionally, these charts provide a convenient point of departure for study in depth.

Value judgments for all the findings reported are hardly feasible. Yet some manner of grouping of the various reports is warranted to assist the reader in weighing the evidence. The well-established custom of differentiating between lower animal and human observations, in our view, is not sufficient. Therefore, an additional, though seldom invoked, method of differentiation is employed, namely a division of the studies into those of a "correlative" nature and those which may be termed "therapeutic." Consequently, some explanation of what is intended by the use of these two terms is indicated. Both correlative and therapeutic observations regarding the influence of diet on disease vary from case reports to sophisticated studies of lower animals and humans in which the very latest biometric tools are employed.

Correlative observations, the discernment of relationships, take many forms. The astute farmer may note a seeming difference in the fertility of animals as their feed source varies with the seasons of the year. The explorer observes an apparent freedom from cancer among primitive peoples in certain environmental situations. Finally, the sophisticated epidemiologist weighs the influence of innumerable variables in determining the statistical significance of relationships between diseases and possible causes. *The most that can be learned from such observations is the frequency with which findings coexist.* They do not establish a cause-and-effect relationship. Many illustrations have been cited by statisticians to underscore this point. For example, the lengths of the middle and index fingers are known to be proportional. The individual with a long middle digit also has a relatively long index finger. However, this correlation does not mean that one caused the other.

Correlations can be tested for their possible cause-and-effect significance. This can be accomplished by adding or withholding nutrients. The discovery of how to prevent scurvy is a classic case in point. First, a correlation was noted: sailors on long voyages during which fresh fruits and vegetables were not available developed scurvy. The significance of this correlation was tested by providing seamen with fresh produce. This experimental approach is not new. Even in biblical antiquity, Shadrach, Meshach, and Abednego demonstrated the superiority of a simple diet of pulse and water over the rich fare provided by King Nebuchadnezzar.

Therapeutic experiments with built-in control groups are of critical importance in the evaluation of diet in disease. Such design has been indicated, where possible, in the forthcoming reviews.

Finally, the section is unique by the notable absence of what is customarily considered to be the relationship of diet and disease. Reports of scurvy, pellagra, beriberi, and other classical deficiency states are glaringly absent from this book because they are uncommon in the developed nations and particularly in the United States. Rather, what we trust will be impressive is the implication of diet in so many allegedly nondietary disorders.

5. INFERTILITY

SINCE CONCEPTION IS THE INITIAL LINK IN LIFE'S CHAIN, IT HAS BEEN selected as the first of the chapters dealing with diet and disease states. The scope of this problem is well-recognized and abundantly reported. As one of the spokesmen on this subject, Doctor Samuel R. Meaker, Emeritus Professor of Gynecology, Boston University School of Medicine, had the following to say *(35)*:

> The exact incidence of involuntary sterility is difficult to determine. Vital Statistics provide a record of births in relation to marriages and to population, but do not distinguish the failure to conceive from the accidents of early pregnancy, and take no account of the use of contraception. A conservative analysis of the best available data indicates that somewhat more than 12 per cent of modern marriages are barren....There are, therefore, in the United States today nearly 3,000,000 childless couples who are still at the age of potential reproduction....

Not only is sterility common, but there is general agreement that its causation is complex and its solution will come only through multidisciplinary study and research. Doctor Meaker continues:

> From ancient times the reproach of barrenness has been visited upon the wife, and the cause has been assumed to be some abnormality of her reproductive organs. Consequently the problem of sterility is assigned by tradition to the gynecologist....The complete investigation and treatment of sterility must involve work in several nongynecologic fields of practice, particularly in urology, internal medicine and endocrinology....

In the opinion of some authorities, the causative mosaic of sterility must include diet and nutrition. For example, Doctor J. Jay Rommer, author of *Sterility, Its Cause and Its Treatment*, states *(47)*:

Since nothing can come out of a human being except from what goes into him, one must assume a close correlation between food and fertility. In general, the more generous the diet, the higher the fertility; the more meager the diet, the lower the fertility. However, it is not simply a matter of gross quantity of food. Wealthier people eat better than poor people, but they have fewer children.

Much has been written about the influence of diet upon the organs of reproduction, and many diverse methods have been used to measure this relationship. Observations regarding degenerative changes in the seminiferous tubules, atrophy of the testes, defective spermatogenesis, and involution of the secondary sex glands have been noted in various male lower animals. These have been ascribed to an excess or deficiency of different dietary factors and cited as indirect evidence of infertility. Analogous findings have also been reported in female lower animals.

The diversity of methods in assessing fertility complicates the data interpretation. In view of the fact that the end product of the various alterations on gonadal function, of concern in infertility, is simply inability to conceive, attention will be limited to those lower animal studies reporting the occurrence or failure of conception. While this approach reduces the number of observations which can be properly reported, it does provide a uniform measurement of the effects of various dietary influences.

CORRELATIVE FINDINGS

Lower Animal Observations: The interest of the animal husbandman in protecting and increasing the source of his livelihood has been a potent stimulus to the exploration of dietary-fertility relationships (Table 5.1). It is clear that fertility has been studied in different lower animals and that numerous nutritional variables may affect conception. Although correlative studies have tended to lend credence to the possible importance of this relationship, some of the evidence appears on the surface to be contradictory.

There is reason to believe that failure to resolve some of these problems may be due less to their complexity than to the fact that they have simply not been explored. Overfeeding is a case in point. Doctor Walter P. Kennedy, Department of

Physiology, University of Edinburgh *(20)*, reported as early as 1926 the favorable results which usually attended the general practice of giving breeding animals extra rations. However, such overfeeding by unskilled husbandmen unquestionably had a detrimental effect upon fertility. He further reported that it was common knowledge among stockmen that "show condition," the stage at which it would seem that stock should be in their prime, was "inimical to efficient breeding." Yet,

Table 5.1
diet and infertility
(lower animal correlative observations)

dietary variable	sex and animal	conclusion	reference
obesity	both, farm	infertility	20, 36
supplementation of hill pasture diet with food concentrates for three weeks before annual estrus	female, sheep	fertility	33, 40
adequate protein (quantity and quality)	male, all both, all	fertility fertility	24 20
vitamin A deficiency	female cattle	infertility	18
vitamin B12 and cobalt deficiency	both, ruminants	infertility	18
calcium deficiency	female, cattle	infertility	20
phosphorus deficiency	female, cattle	infertility	18
adequate manganese	female, cattle	fertility	48

twenty-five years after Kennedy's published observation of the contradictory findings regarding the effects of overfeeding, the matter continued to receive little investigative attention. Such a leading authority as Doctor James H. Leathem, Professor of Zoology at Rutgers University, commenting on the dependence of the reproductive system upon adequate nutrition in the classic text, *Sex and Internal Secretions,* was obliged to state *(25)*:

> ...it is something of a paradox in our culture that much of our effort has been devoted to the investigations of the effects of deficiencies and undernutrition rather than to the effects of ex-

cesses and overnutrition. Much evidence supports the view that in the aggregate the latter are fully as deleterious as the former....

Human Observations: A number of investigators have reported correlations between diet and infertility in humans (Table 5.2). Several items warrant special note. First, it is clear that, of the available observations, the consensus is that diet and infertility are related. Second, there is evidence that unsuccessful conception correlates with different forms of malnutrition. For example, some of the reported data were collected during periods of general or nonspecific

Table 5.2
diet and infertility
(human correlative observations)

dietary variable	sex	conclusion	reference
severe undernutrition as seen in prisoner-of-war camps	male	infertility	22
severe undernutrition in Rotterdam	female	infertility	50
severe undernutrition during Siege of Leningrad	female	infertility	3
period of general undernutrition in Singapore	female	no effect	37
improved diet	both	fertility	46
obesity	both	infertility	20
	female	infertility	31
	male	infertility	27
chronic alcoholism	female	infertility	16
liver cirrhosis and a presumed associated vitamin B deficiency	male	infertility	17
vitamin B complex deficiency may contribute to hepatic cirrhosis	female	infertility	7
pellagra and liver disease	female	infertility	52
vitamin B complex deficiency	both	infertility	7
vitamin E supplementation	female	no effect	15

malnutrition under wartime conditions. In contrast, other studies tend to indict specific nutrients, notably the vitamins and especially the B complex and E fractions. In sharp contrast is the suspicion that obesity, a possible form of overnutrition, may also contribute to sterility in the human.

The explanations are even more incomplete. Generally speaking, the consensus is that, in the male, malnutrition modifies the quantity and the quality of spermatogenesis. In the female, the major attention has been directed to the estrogens and their possible inactivation by the liver.

While much of the recorded literature is difficult to quantitate, there are some interesting, if not conclusive, measurable data. For example, the conception rate was analyzed in Rotterdam during the period December 1944 to May 1945. The evidence suggests *(50)* that one-half of the women reported amenorrhea. Also clearly shown is the fact that the weekly conception rate declined more than 50 per cent from a prewar figure of 206 to 93 during this interval of severe malnutrition (Table 5.2).

Using the frequency of conception within two years after delivery of a previous child as an index of fertility of 939 women *(31)*, the incidence of fertility among 73 women in the heavier weight group (170 pounds and over) was 11.1 per cent, just about half the conception rate in the lower weight range (Table 5.2).

It is well to emphasize that, while these correlative observations in lower animals and the human are interesting, in themselves, they do not prove cause-and-effect. Hence, it is now appropriate to consider the effects of deprivation and supplementation upon the reproductive capacity of lower animals and the human.

THERAPEUTIC FINDINGS

Lower Animal Observations: Examination of Table 5.3 indicates that therapeutic findings seem to confirm and extend the correlations observed in the lower animals. In contrast with the correlative findings, it will be noted that, in practically all of these experiments, small laboratory animals were utilized. All categories of nutrients are represented and it appears that excesses as well as deficiencies of calories and of some nutrients exert a deleterious effect on the ability to conceive.

Table 5.3
diet and infertility
(lower animal therapeutic observations)

dietary variable	species	sex	reference
infertility or reduced fertility			
inanition	mouse	F	30
	rat	F, M	20,34
	rabbit	F	1
alcohol	guinea pig	F	28
20% sucrose for cornstarch	rat	F	57
low protein	rat	M	10
tryptophane free	rat	F	2
low protein	rat	M	10
essential fatty acids removed	rat	F	27
fat free	rat	M	13
high fat	rat	F	14
excess fat	laboratory	F, M	38
vitamin A deficient	mouse	F, M	29,49,54
	rat	F, M	14,43
	bovine	F	18
massive doses vitamin A	rat	F	23
massive doses vitamin B1	rat	F	51
massive doses vitamin B complex	guinea pig	F	31
vitamin C excess	guinea pig	F	39
low phosphorus intake, wide Ca/P ratio	bovine	F	18
manganese free	rat	M	41
sodium deficient	rat	F	42
calcium deficient	rat	F	20
no effect on fertility			
33% reduction normal diet	rat	M	5
massive doses vitamin B1	mouse	F	9
vitamin E deficient	rat, bovine	F	12,18
improved fertility			
diet reduction	obese swine	M, F	21
33% reduction normal diet	rat	F	5
vitamin C supplements	bovine	F	44
copper supplementation in hypocupraemia	bovine	F	18

Viewed as a whole, these studies suggest that a relatively low caloric diet which provides optimal amounts of the essential nutrients is desirable.

The research of Doctor Benjamin N. Berg (Associate Professor, Department of Pathology, College of Physicians and Surgeons, Columbia University) is representative of the numerous experiments in which genetic and other factors have been well controlled. He reported that 24 female rats fed a diet which was adequate nutritionally, but restricted quantitatively by one-third, had 16 successful matings even up to 790 days of age. On the other hand, 33 female rats fed ad libitum had only four successful matings and all occurred under the age of 700 days (Figure 5.1). Parenthetically, it might be added that, while none of the unrestricted group had a second litter, five (20 per cent) of the restricted group did so (5).

Human Observations: It is clear that the human studies are fewer and the nutrient variables more limited (Table 5.4) than in the lower animal group (Table 5.3). Major consideration has been focused on the vitamins, notably B and E. It is very apparent that the male has received practically all of the attention.

The consensus, from these admittedly few studies, appears to be that spermatogenesis is improved both in quantity and in quality by appropriate vitamin supplementation. For example, the administration of alpha-tocopherol acetate (150 to 200 mg. daily by mouth) to patients who demonstrated disturbances in spermatogenesis produced an immediate increase in the sperm count (26). There was some improvement in motility and a reduction in the percentage of abnormal forms. Normal semen values were achieved in 20 of the 55 males and 21 more showed improvement. Seventeen cases proved fertile. However, it should be emphasized that improved spermatogenesis is not a guarantee for conception.

Cervical dysfunction associated with cervical infection is held to be the most common cause of sterility in women over the age of 30 (4). The effect of diet on sterility in overweight women with this problem has been studied. The investigation concerned 88 women in England shortly after the end of World War II, all between 30 and 40 years of age.

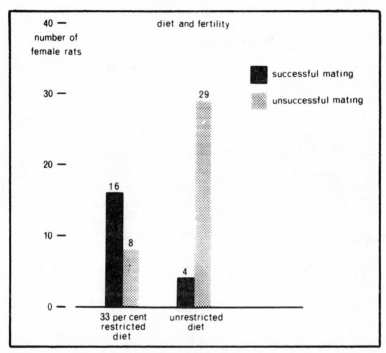

Figure 5.1. Effect on fertility of quantitative changes in the diets of female rats.

The subjects sought advice only because they desired children and not for any clinical complaint. This series included only subjects with no marked departure from the menstrual norm or severe chronic illness. The subjects had proven refractory to the usually effective treatment (antibiotics and estrogen for four to twelve weeks). Initially the intention was to employ reducing diets involving severe caloric restriction or salt balance adjustment; but many subjects were working too hard to be easily placed on a severe reducing diet nor could they afford much unrationed protein. It was decided that lactose (3 oz. daily) would be administered, and ordinary sugar, as the most ready source of fermentable carbohydrate, would be eliminated from the diet. Two reasons were given for this approach: (1) the predominance of infections by intestinal type organisms and reported successes from reorganizing the intestinal flora with lactose in a variety of conditions,

Table 5.4
diet and infertility
(human therapeutic observations)

dietary variable	sex	conclusion	reference
weight reduction by	female	fertility	52
diet in infertile	female	fertility	6
obese patients			
elimination of sugar	female	fertility	4
in obese subjects			
vitamin B complex	male	fertility	45
supplementation			
vitamin E supple-	female	negative	55
mentation		effect	56
vitamin E supple-	male	fertility	11
mentation			
vitamin E supple-	male	fertility	19
mentation			
alpha-tocopherol			
acetate supple-	male	fertility	26
mentation			
vitamin B complex			
alone and with	male	fertility	8
vitamin E			
Tegotina (vitamin T)	male	fertility	53
supplementation			

including genital infections, and (2) reports that sucrose-fed animals developed significantly larger deposits of fat than those receiving lactose.

Treatment resulted in an average loss of one pound a week. Cervical block was resolved in nine of the fourteen subjects (Group I in Figure 5.2) either spontaneously or following a repetition of the previously unsuccessful antibiotic and estrogen therapy. Cervical recovery failed to occur in five cases, three of which had shown no significant reduction of weight.

A second group was then studied in exactly the same manner except that the administration of lactose was omitted (Group II). That lactose had no specific action so far as either the cervical block or weight loss was concerned was demonstrated by the successful response of 47 out of 65 cases in terms of both cervical response and weight loss and weight loss alone in 57 out of 65.

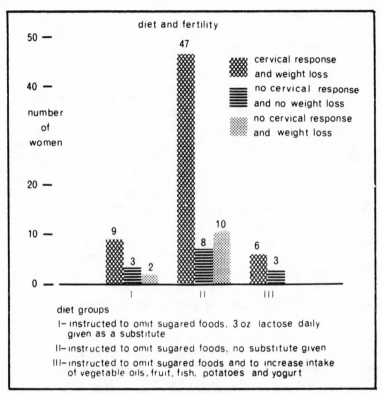

Figure 5.2. The effect of diet on infertility as measured by cervical response and on weight in 88 obese women with cervical dysfunction associated with cervical infection.

It was observed that elimination of sugared foods from the subjects in both Groups I and II resulted in a severe reduction in caloric intake which apparently was compensated by an increased consumption of foods to which no sugar was added.

To verify this observation, a third group of nine subjects was studied (Group III). This group was given the same dietary instructions as Group II except that, in addition to elimination of sugared foods, specific instructions were given to increase consumption of unrationed foods such as vegetable oils, fruit, fish, potatoes, and yogurt. An actual increase in total caloric consumption resulted--an increase of more than 5,000 calories per week in one case cited. The response was essentially the same as in the first two groups; weight loss and restoration of cervical function occurred in six, and neither occurred in three (Figure 5.2).

SUMMARY

Although much remains to be learned about the role of diet in gonadal function, food does seem to be an important determinant of fertility in both sexes. With the exception perhaps of Biskind and Falk (1943), there has been little effort to evaluate the effect of truly comprehensive dieto-therapy under well-controlled conditions. In view of existing dietary habits (Chapter One, The American Diet), such studies seem warranted and perhaps even imperative.

Unfortunately, the clinician cannot defer action indefinitely but is faced with the obligation of functioning within the framework of present knowledge. For him, probably no better general plan for dietotherapy can be suggested than the five-point program recommended by Macomber over thirty-five years ago *(32)*: (1) adequate protein intake, (2) attention to consumption of calcium, phosphorus, iodine, iron, and other mineral salts, (3) high vitamin intake, (4) sufficient water supply, and (5) total caloric intake balance. On the basis of the experience of Barton and Wiesner (1948), the elimination of sugared foods from the diets of at least overweight subjects would also seem justified.

REFERENCES

1. Adams, C. E. *Some aspects of ovulation, recovery and transplantation of ova in the immature rabbit.* In Ciba Foundation Symposium on Mammalian Germ Cell, Eds. Wolstenholme, G. E. W., Cameron, M. P., and Freeman, J. S. 1953. London, Churchill. pp. 198-216.

2. Albanese, A. A., Randall, R. M., and Holt, L. E., Jr. *The effect of tryptophane deficiency on reproduction.* Science 97: #2518, 312-313, April 2, 1943.

3. Antonov, A. N. *Children born during the siege of Leningrad in 1942.* J. Pediat. 30: #3, 250-259, March 1947.

4. Barton, M. and Wiesner, B. P. *The role of special diets in the treatment of female infecundity.* Brit. Med. J. 2: #4584, 847-851, November 13, 1948.

5. Berg, B. N. *Nutrition and longevity in the rat. I. Food intake in relation to size, health and fertility.* J. Nutrit. 71: #3, 242-254, July 1960.

6. Bigsby, F. L. and Muniz, C. *Practical management of the obese patient.* 1962. New York, Intercontinental Medical Book Corporation.

7. Biskind, M. S. *Nutritional therapy of endocrine disturbances.* Vitam. and Horm. 4: 147-185, 1946.

8. Biskind, M. S. and Falk, H. C. *Nutritional therapy of infertility in the male with special reference to the vitamin B complex and vitamin E.* J. Clin. Endocrinol. 3: #3, 148-153, March 1943.

9. Cerecedo, L. R. and Vinson, L. J. *Effect of massive doses of thiamine on fertility and lactation in the albino mouse.* Proc. Soc. Exper. Biol. 55: #7, 139-140, February 1944.

10. Cole, H. H., Guilbert, H. R., and Goss, H. *Further considerations of the properties of the gonad-stimulating principle of mare serum.* Amer. J. Physiol. 102: #1, 227-240, October 1932.

11. Davidson, H. A. *Infertility: Family Planning Association's Conference.* Lancet 2: #6527, 543, October 2, 1948.

12. Evans, H. M. *Vitamin E.* J. A. M. A. 99: #6, 469-475, August 6, 1932.

13. Evans, H. M., Lepkovsky, S., and Murphy, E. A. *Vitamin need of the body for certain unsaturated fatty acids. VI. Male sterility on fat-free diets.* J. Biol. Chem. 106: #2, 445-450, September 1934.

14. French, C. E., Ingram, R. H., Knoebel, L. K., and Swift, R. W. *The influence of dietary fat and carbohydrate on reproduction and lactation in rats.* J. Nutrit. 48: #1, 91-102, September 1952.

15. Garry, R. C. and Wood, H. O. *Dietary requirements in human pregnancy and lactation. A review of recent work.* Nutrit. Abs. Rev. 15: #4, 591-621, April 1946.

16. Gibbons, R. A. *Sterility in women: its causes and treatment.* 1923. London, J. and A. Churchill. P. 23.

17. Glass, S. J., Edmondson, H. A., and Soll, S. N. *Sex hormone changes associated with liver disease.* Endocrinol. 27: #5, 749-752, November 1940.

18. Hignett, S. L. *The influence of nutrition on female fertility in some large domestic animals.* Proc. Nutrit. Soc. 19: #1, 8-15, 1960.

19. Jackson, M. H. *Infertility. Report of Family Planning Association's Conference.* Lancet 2: #6527, 542-544, October 1948.

20. Kennedy, W. P. *Diet and sterility.* Phys. Rev. 6: #3, 485-503, July 1926.

21. Kinsley, A. T. *Sterility in swine practice.* Vet. Med. 17: 67-70, 1922.

22. Klatskin, G., Salter, W. T., and Humm, F. D. *Gynecomastia due to malnutrition. I. Clinical studies.* Amer. J. Med. Sc. 213: #1, 19-30, January 1947.

23. Laschet, U., Hohlweg, W., and Weise, W. *Tierexperimentelle Untersuchungen uber die Wirkung von Vitamin A auf Fertilitat und Foet.* Int. Z. Vitaminforsch. 30: #1 & 2, 77-82, 1959.

24. Leathem, J. H. *Hormones and protein nutrition.* Rec. Prog. Hormone Res. 14: 141-182, 1958.

25. Leathem, J. H. *Sex and internal secretions.* Ed. Young, W. C., Vol. I. *Nutritional effects on endocrine secretions.* 1961. Baltimore, Williams and Wilkins Company. Ch. 8.

26. Lindner, E. *Therapeutische Bedeutung des Vitamins E bei Storungen des Spermatogenese.* Int. Z. Vitaminforsch. 29: #1-2, 33-40, 1958.

27. Lutwak-Mann, C. *The dependence of gonadal function upon vitamins and other nutritional factors.* Vitam. and Horm. 16: 35-75, 1958.

28. MacDowell, E. C. and Lord, E. M. *On the number of corpora lutea produced at successive pregnancies by normal and heavily alcoholized mice.* Anat. Rec. 29: #2, 141, December 1924.

29. McCarthy, P. T. and Cerecedo, L. R. *Vitamin A deficiency in the mouse.* J. Nutrit. 46: #3, 361-376, March 1952.

30. McClure, T. J. *Temporary nutritional stress and infertility in female mice.* J. Physiol. 147: #2, 221-225, September 2, 1959.

31. McKeown, T. and Record, R. G. *An examination of fertility of women following pregnancy according to height and weight.* Brit. J. Prev. and Soc. Med. 11: 102-105, 1957.

32. Macomber, D. *Diet and fertility ratio.* J. Med. Soc. New Jersey 25: #3, 161-171, March 1928.

33. Marshall, F. H. *Fertility in Scottish sheep.* Trans. Highland and Agric. Soc. 5: 20, 1908. As reported by Kennedy (20).

34. Mason, K. E. *Relation of the vitamins to the sex glands.* In *Sex and internal secretions.* 1939. Baltimore, Williams and Wilkins. pp. 1149-1212.

35. Meaker, S. R. *Davis' gynecology and obstetrics.* Ed. Carter, B. Vol. II, Ch. 9 *Sterility.* 1964. W. F. Prior Company, Inc.

36. Millen, J. M. *Nutritional basis of reproduction.* 1962. Springfield, Charles C. Thomas.

37. Millis, J. *A study of the effect of nutrition on fertility and the outcome of pregnancy in Singapore in 1947 and 1950.* Med. J. Malaya 6: #3, 157-177, March 1952.

38. Nelson, V. E., Heller, V. G., and Fulmer, D. I. *Studies on yeast: VII. The dietary properties of yeast.* J. Biol. Chem. 57: #2, 415-424, September 1923.

39. Neuweiler, W. *Die Hypervitaminose und ihre Beziehung zur Schwangerschaft.* Int. Z. Vitaminforsch. 22: #4, 392-396, 1951.

40. Nichols, J. E. *Fertility in sheep.* J. Ministry Agric. 31: 835-843, December 1924. (as reported by Kennedy (20)).

41. Orent, E. R. and McCollum, E. V. *Effects of deprivation of manganese in the rat.* J. Biol. Chem. 92: #3, 651-678, 1931.

42. Orent-Keiles, E., Robinson, A., and McCollum, E. V. *The effects of sodium deprivation on the animal organism.* Amer. J. Physiol. 119: #3, 651-661, July 1937.

43. Parkes, A. S. and Drummond, J. C. *The effects of fat-soluble vitamin A deficiency on reproduction in the rat.* Brit. J. Exper. Biol. 3: #4, 251-273, July 1926.

44. Phillips, P. H., Lardy, H. A., Boyer, P. D., and Werner, G. M. *The relationship of ascorbic acid to reproduction in the cow.* J. Dairy Sc. 24: 153-158, 1941.

45. Pool, T. L. *Infertility in the male.* Proc. Mayo Clinic 20: #7, 97-102, April 4, 1945.

46. Reynolds, E. and Macomber, D. *Fertility and sterility in human marriages.* 1924. Philadelphia, W. B. Saunders Company.

47. Rommer, J. J. *Sterility, its causes and its treatment.* 1952. Springfield, Charles C. Thomas. pp. 54-55.

48. Seekles, L. *Carences reeles et conditionees des oligo-elements.* Rec. Med. vet. 125: 797, 1949.

49. Sherman, H. C. and MacLeod, F. L. *The relation of vitamin A to growth, reproduction and longevity.* J. Amer. Chem. Soc. 47: #6, 1658-1662, 1925.

50. Smith, C. A. *The effect of wartime starvation in Holland upon pregnancy and its produce.* Amer. J. Obstet. & Gynec. 53: #4, 599-608, April 1947.

51. Sure, B. *Influence of massive doses of vitamin B1 on fertility and lactation.* J. Nutrit. 18: #2, 187-194, August 1939.

52. Swyer, G. I. M. *Nutrition and human fertility.* Brit. J. Nutrit. 3: #1, 100-107, 1949.

53. Urgell, J. M. *Vitamin T-komplex bei behandlung mannlicher sterilitat.* Munch. med. Wchnschr. 99: #6, 191-193, 1957. (as reported by Millen (36)).

54. Warkany, J. *Manifestations of prenatal nutritional deficiency.* Vitam. and Horm. 3: 73-103, 1945.

55. Watson, E. M. and Tew, W. P. *Wheat germ oil (vitamin E) therapy in obstetrics.* Amer. J. Obstet. and Gynec. 31: #2, 352-358, February 1936.

56. Watson, E. M. *Clinical experiences with wheat germ oil (vitamin E).* Canad. Med. Assn. J. 34: #2, 134-140, February 1936.

57. Whitnah, G. H. and Bogart, R. *Reproductive capacity in female rats as affected by kinds of carbohydrate in the ration.* J. Agric. Res. 53: #7, 527-532, October 1, 1936.

6. OBSTETRICAL COMPLICATIONS

ON THE ASSUMPTION THAT CONCEPTION OCCURS (CHAPTER FIVE), the next possible weak link in the chain of life's experiences is difficulty during gestation. The problem is immense whether measured in terms of mortality, morbidity, socioeconomic distress, or emotional and mental trauma.

More than 10 per cent of the deaths in the United States occur during or immediately after gestation. Fetal fatality or stillbirths and neonatal mortality accounted for 175,000 deaths in 1958. It has been concluded that over 50 per cent of these deaths could have been prevented with the application of present knowledge *(40)*. These preventable deaths occurred chiefly among the nonwhite. Dietary deficiencies were among the most important environmental factors cited.

By far the most important cause of stillbirths and neonatal deaths is premature birth. However, the causative factors of prematurity are incompletely understood in 60 per cent of the cases. Exceeding stillbirths and neonatal mortality as a cause of fetal wastage is spontaneous abortion, many of which are of unknown etiology. It is estimated that about 10 per cent or 400,000 pregnancies in the United States abort spontaneously *(40)*.

In the same year 1,581 women died in the course of 4,203,812 live births. Hemorrhage, toxemias of pregnancy, and puerperal infection account for about 75 per cent of all maternal deaths. Hemorrhage is listed as the most common cause (29.8%), but its importance is even greater when the frequency with which it acts as a predisposing cause of death is considered.

After citing the above figures in their textbook on obstetrics, Doctor Nicholson J. Eastman, Emeritus Professor of Obstetrics at Johns Hopkins University, and Doctor Louis M. Hellman, Professor and Chairman of the Department of Obstetrics and Gynecology at the State University of New York, emphasize the important relationship that exists between their specialty and other disciplines. They point out that obstetrics "owes much to the science of nutrition and in time will probably owe more, since many disturbances of pregnancy are suspected of being dietary in origin." They conclude the introductory chapter of their textbook with the following challenge (40):

> But with our knowledge in its present state, the outlook for reducing the 175,000 infant deaths associated with birth each year and the 400,000 spontaneous abortions -- all potential American lives -- is less promising. Here new knowledge must be forthcoming if any substantial inroads are to be made....To unearth the etiologic factors responsible for these many premature labors, these many abortions, and the many other complications which threaten the infant as well as the mother, is a Herculean charge, but one which must be met if any great reduction in our fetal losses is to be anticipated. Only with the advent of such knowledge can any true millennium be promised for maternity.

Doctor Ashley Montagu, the famous social biologist and former Chairman of the Department of Anthropology at Rutgers, emphasizes in his book, *Prenatal Influences (111)*, the potential role of nutrition as an etiologic factor:

> ...apart from the genetic factor, the principal condition involved in producing the differences in height, weight, general development, morbidity rates, and the like, is the nutritional history of the individual.

CORRELATIVE FINDINGS

Lower Animal Observations: It is apparent from Table 6.1 that reported observations regarding the relation of diet to obstetrical complications are limited to livestock in the medical literature. Most of the observations are concerned with a correlation between vitamin or iodine deficiency and reproductive disorders. On the basis of these studies, it would appear that interrelationships exist between diet and obstetrical complications in farm animals.

Human Observations: The almost complete concurrence regarding the importance of diet in obstetrical complications in Tables 6.2 and 6.3 is remarkable. It will be noted that the findings are largely in agreement regarding this relationship as it pertains to fetal complications (Table 6.2) and maternal disorders (Table 6.3). The findings in toxemia, pre-eclampsia, and eclampsia are in agreement except for the reports emanating from the Philadelphia *(176)* and Vanderbilt *(32,33, 101,102)* studies and some of the reports on wartime under-nutrition (20,84,99,151).

Table 6.1
diet and obstetrical complications
(lower animal correlative observations)

dietary variable	animal	obstetrical complications	references
vitamin A deficiency	cow	premature births, stillborn, weakly young	64 112 104
low blood serum levels of B12	swine	reproductive failure	51
estrogen from the bioflavonoid, genistin, in clover	sheep	reproductive disturbances associated with cystic hyperplasia of the endometrium	11
iodine deficiency	swine	one million neonatal deaths in U. S. in 1917	152
	farm animals	stillborn	95
	cow	abortion, stillborn	173
	sheep	weakly offspring	143
diet low in calcium	cow, swine	no effect	105

Table 6.2
diet and fetal obstetrical complications
(human correlative observations)

dietary variable	complication	reference
increase		
poor quality diet		
216 gravidas, Boston, 1930-1942	premature babies, stillborn, neonatal deaths, other	21
300 deliveries, Glasgow	premature babies, stillborn	23
low socio-economic groups, Aberdeen	premature babies, stillborn	6
404 low income gravidas	premature babies	76
838 low socio-economic gravidas, North Carolina	fetal deaths, neonatal deaths	172
defective maternal diet, England	stillborn, neonatal deaths	139
186 Australian gravidas, 1948-1950	premature babies	179
polished rice and vegetables, Burma	neonatal deaths	133
wartime undernutrition	fetal deaths, still-	71,
Russian famine in World War I	born, neonatal deaths	153
Siege of Leningrad, 1942	fetal deaths, still-born, neonatal deaths	3
Rotterdam & The Hague, 1944-1945	premature babies	150
680 Naples gravidas, 1945	abortions, stillborn	84
obesity		
pregnancy & postpartum in obese women	stillborn, neonatal deaths	128
gravidas weighing over 200 pounds	neonatal deaths, other	100
specific nutrients		
low ratios reduced to oxidized plasma ascorbic acid	abruptio placentae	27
low vitamin C serum levels	premature babies	97
low vitamin C plasma levels, 288 gravidas	other	174
deficiencies of vitamins B1 & E	premature babies	145
prothrombin deficiency in pregnancy	abortions	75, 82
macrocytic hypochromic anemia in India	neonatal deaths	117
decrease		
general dietary improvement		
world-wide, World War II	stillborn	37
post-depression, England & Wales	stillborn	157
no effect		
poor quality diet	abortions, premature	176
514 gravidas in Philadelphia	babies	

Table 6.3
diet and maternal obstetrical complications
(human correlative observations)

dietary variable	complication	reference
increase		
poor quality diet		
Boston study	preeclampsia	22
Australian study	toxemia	179
poor diets seasonally	toxemia	83
obesity		
pregnancy & postpartum in 641 obese women	toxemia, preeclampsia, eclampsia, maternal deaths, other	128
200 gravidas weighing over 200 pounds	toxemia, preeclampsia, eclampsia, other	100
increased initial weight & rate of gain	preeclampsia	175
obese patients, Vanderbilt study	preeclampsia, eclampsia	101
specific nutrients		
less than 54 g. protein daily	toxemia	4
beriberi	toxemia	81
subclinical thiamine (B1) deficiency	toxemia	126
low thiamine intake	nausea & vomiting	176
thiamine deficiency	nausea & vomiting	103,123 134,177
niacin deficiency	toxemia	130
low niacin values	preeclampsia, eclampsia	102
pellagra	eclampsia	148
niacin deficiency	toxemia	67
choline deficiency	toxemia	110
low ratios reduced to oxidized plasma ascorbic acid	preeclampsia	27
macrocytic hypochromic anemia	maternal deaths	117
decrease		
wartime undernutrition		
Amsterdam, World Wars I & II	toxemia, eclampsia	99
Rotterdam & The Hague, 1944-45	toxemia	151
680 Naples gravidas, 1945	toxemia	84
Germany, World Wars I & II	toxemia	20
specific nutrients		
high plasma A levels	other	91
no effect		
poor quality diet		
Vanderbilt study	preeclampsia, eclampsia	32,33 101,102
Philadelphia study	toxemia	176
specific nutrients		
less than 50 g. protein daily	preeclampsia, eclampsia	102
high plasma A levels	toxemia	91

Typical of the findings in the majority of these reports were those cited in the carefully designed and similar Harvard *(21,22)* and Australian *(179)* studies carried out half a world apart. In the Harvard study, Burke and her collaborators investigated the obstetrical histories of 216 middle class women between 1930 and 1942. A complete record was made of the diet of each woman for the twenty-four hours previous to her first visit, and the nutritional value of the diet consumed was rated by a scoring system based on the recommended allowance of the Food and Nutrition Board of the National Research Council (1945). The women were seen monthly through the seventh month, and at least once each trimester a three-day consecutive record of the food intake was made. One-third of the women were observed for at least the last six months of pregnancy. Of the 216 women studied, only 14 per cent consumed a diet rated as "excellent" or "good" and only 10 per cent ingested the optimal amount of protein (85 grams). Two hundred babies were born at full term, nine were premature, five were stillborn, and two died within a few hours after birth. All the stillborn and all but one of the premature infants were born to mothers on the poorest diets. Complications of pregnancy were fewer in mothers who consumed a good diet. No mother on a "good" and "excellent" diet suffered from preeclamptic toxemia as compared with 44 per cent of the women on "poor" or "very poor" diets.

The same methods of collection and rating of dietary data were also employed in the Australian study. However, in addition to obtaining dietary data for the first and second halves of pregnancy, dietary information was also recorded for the period previous to pregnancy — an important but neglected area of research in the great majority of studies.

There were 186 middle-class women included in this program which extended from 1948 to 1950. The incidence of toxemia in relation to overall maternal diet was 42.1 per cent in the "very poor," 21.2 per cent in the "poor," 9.7 per cent in the "fair," 7.0 per cent in the "good," and 5.6 per cent in the "excellent" diet groups. The relationships in all three periods (before pregnancy, the first half, the second half, and the mean) revealed a high statistical significance.

During this study there were 15 prematurely born infants.

No statistically significant relationship could be demonstrated between diet previous to pregnancy and incidence of prematurity. For the first half of pregnancy a relationship significant at the 6 per cent level was shown, and for the second half of gestation a relationship significant at the 1 per cent level. The correlation between maternal diet during the latter part of pregnancy and both toxemia and prematurity is shown graphically in Figure 6.1. It was concluded that a definite relationship existed between both toxemia and prematurity and the maternal diet. They added "that control of the nutritional state of the pregnant woman is an important factor in relation to the prevention and treatment of toxemia." Finally, they noted that toxemia was related to prepregnancy obesity.

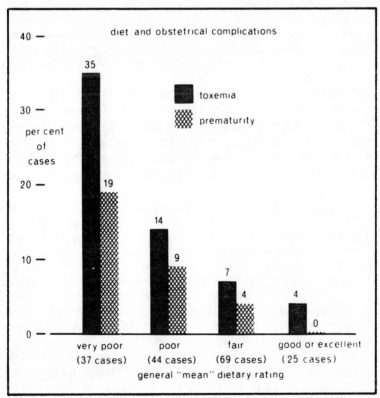

Figure 6.1. Maternal diets in the latter half of pregnancy related to toxemia and prematurity in 186 middle-class Australian women (Sydney, 1948-1950).

While the correlation of the B vitamins to toxemia, eclampsia, and preeclampsia seems rather strong, there is less agreement regarding the role of undernutrition in general and protein in particular. Millen *(105),* in his excellent monograph, points out that the difficulty is at least partly due to the diverse criteria for the diagnosis of toxemia used by different workers. Dalderup *(31)* of the Netherlands Institute of Nutrition (1959) has commented on the paradoxical effect of wartime diets in actually causing a reduction of toxemia:

> ...it might be suggested that the reduced frequency was partly due to extra food rations, for instance, milk and vitamin supplements given to pregnant women. But...the sudden greatly increased availability of food after the liberation produced at once a higher frequency....In any case, the food consumed during the war had much in common with the food of primitive people: it was less refined, contained less animal fat and proteins, more fruit and vegetables....and was a low fat, and often a low calorie diet, distinctly richer in vitamin and mineral content than at other times.

Doctor Dalderup goes on to explain that, in some instances, toxemia might increase in the presence of actual famine.

The Vanderbilt findings, in a comprehensive and carefully organized study involving 2,046 pregnant women, were by no means completely negative in regard to the relationship between diet and obstetrical complications, as they point out *(102):*

> The intake of one or more nutrients was lowered significantly in women with associated medical disorders, anemia, pre-eclampsia and eclampsia, and in mothers who delivered premature offspring. Hematologic and serum values during one or more periods of gestation were decreased among women with anemia, twins, puerperal complications, and excessive degrees of blood loss. The rating of obesity was increased in the preeclamptics and mothers of stillborn infants; edema in women with associated medical diseases, acute toxemia, and twins; and undernutrition in mothers who delivered premature infants....
>
> We recognize that with a sufficiently low level of nutriture, *nutritional* complications may arise from dietary inadequacies. We do not wish to be interpreted as concluding that nutrition is unimportant in pregnancy....Can we not liken the differences between our findings and those of some others to one's perspective? It is commonly stated that of one hundred congenitally

malformed infants, 40 per cent of the mothers will give a history of acute viral infection during the first trimester. However, when 100 cases of viral infection during the first trimester are followed, the resultant congenital defects occur in only about 10 per cent. We feel the Vanderbilt Cooperative Study has developed this latter perspective.

THERAPEUTIC EXPERIMENTAL FINDINGS

Lower Animal Observations: Tables 6.4 and 6.5 reveal the abundant number of reported observations following therapy. They are concerned primarily with fetal complications. Inanition in the small experimental animal was noted to result in abortion or fetal resorption, but cows did not seem affected until the inanition was extreme. Total resorption occurred on low protein diets in rats. Carbohydrate deprivation did not appear to affect the incidence of obstetrical complications.

Of the vitamins, A has been studied most intensively and in the widest variety of animals. Its deficiency, reportedly, produces fetal resorptions, stillbirths, and the birth of premature weakly offspring. More recently, massive doses have resulted in fetal death.

Many of the B complex vitamins seem to be essential for normal pregnancy. Deficiencies of thiamine (B1), riboflavin (B2), pyridoxine (B6), pantothenic acid, biotin, folic acid, and vitamin B12 are all reported to cause fetal loss. Niacin deficiency seemed to exert little effect on reproduction in the rat, but it may prevent lactation. No adverse effects have been reported from excessive dosage of any of the B complex fractions.

Both a deficiency and an excess of vitamin C have been noted to affect adversely reproduction in the guinea pig. Abortion or fetal absorption were reported when a deficiency occurred early in pregnancy and stillborn or premature young when it developed late. Abortions also have been described in cases of excessive intake. An interesting dietary inter-relationship (Chapter Four) is the finding that the reproductive performance of pantothenic acid deficient rats was enhanced by ascorbic acid supplementation. This is particularly noteworthy in view of the fact that the rat is known to be capable of synthesizing its daily ascorbic acid requirement.

Table 6.4

diet (deficiencies) and obstetrical
complications (lower animal
therapeutic observations)

dietary variable	animals	references
	adverse effects (failure of implantation, fetal resorption, abortion, stillborn, premature birth, neonatal deaths, weakly, anemic or stunted progeny)	
inanition	albino rat, rabbit	9, 77
	guinea pig, cow	42, 88
		26
protein deprivation	rat	30, 57
		93,118
vitamin A deficient	rat	98
	rabbit	85,107
	sheep	108
	swine	60, 61,
		68, 69
	cow	58, 59
thiamine deficient	rat	28
	swine	29, 44
riboflavin deficient	rat	53, 54
pyridoxine deficient	rat	138
pyridoxine antagonist	rat	120
pantothenic acid deficient	rat	8, 16,
		121
biotin deficient	rat	79
folic acid deficient	rat	122
folic acid antagonist (aminopterin)	mouse	164
vitamin B12 deficient	rat	87
vitamin C deficient	guinea pig	70
vitamin E deficient	rat	25, 46
vitamin K deficient	rabbit	113
calcium deficient	rat	94
phosphorus deficient	rat, cow	43,167
iron deficient	mouse, rat	142
copper deficient	rat	38
manganese deficient	rat	17

no adverse effects (except as noted)

carbohydrate deprivation	rat	49
niacin deficient	rat (failure to lactate)	47
vitamin E deficient	large farm animals	14
low calcium diet	cow, swine	105
manganese deficient	rat (young did not suckle)	129

Table 6.5
diet (supplements and excesses) and
obstetrical complications (lower
animal therapeutic observations)

dietary variable	animals	references
adverse effects (failure of implantation, fetal resorption, abortion, stillborn, premature birth, neonatal deaths, weakly, anemic or stunted progeny)		
pure sucrose and tap water	rat	39
erucic acid 15%	rat	24
vitamin A excess	rat	106
	mouse, guinea pig	55
	rabbit	119
vitamin C excess	guinea pig	115
vitamin B & C excess	guinea pig	124
1200 I.U. vitamin D daily	guinea pig	125
favorable effects (larger litters, improved reproductive and lactation performance or survival rate)		
pantothenic acid supplement stock diet	mouse, rat	159
biotin added to highly purified diet	mouse	109
addition of either vitamin	mouse	73
B12 or cobalt chloride to a B12 deficient diet	rat	135,156
vitamin C added to pantothenic acid deficient diet	rat (dietary vitamin C not required)	50
calcium content of diet increased	rat	144
no adverse effects		
massive doses of thiamine	rat	114
massive doses of para-aminobenzoic acid and inositol	rat	48
massive doses of B12	rat	135

While vitamin E is essential for the maintenance of pregnancy in rats, it is apparently not necessary in large farm animals. Vitamin K lack in rabbits has resulted in abortions. Calcium and copper deficiencies seem to increase fetal mortality rates. Phosphorus deficit is reported to contribute to abortions in cows and fetal resorption in the rat. Lack of iron does not appear to exert any adverse effects on maintenance of pregnancy in mice and rats, but the young may develop anemia. The findings regarding the effect of manganese deprivation are somewhat uncertain. It is thought that the failure of some investigators *(129)* to find adverse effects was due to lack of a sufficient degree of manganese deficiency *(111)*. Nelson and Evans *(118)* demonstrated quite clearly how this could occur.

In a study on the influence of protein on pregnancy in the rat, diets containing no protein, 2.5, 5, 10, 15, 20, and 25 per cent protein were administered. With a protein deficient diet or one with only 2.5 per cent protein, there was almost total fetal resorption. At the 5 per cent level, almost one-third of the implanted ova underwent resorption. Above 5 per cent no effect on the litters was produced. They *(118)* also demonstrated an interesting nutrient interrelationship (Chapter Four). When vitamin B12 was added to diets low in protein, the number of resorptions was decreased; but the added vitamin B12 had no effect if the diet was completely protein-free.

Human Observations: The numerous obstacles which beset the path of one who desires to study the effect of diet on the outcome of human pregnancy have failed to deter many investigators (Tables 6.6 and 6.7). There is an admitted variation in the quality of the studies. Nevertheless, the number of well-designed and carefully executed investigations revealing important therapeutic relationships between diet and obstetrical complications is quite impressive. Their quality, number, and scope make it difficult to escape the conclusion that diet is a most important determinant of the eventfulness of pregnancy.

One of the most carefully designed and executed therapeutic studies was conducted by Ebbs, Tisdall, and Scott of the Departments of Obstetrics and Pediatrics, University of Toronto *(41)*. The diets of 380 patients who had not reached the sixth month of pregnancy were carefully analyzed by means of a seven-day diet record. Each detail on the record was checked by means of questioning and comparison with amounts bought and served at each meal to the whole family. Recipes and cooking methods were also discussed. In some instances the homes were visited and the food weighed after the subjects had estimated and recorded the amount.

The patients were divided into three groups (Table 6.8). Group A was composed of 120 low-income, poor-diet patients who remained on their poor diets and were given placebo

Table 6.6
diet and fetal obstetrical complications
(human therapeutic observations)

dietary variable	complication	reference
	increase	
folic acid antagonist	abortion (therapeutic)	162
	decrease	
good quality diet		
added food & vitamins and/or diet instruction*	abruptio placentae, premature babies, stillborn, neonatal deaths	41
milk, chocolate, vitamin B*	stillborn, neonatal deaths	7
dietary advice	premature babies, stillborn, neonatal deaths	158
dietary instructions*	premature babies, stillborn, neonatal deaths	23
dietary instructions*	premature babies	12
dietary regime	stillborn	116
high protein & green vegetable diet (weight restriction stressed, thyroid when pulse rate low)*	fetal deaths	90
vitamin & mineral supplementation		
vitamin & mineral supplement	premature babies	127
folic acid deficient gravidas (lymphocyte count <1500/cmm) supplemented*	fetal deaths	86
vitamin C & bioflavonoids	fetal deaths due to erythroblastosis fetalis	137
vitamin C & bioflavonoids*	stillborn & neonatal deaths due to erythroblastosis fetalis	72
large amounts of vitamin C or bioflavonoids	habitual or threatened abortion	1, 36, 56, 74, 80,160
20-200 mg. of vitamin E	habitual or threatened abortion	5, 10, 15, 52, 89,140, 146,147, 165,168
2-3 minims sodium or potassium iodide (weekly)*	stillborn	136
	no effect	
vitamin C & hesperidin for 5 weeks in gravidas on multivitamins including 50 mg. vitamin C*	abortions	18
20-200 mg. vitamin E	abortions	96

*compared with control group

Table 6.7
diet and maternal obstetrical complications
(human therapeutic observations)

dietary variable	complication	reference
increase		
16 g. NaCl to gravidas	preeclampsia	35
decrease		
good quality diet		
milk, chocolate, vitamin B*	maternal deaths	7
high protein & green vegetable diet (weight restriction stressed, thyroid if pulse rate low)*	toxemia, preeclampsia, eclampsia	90
110-120 g. protein daily*	toxemia	66
3,000 calorie, 90 g. protein diet	toxemia	92
120 g. protein diet*	toxemia	2
high protein, high vitamin, restricted salt intake diet	preeclampsia, eclampsia	62
110 g. protein diet	toxemia	163
amino acid (cystine) therapy of gravidas with low blood cystine levels	toxemia	141
thiamine injections & 260 g. protein	toxemia	154
vitamin & mineral supplementation		
vitamin & mineral supplement	toxemia, preeclampsia	127
injection of vitamins A, B1, B2, C & D	nausea & vomiting	169
vitamins A & B & calcium lactate*	toxemia	161
vitamin B complex & wheat germ oil	toxemia	13
thiamine, niacin & Brewer's yeast	polyneuritis	132
whole liver extract & thiamine	nausea & vomiting	45
50-100 mg. pyridoxine with or without thiamine	nausea & vomiting	63
pyridoxine or thiamine	nausea & vomiting	178
pyridoxine (10 mg. to 160 mg.)	toxemia	166
	nausea & vomiting	149,170, 171
vitamin C & bioflavonoids plus usual treatment	varicose veins	131
low salt diet	eclampsia	82
alkaline diet	eclampsia	155
supplementation with salt	toxemia	34
no effect		
good quality diet		
added food & vitamins and/or diet instructions*	preeclampsia	41
vitamin & mineral supplementation		
vitamin B1	polyneuritis	103
thiamine (3 mg.)	toxemia	19
pyridoxine therapy*	nausea & vomiting	65

*compared with control group

capsules and no dietary advice. Group B included 90 similar patients selected on an alternate basis who were sent 30 ounces of milk, 1 egg, and 1 orange daily, and 32 ounces of canned tomatoes and a half pound of cheddar cheese weekly. Dried wheat germ, containing malt and added iron, and vitamin D capsules were distributed at the clinic. Detailed advice regarding the use of the supplemental food and in planning the diet from the family income was given. Many of the homes in this group were visited in order to check on food consumption. Supplementation was initiated in the fourth or fifth month. One hundred and seventy patients on moderately good diets and deemed financially able to obtain a satisfactory diet if given suitable advice were placed in Group C and supplied with detailed dietary instructions also beginning in the fourth or fifth month. The seven-day diet analysis was repeated two months later in all three groups.

The effects of these dietary regimes on nutrient consumption as measured by the second dietary analysis can be seen in Table 6.8. Both supplementation and education resulted in marked improvement in nutrient intake. Parenthetic mention should be made that these results do not substantiate the frequently expressed opinion that a significant number of patients will not follow dietary advice.

Figure 6.2 reveals a marked decrease in obstetrical complications experienced by the two groups (B and C) receiving dietotherapy as compared to the control group (A). For example, there were no neonatal deaths in either of the experimental groups in contrast to a 2.5 per cent mortality in the control category. Similar findings were reported for anemia, threatened miscarriage, endometritis, breast abscess, and hemorrhage during both the prenatal period and labor. The postnatal infant findings of this study are appropriately reported in Chapter Seven (Congenital Defects).

The obstetrician in charge of the patients rated their condition and progress during the prenatal period, labor, and convalescence without prior knowledge of the group to which each belonged. The condition and progress of Group B (poor diet with dietary instructions and supplements) was always best in all three periods, Group C (good diet with dietary instructions) was always intermediate, and Group A (poor

Table 6.8
effect of dietotherapy on consumption
of protein, fat, carbohydrate.
calcium and calories

	Group A			Group B			Group C		
	initial	final	% in-crease	initial	final	% in-crease	initial	final	% in-crease
protein (gm.)	56	62	11	56	94	68	81	92	14
fat (gm.)	66	75	14	67	111	66	95	113	19
carbohy-drate (gm.)	213	232	9	212	283	34	261	293	12
calcium (gm.)	0.54	0.75	39	0.56	1.61	188	0.89	1.30	46
iron (mg.)	10.7	11.6	8	10.5	24.3	131	14.2	18.3	29
calories	1700	1800	6	1700	2400	41	2200	2500	14

diet with placebo capsules) always worst.

From the findings noted in Figure 6.2, it appears that this type of dietotherapy, when not instituted until relatively late in pregnancy, does not affect preeclampsia. This is not inconsistent with the findings of Hamlin *(62)* in the Sydney Women's Hospital in Australia. The cases of eclampsia entirely disappeared, and the incidence of severe preeclampsia was greatly reduced in a three-year period when a regime which included a relatively high-protein and vitamin diet, and restricted salt intake for all women with digital edema, was instituted (Figure 6.3) at the start of pregnancy and intensified between the 20th and 30th weeks.

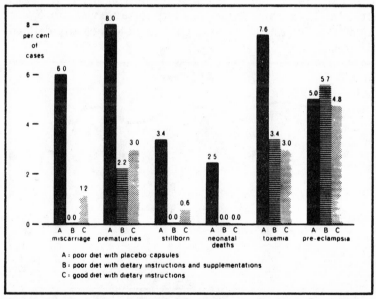

Figure 6.2. The effect of dietotherapy upon complications of pregnancy.

Reexamination of thousands of outpatient records revealed the need for extremely close regulation of weight gain between the 20th and 28th weeks. Hamlin subsequently concluded:

The bad high-carbohydrate, low-protein diet was changed on a wholesale scale in thousands of patients to a low-carbohydrate, high-protein, high-vitamin diet before mid-pregnancy. The successful result of this campaign suggests that it may be possible to reduce preeclamptic toxaemia to a minimum in this country by the adoption of two simple measures:

The giving of correct diet education in the early weeks of pregnancy.

The critical study of every patient's weight chart between the 20th and 28th weeks, so that the warning evidence of eclampsia-in-the-making may be seen in time.

A sizable number of studies have involved specific nutrients. The number of subjects and the use of controls in many instances have not appeared to be sufficient. However, where these factors have been adequate, the findings have largely confirmed the observations of the less well controlled studies regarding the importance of the various nutrients. Thus, it would appear that in addition to protein, the B vitamins, vitamin C, the bioflavonoids, iodine, and vitamin E are important. The role of low sodium diets is less clearly defined experimentally.

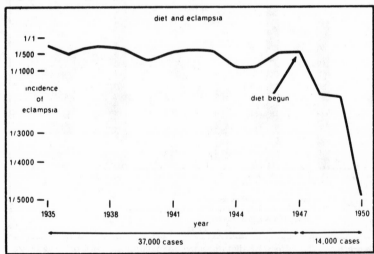

Figure 6.3. The effect of a regime instituted in 1947, which included a high protein diet, with restricted salt intake for all women with digital edema, on eclampsia at Women's Hospital, Sydney, Australia.

Rather exciting is the finding of a reduction in the stillborn and neonatal death rate from erythroblastosis fetalis by vitamin C and bioflavonoid supplementation (72,137). This is especially so in view of the fact that the disorder is regarded as being genetic in origin and because bioflavonoids are seldom included in prenatal supplements. The evidence regarding the positive role of vitamin E in the prevention of habitual or threatened abortion is also becoming increasingly convincing. There is suggestive but less convincing evidence of a similar role for vitamin C and the bioflavonoids.

SUMMARY

When considered as a whole, the lower animal and human studies present a rather impressive picture of the role of diet in obstetrical complications. As might be expected, there is a difference of opinion as to the clinical significance of this knowledge and its manner of application.

The lower animal studies have been concerned primarily with the role of specific factors. While there has been interest in the effects of isolated factors in humans, the larger studies have been more concerned with multiple dietary variables.

A second important difference in the human and lower animal studies rests in the homogeneity of the samples and timing of the beginning of the studies. In lower animals the observation period usually begins almost immediately after mating, and relatively complete knowledge regarding the preconceptual diet, other environmental factors, and the genetic background are available. Human observation periods are usually not started before the second trimester. Pertinent information about the preobservation period has been limited and seldom exploited even to the limited extent possible. Considering the degree of fetal development by the second trimester and the alterations which have occurred in the mother at this point, it is remarkable that correlative and therapeutic studies of diet and obstetrical complications in humans have achieved the degree of reported significance.

The scarcity of truly *excellent* diets in the human studies where the food intake has been carefully measured and classified is an interesting phenomenon. Doctor Montagu *(111)* has summarized the importance of nutrition during the preconceptual period.

> Were they called upon to name the most important factor in contributing to the health development of the human conceptus, most authorities would unhesitatingly declare for the good nutritional status of the mother. This means not merely that her

nutritional welfare during pregnancy is the important requisite, but that her own nutrition during her whole life, including the period of her sojourn in her own mother's womb, shall have been adequate.

If the contents of the mother's ovaries have been affected by some serious nutritional disturbance during her own development, good nutrition during pregnancy will certainly not repair the damage done, although poor nutrition will almost certainly worsen it. Good nutrition will, at least, ensure that development occurs as well as other conditions permit....Rickets acquired in infancy or in childhood may so affect the development of the pelvis of a female that her later reproductive history and the fate of her children may be seriously affected. Rickets is largely a nutritional disorder....Can women who have always lived on a nutritionally inadequate plane, with no nutritional training, and their own nutritional stores depleted, provide a satisfactory environment and an adequate nutrition for the healthy building of another body? As we might expect, the answer is that they cannot.

It would appear that the need for a fresh approach to the problem of obstetrical complications may be found, at least in part, in the field of dietotherapy. Indeed, it would seem from the experience of many of the investigators cited in this chapter that scrupulous attention to established methods of dietotherapy would yield impressive results.

Finally, one of the ironies of medical science is the persistent report of superior health among isolated primitive peoples obtained without benefit of our vast medical knowledge. For example, Kemp *(78)* noted that the incidence of stillbirth among the Indians of British Columbia from 1925 to 1929 was 1.26 per cent compared to 2.73 per cent for the white population of British Columbia and 2.09 per cent for all of Canada during the same period. This low incidence occurred despite the fact that the great majority of the squaws delivered themselves unaided by medical assistance. The food of these Indians was almost entirely salmon, salmon eggs, and seaweed.

REFERENCES

1. Ainsle, W. H. *Treatment of habitual abortion.* Obstet. and Gynec. 13: #2, 185-188, February 1959.

2. Ajzenberg, M. F. *K voprosu o pitani beremennyh.* Akush Ginek. No. 1: #16, 1960. Quoted by Millen (1962).

3. Antonov, A. N. *Children born during the siege of Leningrad in 1942.* J. Pediat. 30: #3, 250-259, March 1947.

4. Arnell, R. E., Goldman, D. W. and Bertucci, F. J. *Protein deficiencies in pregnancy.* J. A. M. A. 127: #17, 1101-1109, 28 April 1945.

5. Bacharach, A. L. *Vitamin E and habitual abortion.* Brit. Med. J. 1: #4143, 890, 1 June 1940.

6. Baird, D. *The influence of social and economic factors on stillbirths and neonatal deaths.* J. Obstet. Gynec. Brit. Emp. 52: #3, #4, 217-234, 339-366, June and August 1945.

7. Balfour, M. I. *Supplementary feeding in pregnancy.* Lancet 1: #6285, 208-211, 12 February 1944.

8. Barboriak, J. J., Krehl, W. A., Cowgill, G. R. and Whedon, A. D. *Effect of partial pantothenic acid deficiency on reproductive performance of the rat.* J. Nutrit. 63: #4, 591-599, 10 December 1957.

9. Barry, L. W. *The effects of inanition in the pregnant albino rat, with special reference to the changes in the relative weights of the various parts, systems, and organs of the offspring.* Contr. Embryol. Carnes Instn. 11: #53, 91-136, 1920.

10. Bayer, R. *Results of pretreatment with vitamin E for control of primary and secondary essential infertility; reports on studies with 100 married couples.* Wein. Med. Wochschr. 109: #13, 271-275, 28 March 1959.

11. Bennett, H. W., Underwood, E. J. and Shier, F. L. Australian Vet. J. 22: #2, 1946. Cited by Clemetson, C. A. B., Blair, L. and Brown, A. B. *Capillary strength and the menstrual cycle.* Annals N. Y. Acad. Sci. 93: #7, 277-300, 15 April 1962.

12. Berry, K. and Wiehl, D. G. *An experiment in diet education during pregnancy.* Milbank Mem. Fund Quar. 30: #2, 119-151, April 1952.

13. Bijdendijk, A. and van Assen, F. J. J. *Een methode ter behandlung van zwangerschaps-toxaemieen met vitamins.* Ned. Tijdscr. Geneesk. 93: 243-248, 22 January 1949. Quoted by Millen (1962).

14. Blaxter, K. L. and Brown, F. *Vitamin E in the nutrition of farm animals.* Nutrit. Abst. Rev. 22: #1, 1-21, July 1952.

15. Boileau, P. A. *Treatment of varicose veins of pregnancy with water-soluble citrus bioflavonoids.* Clin. Med. 44: #4, 1383-1387, July 1960.

16. Boisselot, J. *Malformations congenitales provoquees chez le rat par une insuffisance en acide pantothenique du regime maternel.* C. R. Soc. Biol. Paris, 142: #13 & 14, 928-929, July 1948.

17. Boyer, P. D., Shaw, J. H., and Phillips, P. H. *Studies on manganese deficiency in the rat.* J. Biol. Chem. 143: #2, 417-425, April 1942.

18. Briscoe, C. C. *The role of vitamin C-hesperidin in the prevention of abortion.* Obstet. and Gynec. 14: #3, 288-290, September 1959.

19. Browne, F. J. *On the value of vitamin B in prevention of toxaemia of pregnancy.* Brit. Med. J. i: #4292, 445-446, April 10, 1943.

20. Burger, H. *Ist die Eklampsie auch im letzten Krieg (1939-1945) zuruckgegangen?* Zbl. Gynak. 72: 551-555, 1950.

21. Burke, B. S., Beal, V. A., Kirkwood, S. B. and Stuart, H. C. *The influence of nutrition during pregnancy upon the condition of the infant at birth.* J. Nutrit. 26: #6, 569-583, December 1943.

22. Burke, B. S., Beal, V. A., Kirkwood, S. B. and Stuart, H. C. *Nutrition studies during pregnancy.* Amer. J. Obstet. Gynec. 46: #1, 38-52, July 1943.

23. Cameron, C. S. and Graham, S. *Antenatal diet and its influence on stillbirths and prematurity.* Glasg. Med. J. 24: #1, 1-7, July 1944.

24. Carroll, K. K. and Noble, R. L. *Influence of a dietary supplement of erucic acid and other fatty acids on fertility in the rat.* Canad. J. Biochem. Physiol. 35: #11, 1093-1105, November 1957.

25. Cheng, D. W., Chang, L. F., and Bairson, T. A. *Gross observations on developing abnormal embryos induced by maternal vitamin E deficiency.* Anat. Rec. 129: #2, 167-185, October 1957.

26. Chow, B. F. *Growth of rats from normal dams restricted in diet in previous pregnancies.* J. Nutrit. 83: #4, 289-292, August 1964.

27. Clemetson, C. A. B. and Anderson, L. *Ascorbic acid metabolism in preeclampsia.* Obst. & Gynecol. 24: #5, 774-782, November 1964.

28. Coward, K. H. and Morgan, B. G. E. *The determination of vitamin B1 by means of its influence on the vaginal contents of the rat.* Biochem. J. 35: #849, 974-978, September 1941.

29. Coward, K. H., Morgan, B. G. E. and Waller, L. *The influence of a deficiency of vitamin B1 and riboflavin on the reproduction of the rat.* J. Physiol. 100: #4, 423-431, March 1942.

30. Curtiss, C. *Effect of a low protein intake on the pregnant rat.* Metabolism 2: #4, 344-353, July 1953.

31. Dalderup, L. M. *Atherosclerosis and toxemia of pregnancy in relation to nutrition and other physiological factors.* Vitam. and Horm. XVII, 224-324, New York, Academic Press. 1959.

32. Darby, W. J., Densen, P. M., Cannon, R. O., Bridgforth, E., Martin, M. P., Kaser, M. M., Peterson, C., Christie, A., Frye, W. W., Justus, C. W., Carothers, E. L. and Newbill, J. A. *The Vanderbilt cooperative study of maternal and infant nutrition. 1. Background, 2. Methods, 3. Description of sample and data.* J. Nutrit. 51: #4, 539-563, 10 December 1953.

33. Darby, W. J., McGanity, W. J., Martin, M. F., Bridgforth, E., Denson, P. M., Kaser, M. M., Ogle, P. J., Newbill, J. A., Stockell, A., Ferguson, M. E., Touster, O., McClellan, G. S., Williams, C., and Cannon, R. O. *The Vanderbilt cooperative study of maternal and infant nutrition. IV. Dietary, laboratory and physical findings in 2,129 delivered pregnancies.* J. Nutrit. 51: #4, 565-597, 10 December 1953.

34. De Raadt, O. L. E. *Behandlung en prophylaxis van eclampsia.* Geneesk. Tijdschv. Ned. Ind. 78: 1401-1404, 7 June 1938.

35. De Snoo, K. *The prevention of eclampsia.* Amer. J. Obstet. and Gynec. 34: #6, 911-939, December 1937.

36. Dill, L. V. *Therapy of late abortion.* M. Ann. District of Columbia 23: #12, 667-669, December 1954.

37. Duncan, E. H. L., Baird, D., and Thomson, A. M. *The cause and prevention of stillbirths and first-week deaths.* J. Obstet. Gynaec. Brit. Emp. 59: #2, 183-196, April 1952.

38. Dutt, B. and Mills, C. F. *Reproductive failure in rats due to copper deficiency.* J. Comp. Path. and Therapeutics 70: #1, 120-125, January 1960.

39. Dyban, A. P., Demkiv, L. P. and Avgustinovic, M. S. *Inhibition of implantation dispause in rats maintained on a deficient sucrose diet.* (Dokl. Akad. Nauk SSSR, 1963, 149, 1453-1456, Gosud. med. Univ., Lwow.) Russian. Cited in Nutrit. Abst. & Rev. 33: #4, 1074, Art. 6490, October 1963.

40. Eastman, N. J. and Hellman, L. M. *Williams Obstetrics.* 12th edition. 1961. New York, Appleton-Century-Crofts.

41. Ebbs, J. H., Tisdall, F. F., and Scott, W. A. *The influence of prenatal diet on mother and child.* J. Nutrit. 22: #5, 515-526, November 1941.

42. Eckles, C. H. *A study of the birth weight of calves.* University Missouri Agr. Exp. Sta. Res. Bull. #35, 1919.

43. Eckles, C. H., Palmer, L. S., Gullickson, T. W., Fitch, C. P., Boyd, W. L., Bishop, L., and Nelson, J. W. Cornell Vet., 25: 22, 1935. (Quoted by Warkany, J.) *Manifestations of prenatal nutritional deficiency.* Vitamins and Hormones, 3: 73-103, 1945.

44. Ensminger, M. E., Bowland, J. P., and Cunha, T. J. *Observations on the thiamine, riboflavin and choline needs of sows for reproduction.* J. Anim. Sci. 6: 409, 1947.

45. Epstein, B. *The treatment of vomiting of pregnancy with injections of whole liver and thiamine chloride.* S. Afr. Med. J. 19: #9, 150-151, 12 May 1945.

46. Ershoff, B. H. *Degeneration of the corpora lutea in the pregnant vitamin E-deficient rat.* Anat. Rec. 87: #3, 297-301, November 1943.

47. Ershoff, B. H. *Dispensability of dietary niacin for reproduction and lactation in the rat.* Arch. Biochem. 9: #1, 81-84, January 1946.

48. Ershoff, B. H. *Effects of massive doses of p-aminobenzoic acid and inositol on reproduction in the rat.* Proc. Soc. Exp. Biol. & Med., 63: #2, 479-483, November 1946.

49. Evans, H. M. and Bishop, K. S. *On the relations between fertility and nutrition. II. The ovulation rhythm in the rat on inadequate nutritional regimes.* J. Metab. Res. 1: #3, 335-356, March 1922.

50. Everson, G., Northrop, L., Chung, N. Y., and Getty, R. *Effect of ascorbic acid on rats deprived of pantothenic acid.* J. Nutrit. 54: #2, 305-311, October 1954.

51. Frederick, G. L. *A relationship between B12 and reproduction, and a method of diagnosing vitamin B12 deficiency in individual swine.* Am. J. Vet. Res. 21: 478-481, May 1960.

52. Garry, R. C. and Wood, H. O. *Dietary requirements in human pregnancy and lactation: a review of recent work.* Nutrit. Abst. Rev. 15: #4, 591-621, April 1946.

53. Gilman, J. P. W., Perry, F. A., and Hill, D. C. *Some effects of a maternal riboflavin deficiency on reproduction in the rat.* Canad. J. Med. Sci. 30: #3, 383-389, October 1952.

54. Giroud, A., Levy, G., Lefebvres, J., and Dupuis, R. *Chute du taux de la riboflavine au stade ou se determinant les malformations embryonnaires.* Int. Z. Vitaminforsch. 23: 490-494, 1952.

55. Giroud, A. and Martinet, M. *Extension a plusieurs especes de mammiferes des malformations embryonnaires par hypervitaminose A.* C. R. Soc. Biol. Paris, 153: #2, 201-202, 10 June 1959.

56. Greenblatt, R. B. *Habitual abortion: possible role of vitamin P in therapy.* Obstet. and Gynec. 2: #5, 530-533, November 1953.

57. Guilbert, H. R. and Goss, H. *Some effects of restricted protein intake on the estrous cycle and gestation in the rat.* J. Nutrit. 5: #3, 251-265, May 1932.

58. Guilbert, H. R. and Hart, G. H. *Storage of vitamin A in cattle.* J. Nutrit. 8: #1, 25-44, July 1934.

59. Guilbert, H. R. and Hart, G. H. *Minimum vitamin A requirements with particular reference to cattle.* J. Nutrit. 10: #4, 409-427, October 1935.

60. Hale, F. *Pigs born without eyeballs.* J. Hered. 24: #3, 105-106, March 1933.

61. Hale, F. *The relation of vitamin A deficiency to anophthalmia in pigs.* Amer. J. Ophthal. 18: #12, 1087-1093, December 1935.

62. Hamlin, R. H. J. *The prevention of eclampsia and pre-eclampsia.* Lancet 1: #6698, 64-68, January 1952.

63. Hart, B. F., McConnell, W. T. and Pickett, A. N. *Vitamin and endocrine therapy in nausea and vomiting of pregnancy.* Amer. J. Obstet. Gynec. 48: #2, 251-253, August 1944.

64. Hart, G. H. and Guilbert, H. R. *Vitamin A deficiency as related to reproduction in range cattle.* California Agri. Exp. Sta. Bull. #560, 3, 1933.

65. Hesseltine, H. C. *Pyridoxine failure in nausea and vomiting of pregnancy.* Amer. J. Obstet. Gynec. 51: #1, 82-86, January 1946.

66. Holmes, O. M. *Protein diet in pregnancy.* West J. Surg. 49: #1, 56-60, January 1941.

67. Holson, W. *A dietary and clinical survey of pregnant women with particular reference to toxaemia of pregnancy.* J. Hyg. 46: #2, 198-216, July 1948.

68. Hughes, E. H. *Some effects of vitamin-A-deficiency diets on reproduction in sows.* J. Agri. Res. 49: 943, 1934.

69. Hughes, J. S., Aubel, C. E. and Lienhardt, H. F. *The importance of vitamin A and vitamin C in the ration of swine, concerning especially their effect on growth and reproduction.* Kansas Agri. Exp. Sta. Bull. #23, 1, 1928.

70. Ingier, A. *A study of Barlow's disease experimentally produced in fetal and newborn guinea pigs.* J. Exp. Med. 21: #6, 525-538, June 1915.

71. Ivanovsky, A. *Physical modifications of the population of Russia under famine.* Amer. J. Phys. Anthrop. 6: #4, 331-353, October-December 1923.

72. Jacobs, W. M. *Citrus bioflavonoid compounds in Rh-immunized gravidas.* Obstet. & Gynec. 25: #5, 648-649, May 1965.

73. Jaffe, W. G. *Influence of cobalt on reproduction in mice and rats.* Science 115: #2984, 265-267, 7 March 1952.

74. Javert, C. T. *Repeated abortion.* Obstet. & Gynec. 3: #4, 420-434, April 1954.

75. Javert, C. T. and Stander, H. J. *Plasma vitamin C and prothrombin concentration in pregnancy and in threatened, spontaneous and habitual abortion.* Surg. Gynec. Obstet. 76: #1, 115-122, January 1943.

76. Jeans, P. C., Smith, M. B. and Stearns, G. *Incidence of prematurity in relation to maternal nutrition.* J. Amer. Diet A. 31: #6, 576-581, June 1955.

77. Jonen, P. *Tierexperimentelle untersuchungen uber intrauterine fruchtschadigung.* Z. Geburtsh. Gynak. 101: 50-115, 1931.

78. Kemp, W. N. *Iodine deficiency in relation to stillbirth problem.* Canad. Med. A. J. 41: #4, 356-361, October 1939.

79. Kennedy, C. and Palmer, L. S. *Biotin deficiency in relation to reproduction and lactation.* Arch. Biochem. 7: #1, 9-13, June 1945.

80. King, A. G. *Threatened and repeated abortion: present status of therapy.* Obstet. & Gynec. 1: #1, 104-114, January 1953.

81. King, G. and Ride, L. T. *The relation of vitamin B1 deficiency to the pregnancy toxaemias.* J. Obstet. Gynaec. Brit. Emp. 52: #2, 130-147, April 1945.

82. King, W. E. *Vitamin studies in abortions.* Surg. Gynec. Obstet. 80: #2, 139-142, February 1945.

83. Kooser, J. H. *Observations on the possible relationship of diet to the late toxemia of pregnancy.* Amer. J. Obstet. Gynec. 41: #2, 288-294, February 1941.

84. Kyhos, E. D., Vaglio, N., Sevringhaus, E. L., Nutley, N. J., Hagedorn, D., Knowlton, M. *Effects of malnutrition upon mothers and infants in Naples 1945.* Amer. J. Dig. Dis. 16: #12, 436-441, December 1949.

85. Lamming, G. E., Salisbury, G. W., Hays, R. L., and Kendall, K. A. *Effect of incipient vitamin A deficiency on reproduction in the rabbit. II. Embryonic and fetal development.* J. Nutrit. 52: #2, 227-240, February 1954.

86. Lawson, D. F., De Garis, C. N. and Bolton, J. H. *Folic acid and reproductive efficiency.* Med. J. Aus. 1: #24, 848, 13 June 1953.

87. Lepkovsky, S., Borson, H. J., Bouthilet, R., Pencharz, R., Singman, D., Dimick, M. K., and Robbins, P. *Reproduction in vitamin B-deficient rats with emphasis on intrauterine injury.* Amer. J. Physiol. 165: #1, 79-86, April 1951.

88. Loeb. L. *The experimental production of hypotypical ovaries through underfeeding. A contribution to the analysis of sterility.* Biol. Bull., Wood's Hole 33: 91, 1917.

89. Lubin, S. and Waltman, R. *The use of synthetic vitamin E in the treatment of abortion.* Amer. J. Obstet. Gynec. 41: #6, 960-970, June 1941.

90. Luikurt, R. *High-protein low calorie diet for the prevention of toxaemia of pregnancy.* Amer. J. Obstet. & Gynec. 52: #3, 428-434, September 1946.

91. Lund, C. J. and Kimble, M. S. *Vitamin A during pregnancy, labor and the puerperium.* Amer. J. Obstet. Gynec. 46: #4, 486-501, October 1943.

92. Lu've, A. *Ju K voprosu o vacional nom pitani beremennyh zenscin.* A kush. Ginek. 1: #10, 1960. Quoted by Millen (1962).

93. Macomber, D. *Studies of reproduction in the rat. 1. The effect of changes in the protein upon fertility, pregnancy, and lactation.* New England J. Med. 209: #22, 1105-1109, 30 November 1933.

94. Macomber, D. *Effect of a diet low in calcium on fertility, pregnancy, and lactation in the rat.* J. A. M. A. 88: #1, 6-13, January 1927.

95. Madsen, L. L. *Nutritional diseases of farm animals.* In Keeping livestock healthy. 1942. Yearbook of Agric., Washington, D. C.

96. Malpas, P. *The incidence of human malformations.* J. Obstet. Gynec. Brit. Emp. 44: #3, 434-454, 1937.

97. Martin, M.P., Bridgforth, E., McGanity, W. J. and Darby, W. J. *The Vanderbilt cooperative study of maternal and infant nutrition. X. Ascorbic acid.* J. Nutrit. 62: #2, 201-223, June 1957.

98. Mason, K. E. *Fetal death, prolonged gestation, and difficult parturition in the rat as a result of vitamin A deficiency.* Amer. J. Anat. 57: #2, 303-344, September 1935.

99. Mastboom, J. L. *Defrequentic van eclampsie in corlogstijd.* Ned. Tijdschr. Geneesk. 92: #45, 3604-3616, November 6, 1948.

100. Matthews, H. B. and der Brucke, M. G. *Normal expectancy in the extremely obese pregnant woman.* J. A. M. A. 110: #8, 554-559, February 19, 1938.

101. McGanity, W. J., Cannon, R. O., Bridgforth, E. B., Martin, M. P., Densen, P. M., Newbill, J. A., McClellan, G. S., Christie, A., Peterson, J. C., and Darby, W. J. *The Vanderbilt cooperative study of maternal and infant nutrition. 6. Relationship of obstetric performance to nutrition.* Amer. J. Obstet. Gynec. 67: #3, 501-527, March 1954.

102. McGanity, W. J., Cannon, R. O., Bridgforth, E. B., Martin, M. P., Newbill, J. A., and Darby, W. J. *The Vanderbilt cooperative study of maternal and infant nutrition. VIII. Some nutritional implications.* J. Amer. Diet. Assn. 31: #5, 582-588, June 1955.

103. McGoogan, L. S. *Severe polyneuritis due to vitamin B deficiency in pregnancy.* Amer. J. Obstet. Gynec. 43: #5, 752-762, May 1942.

104. Meigs, E. B. and Converse, H. T. *The vitamin A requirements of dairy cows for reproduction and lactation under practical conditions.* J. Dairy Sc. 19: 438, 1936.

105. Millen, J. W. *The nutritional basis of reproduction.* 1962. Springfield, Charles C. Thomas.

106. Millen, J. W. and Woollam, O. H. M. *Influence of cortisone on teratogenic effects of hypervitaminosis A.* Brit. Med. J. 11: #5038, 196-197, July 27, 1957.

107. Millen, J. W., Woollam, O. H. M., and Lamming, G. E. *Congenital hydrocephalus due to experimental hypovitaminosis A.* Lancet 11: #14, 679-683, October 2, 1954.

108. Miller, R. F., Hart, G. H., and Cole, H. H. *Fertility in sheep as affected by nutrition during the breeding season and pregnancy.* California Agri. Exp. Sta. Bull. 672, 1942.

109. Mirone, L. and Cerecedo, L. R. *The beneficial effect of xanthopterin on lactation, and of biotin in reproduction and lactation, in mice maintained on highly purified diets.* Arch. Biochem. 15: #2, 324-326, November 1947.

110. Mischel, W. *Uber den cholingehalt der menschlichen plazenta, seine aufgabe und seine bedeutung fur die atiologie der toxikose.* Z. Geburtsh. Gynak. 141: 334-345, 1954. Cited by Millen, J. W. *The nutritional basis of reproduction.* 1962. Springfield, Charles C. Thomas.

111. Montagu, M. F. A. *Prenatal influences.* 1962. Springfield, Charles C. Thomas.

112. Moore, L. A., Huffman, C. F. and Duncan, C. W. *Blindness in cattle associated with a constriction of the optic nerve and probably of nutritional origin.* J. Nutrit. 9: #5, 533-551, May 1935.

113. Moore, R. A., Bittenger, I., Miller, M. L., and Hellman, L. M. *Abortion in rabbits fed a vitamin K deficient diet.* Amer. J. Obst. Gynec. 43: #6, 1007-1012, June 1942.

114. Morrison, A. B. and Sarett, H. P. *Effects of excess thiamine*

and pyridoxine on growth and reproduction in rats. J. Nutrit. 69: #2, 111-116, October 1959.

115. Mouriquand, G. and Edel, V. *Sur l'hypervitaminose C.* C. R. Soc. Biol., Paris 147: #13-14, 1432-1434, July 1953.

116. Mullins, A. *Overweight in pregnancy.* Lancet 1: #7116, 146-147, 16 January 1960.

117. Napier, L. E. and Neal-Edwards, M. I. *Anaemia in pregnancy in Calcutta. An analysis of haematological and other data from 529 pregnant women.* Indian Med. Res. Mem. 33. 1941. Cited by Millen, J. W. *The nutritional basis of reproduction.* 1962. Springfield, Charles C. Thomas.

118. Nelson, M. M. and Evans, H. M. *Relation of dietary protein levels to reproduction in the rat.* J. Nutrit. 51: #1, 71-84, September 1953.

119. Nelson, M. M. and Evans, H. M. *Relation of thiamine to reproduction in the rat.* J. Nutrit. 55: #1, 151-163, January 1955.

120. Nelson, M. M. and Evans, H. M. *Effect of pyridoxine deficiency on reproduction in the rat.* J. Nutrit. 43: #2, 281-294, 10 February 1951.

121. Nelson, M. M. and Evans, H. M. *Pantothenic acid deficiency and reproduction in the rat.* J. Nutrit. 31: #4, 497-507, 10 April 1946.

122. Nelson, M. M., Wright, H. V., Baird, C. D. V., and Evans, H. M. *Effect of a 36-hour period of pteroylglutamic acid deficiency on fetal development in the rat.* Proc. Soc. Exp. Biol., New York, 92: #3, 554-556, July 1956.

123. Neuweiler, W. *Polyneuritis in der Schwangerschaft.* Med. Klin. 36: #43, 1179-1181, 25 October 1940.

124. Neuweiler, W. *Die hypervitaminose und ihre beziehung zur schwangerschaft.* Int. Z. Vitaminforsch 28: #4, 392-396, 1951.

125. Neuweiler, W. *Vitamin D-hypervitaminose und schwangerschaft.* Int. Z. Vitaminforsch 25: #2, 203-205, 1954.

126. Nixon, W. C. W., Wright, M. D. and Fieller, E. C. *Vitamin B1 in the urine and placenta in toxaemia of pregnancy.* Brit. Med. 1: #4245, 605-607, 16 May 1942.

127. *The nutrition of expectant and nursing mothers in relation to maternal and infant mortality and morbidity.* The People's League of Health. J. Obst. & Gynec. Brit. Emp. 53: 498-509, December 1946.

128. Odell, L. D. and Mengert, W. F. *The overweight obstetric patient.* J. A. M. A. 128: #2, 87-89, 12 May 1945.

129. Orent, E. R. and McCollum, E. V. *Effects of deprivation of manganese in the rat.* J. Biol. Chem. 92: #3, 651-678, August 1931.

130. Pai, M. L. *Urinary excretion of miotinic acid in toxemia of pregnancy.* J. Anim. Morph. Physiol. 3: 79, 1956.

131. Pearse, H. E. and Trisler, J. D. A. *Rational approach to the treatment of habitual abortion and menometrorrhagia.* Clin. Med. 4: #9, 1081-1084, September 1957.

132. Posner, A. C. and Hecht, E. L. *Gestational neuronitis deficiency disease.* Amer. J. Obstet. Gynec. 46: #5, 700-707, November 1943.

133. Postmus, S. *Beriberi of mother and child in Burma.* Trop. Geogr. Med. 10: 363-370, 1958.

134. Randall, L. M. and Wagener, H. P. *Vitamin deficiency associated with vomiting of pregnancy: report of a case.* Proc. Mayo Clinic 12: #20, 305-308, 19 May 1937.

135. Richardson, L. R. and Brock, R. *Studies of reproduction in rats using large doses of vitamin B12 and highly purified soybean products.* J. Nutrit. 58: #1, 135-145, 10 January 1956.

136. Robinson, M. *Salt in pregnancy.* Lancet 1: #4, 178-181, 25 January 1958.

137. Rogers, G. C. and Fleming, J. M. *Therapeutic evaluation of citrus bioflavonoids in the prevention of erythroblastosis.* West J. Surg., Obstet. & Gynec. 63: #6, 386-388, June 1955.

138. Ross, M. L. and Pike, R. L. *The relationship of vitamin B6 to protein metabolism during pregnancy in the rat.* J. Nutrit. 58: #2, 251-268, 10 February 1956.

139. Royal College of Obstetricians and Gynaecologists, *Report on National Maternity Service,* 1944.

140. Schafer, L. *Weitere Erfahrungen mit der vitamin E- behandlung.* Klin. Wschr. 21: 991, 1942. Cited by Millen (1962).

141. Schuck, J. *Aminosaureanalysen im plasmaeiweiss bei schwangerschaftstoxikosen.* Arch. Gynak. 178: Supp. 23, 217-220, February 1950.

142. Scott, J. M. D. *Studies in anemia.* Biochem. J. 17: #2, 166-173, February 1923.

143. Shand, A. B. V. A. Publ. No. 23, 58, 1952. Cited by Highnett, S. L. *The influence of nutrition on female fertility in some large domestic animals.* Proc. Nutrit. Soc. 19: #1, 8-14, 1960.

144. Sherman, H. C. and Campbell, H. L. *Effects of increasing the calcium content of a diet in which calcium is one of the limiting factors.* J. Nutrit. 10: #4, 363-371, October 1935.

145. Shute, E. *The association of deficiency of vitamin B1 and E during pregnancy.* Canad. Med. A. J. 47: #4, 350-351, October 1942.

146. Shute, E. *Vitamin E and premature labour.* Am. J. Obstet. & Gynec. 44: #2, 271-273, August 1942.

147. Shute, E. *Vitamin E in habitual abortion and miscarriage.* J. of Obstet. & Gynec. Brit. Emp. 49: #5, 534-541, October 1942 (A).

148. Siddall, A. C. *Vitamin B1 deficiency as an etiological factor in pregnancy toxemias.* Amer. J. Obstet. Gynec. 39: #5, 818-821, May 1940.

149. Silbernagel, W. M. and Burt, O. P. *Effects of pyridoxine on nausea and vomiting of pregnancy: results of treatment of 40 patients.* Ohio St. Med. J. 39: #12, 1113-1114, December 1943.

150. Smith, C. A. *Effects of maternal undernutrition upon the new-born infant in Holland. (1944-1945).* J. Pediatrics 30: #3, 229-243, March 1947.

151. Smith, C. A. *The effect of wartime starvation in Holland upon pregnancy and its product.* Am. J. Obst. & Gynec. 53: #4, 599-608, April 1947.

152. Smith, G. E. *Fetal athyrosis. A study of the iodine requirements of the pregnant sow.* J. Biol. Chem. 29: #2, 215-225, 1917.

153. Sorokin, P. A. *The sociology of revolution.* 1925. Philadelphia, Lippincott.

154. Strauss, M. B. *Observations on the etiology of the toxemias of pregnancy.* Amer. J. Med. Sci. 190: #6, 811-824, December 1935.

155. Strauss, M. B. *Observations of the etiology of the toxemias of pregnancy. 2. Production of acute exacerbation of toxemia by sodium salts in pregnant women with hypoproteinemia.* Amer. J. Med. Sci. 194: #6, 772-783, December 1937.

156. Sure, B. *Vitamin B12 in reproduction and lactation.* J. Am. Diet. A. 27: #7, 564-567, July 1951.

157. Sutherland, I. *The stillbirth rate in England and Wales in relation to social influences.* Lancet 11: #18, 953-956, 28 December 1946.

158. Taverud, K. U. *Buetning om de Forste 6 ars arbeid ved Oslo kommunes helsestasjor for morog barn pa Saegene (1939-1944).* 1945. Oslo, Fabritius and Sonner.

159. Taylor, A., Pennington, D., and Thacker, J. *The effect of high levels of pantothenic acid on reproduction in the rat and mouse.* J. Nutrit. 25: #4, 389-393, April 1943.

160. Taylor, F. A. *Habitual abortion: therapeutic evaluation of citrus bioflavonoids.* West J. Surg., Obstet. & Gynec. 64: #5, 280-283, May 1956.

161. Theobald, G. W. *Effect of calcium and vitamin A and D on incidence of pregnancy toxaemia.* Lancet 1: #27, 1397-1399, 12 June 1937.

162. Thiersch, J. B. *Therapeutic abortions with a folic acid antagonist 4-aminopteroylglutamic acid (4-amino P. G. A.) administered by the oral route.* Amer. J. Obstet. Gynec. 63: #6, 1298-1304, June 1952.

163. Tompkins, W. T. *Significance of nutritional deficiency in pregnancy: preliminary report.* J. Int. Coll. Surg. 4: #2, 147-154, April 1941.

164. Tuchmann-Duplessis, H. and Mercier-Parot, L. *Production de malformations chez la souris par administration de l'acide x-methylfolique.* C. R. Soc. Biol., 151: #11, 1855-1857, November 1957.

165. Vogt-Moller, P. *Treatment of habitual abortion with wheat germ oil.* Lancet 11: #5630, 182-183, July 25, 1931.

166. Wachstein, M. and Graffeo, L. N. *Influence of vitamin B6 on the incidence of pre-eclampsia.* Obstet. Gynec. 8: #2, 177-180, August 1956.

167. Warkany, J. *Manifestations of prenatal nutritional deficiency.* Vitam. & Horm. 3: 73-103, 1945.

168. Watson, E. M. and Tew, W. P. *Wheat germ oil (vitamin E) therapy in obstetrics.* Am. J. Obstet. & Gynec. 31: #2. 352-358, February 1936.

169. Watt, L. O. *Hyperemesis gravidarum and high vitamin therapy.* J. Obstet. Gynaec. Brit. Emp. 48: #5, 619-626, October 1941.

170. Weinstein, B. B., Mitchell, G. J., and Sustendal, G. F. *Clinical experience with pyridoxine hydrochloride in treatment of nausea and vomiting of pregnancy.* Amer. J. Obstet. Gynec. 46: #2. 283-285, August 1943.

171. Weinstein, B. B., Wohl, Z., Mitchell, G. J. and Sustendal, G. F. *Oral administration of pyridoxine hydrochloride in treatment of nausea and vomiting of pregnancy.* Amer. J. Obstet. Gynec. 47: #3, 389-394, March 1944.

172. Wells, H. B. Greenberg, B. G., and Donnelly, J. F. *North Carolina foetal and neonatal death study. 1. Study design and some preliminary results.* Amer. J. Pub. Health 48: #12, 1583-1595, December 1958.

173. White, J. H. B. V. A. Publ. No. 24, 43, 1954. Cited by Hignett, S. L. *The influence of nutrition on female fertility in some large domestic animals.* Proc. Nutrit. Soc. 19: #1, 8-14, 1960.

174. Wideman, G. L., Baird, G. H. and Bolding, O. T. *Ascorbic acid deficiency and premature rupture of fetal membranes.* Amer. J. Obstet. Gynec. 88: #5, 592-595, March 1, 1964.

175. Williams, C. D. *Weight in relation to pregnancy toxemia.* Brit. Med. J. 11: #5057, 1338-1340, December 7, 1957.

176. Williams, P. F. and Fralin, F. G. *Nutrition study in pregnancy.* Amer. J. Obstet. Gynec. 43: #1, 1-20, January 1942.

177. Williams, P. F., Griffith, G. C., and Fralin, F. G. *The relation of vitamin B1 to the reproductive cycle.* Amer. J. Obstet. Gynec. 40: #2, 181-193, August 1940.

178. Willis, R. S., Winn, W. W., Morris, A. T., Newsom, A. A., and Massey, W. E. *Clinical observations in treatment of nausea and vomiting in pregnancy with vitamins B1 and B6. A preliminary report.* Amer. J. Obstet. Gynec. 44: #2, 265-271, August 1942.

179. Woodhill, J. M., Van Den Berg, A. S., Burke, B. S., and Stare, F. J. *Nutrition studies of pregnant Australian women.* Amer. J. Obstet. Gynec. 70: #5, 987-1003, November 1955.

7. CONGENITAL DEFECTS

FOLLOWING CONCEPTION AND GESTATION, THERE IS STILL THE possibility of congenital defects. In a summary presented at the Second International Conference on Congenital Malformations held in 1964 at New York City, Doctor James L. Wilson, Professor and Chairman of the Department of Pediatrics and Communicable Diseases of the University of Michigan Medical Center, crystallized the graveness of the congenital defect problem in the following words *(147)*:

> The precise statistics of incidence are not of importance, I think, because the definition of a congenital anomaly can be as broad as we choose. Suffice it to say that it is a relatively rapidly growing part of our burden in the practice of medicine. In almost any hospital ward for infants, almost 50% of the babies are there because of congenital anomalies, and if we take the wards in the big university hospitals, the great referral centers, it can go up to 90%. If we add mental deficiency to the list of birth defects, as has seemed to be the habit in this meeting (and why not?), the problem becomes far greater.

The increasing magnitude of this problem is further reflected in the death rates for congenital malformations (Figure 7.1) reported by the National Center for Health Statistics *(91)*.

> Malignant neoplasms and congenital malformations assumed greater relative importance in terms of frequency of deaths in 1960. This is because of the rising mortality from these diseases and the declining mortality from the infectious diseases....The death rate for congenital malformations increased slowly until 1953 or 1954 and then leveled off. This may be related to the possible prolongation of life of those with congenital defects, as is suggested by the corresponding rise in the death rate for congenital malformations in the following age group, 5-14 years.

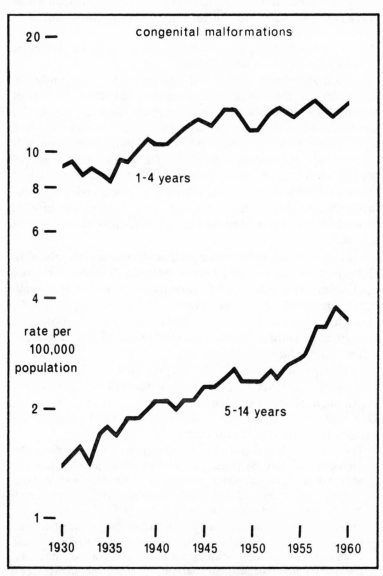

Figure 7.1. Death rates for congenital malformations, age groups 1-4 and 5-14 years: United States, 1930-1960.

The famous pioneer in teratologic research, Doctor Josef Warkany, best sums up the impact of this problem on pediatric care (66):

...today ten times as many children die of congenital malformations as of five contagious diseases once greatly feared.

Such sobering statistics still fail to reveal adequately the dimensions of the problem. The tremendous financial cost of supporting a defective child can be projected; but how is the emotional anguish of the parents and, later, of the offspring as he finds himself in a world not for his kind, to be measured?

Though the defects apparent at birth may have been recorded with reasonable accuracy, obtaining data on latent congenital deviations is more difficult. Certain malformations, for example cerebral palsy, may not be picked up for months or even years. Some may be finally diagnosed at autopsy at age 80.

In this chapter the relationships of dietary variables to malformations per se will be considered. The effect of diet upon some other attributes frequently employed in the qualitative appraisal of the newborn will not be reported. Although mental acuity is certainly such an attribute, its importance justifies separate consideration in Chapter Eight (Mental Retardation).

Writing in a special 1964 supplement of the American Journal of Obstetrics and Gynecology devoted to a Symposium on Congenital Defects, Doctor James G. Wilson (142) of the University of Florida College of Medicine, noted among other factors the role of diet and nutrition:

The agents now known to have a teratogenic capacity are multitudinous and may be generally categorized as follows: physical agents, infections, endocrine substances and states, vitamin deficiencies, analogues and antimetabolites, alkylating agents, antibiotics, and miscellaneous agents....

Several promising but relatively unexplored new areas of investigation may lead to early advances in analytical teratology. These include: (1) protein specificity and immune-like reactions, (2) chemical and cytochemical analysis of abnormal embryos, (3) teratogenic interaction of two or more agents, (4) embryo transplants and explants, and (5) time-limited exposure to teratogens using specific antagonists followed by appropriate supplements.

It will be observed that diet is potentially a factor in at

least three of these five relatively unexplored new areas of investigation.

If further evidence is needed to justify intensive investigation of dietary implications in congenital defects, the following excerpts from the Proceedings of the Second Scientific Conference of the Association for the Aid of Crippled Children in 1954 should be considered *(148)*:

...no disease that I know of has been controlled by modifying either the genetics or embryology of human beings; such an objective is impractical and unrealistic. Attention is more logically directed to, and success more to be expected from, protecting the conceptus from antenatal stresses. This means devoting more attention to the study of the mother and her gestational diseases and other events of her reproductive life. (Dr. Theodore Ingalls, Associate Professor of Epidemiology in the School of Public Health, Harvard University).

It would seem that when the patient first reports to her obstetrician at the second month of pregnancy, the pattern of behaviour during pregnancy with regard to...gross fetal deformity, is in great part already determined.

It is obvious that the most dramatic fall in the incidence...of deaths from deformity, will follow improvement in the health, physique and nutrition of mothers. Meanwhile, however, intensive research into the problems of nutrition of the early embryo and the physiology and pathology of early pregnancy in the human will perhaps allow us, in part at least, to mitigate the effects of years of defective environment. (Dr. James Walker, senior lecturer in the Department of Obstetrics and Gynecology of the University of Aberdeen).

Dr. Walker has demonstrated that good obstetrical care is a very broad type of care that must start with the birth of the future mother, or even before that, with her mother who is the grandmother of the baby we are discussing....

We found that if the mother had been prenatally on a diet that was good, according to standards we set up, she had the best chance of having a baby in good physical condition. All of the stillbirths, all of the neonatal deaths save one, all of the babies that were labelled functionally immature, all of the babies with major congenital defects, were of mothers who had been on a poor diet.

This was not a strict cause and effect relationship, but certainly nutrition was one of the factors involved.... we felt that here was a means by which some influence could be brought to bear on the prenatal period. Our studies suggested to us that the nutritional state in which the mother entered pregnancy was of prime importance so that we were pushed back into the period before conception, into the premarital state, into adolescence, into the birth of the mother. (Dr. Samuel Kirkwood of the School of Public Health, Harvard University, and Commissioner of Health for the State of Massachusetts).

CORRELATIVE FINDINGS

Lower Animal Observations: It is of interest to note that correlative animal studies or reports are not cited in the medical teratologic literature. Perhaps the complex nature of the problem is such as to simply not lend itself to this type of investigation. It is more likely that the plethora of clinical trials have negated the need for correlative observations.

Human Observations: By contrast, human correlative data seem to be more numerous than their counterpart, human experimental studies. Almost two-thirds of these correlative studies (Table 7.1) are concerned with congenital malformations, and a like proportion report a positive correlation between major congenital malformations and diet. Three of the six failing to find a significant relationship were war-related undernutrition studies. These three report an actual decrease in the number of major congenital defects with a presumably poor diet. It may well be that Dalderup's comments on the beneficial effect of wartime food restriction on toxemia (Chapter Six, Obstetrical Complications) are also apropos to this problem. Table 7.2 outlines the relationships of diet to relatively minor congenital defects. With but one exception, all studies underscore the positive effect of diet upon optimal development.

Certainly the most dramatic contribution of a human correlative study was the linking of iodine deficiency to cretinism. This relationship is perhaps the only unequivocally clear-cut evidence of the effect of the mother's diet on the development of the fetus *(87)*. Doctor Josef Warkany *(132)* has drawn attention to the significance of this event.

Investigators who have studied endemic cretinism with its social and economic problems and its eradication within one generation,

Table 7.1
diet and major congenital defects
(human correlative findings)

dietary variable	reference
increase in congenital defects	
poor quality diet	
poor diet	15,16
short structure and "poor circumstances" as indicators	10
low socio-economic level as indicator	40
study involving 37,585 single births	6
malnutrition	24
war-related undernutrition	
famine conditions in Russia, World War I	60
Rotterdam and The Hague, 1944-1945	120
Germany during and immediately after World War II	8,39, 101
specific nutrients	
deficiency of vitamin A and riboflavin (case report)	58
iron deficiency	112
decrease in congenital defects	
war-related undernutrition	
Japan during and immediately after World War II	86
good maternal diet during pregnancy preceded several years previously by malnutrition in German concentration camp in group of Jewish women	69
Italy during and immediately after World War II	41
no effect on congenital defects	
poor quality diet	
poor housing as criterion	109
low socio-economic status as index	20
Vanderbilt Cooperative Study of 2,046 gravidas and their offspring	75
low social class as indicator	38
specific nutrients	
retrospective study of mothers who gave birth to cleft lip and/or palate infants and who reported taking a prescribed nutritional supplement during pregnancy	42

have a sincere appreciation of the influence of the maternal diet upon the physical and mental make-up of children.

For many years Sir Dugald Baird and his staff in the Department of Obstetrics at the University of Aberdeen have studied the effects of physical and environmental factors upon the incidence of stillbirth, neonatal death, and pre-

Table 7.2
diet and minor congenital defects
(human correlative defects)

dietary variable (related defect in parentheses)	reference
increase in congenital defects	
poor quality diet	
poor diet (poor physical condition & low birth weight)	15,16
short stature & "poor circumstances" as indicators (low birth weight)	10
poor diets, 365 Philippine women (low birth weight)	1
poor diets due to extreme inflation, Singapore gravidas (low birth weight)	85
inadequate diet during pregnancy (retarded bone growth)	121
poor maternal diets during pregnancy (defective teeth)	11,14, 73,129
war-related undernutrition	
Rotterdam & The Hague, 1944-1945 (low birth weight)	120
Siege of Leningrad (poor physical condition, low birth weight)	7
summary of 29 studies of births during World War I, 19 of which involved a total of approximately 90,000 offspring & 10 additional studies where number of offspring involved not reported (low birth weight)	115
Vienna during & immediately after World War I (low birth weight, retarded growth)	105
Wuppertal & Hamburg, 1945 (low birth weight)	29
specific nutrients	
protein intake less than 75 g. daily (poor physical condition, low birth weight)	17
lowered protein and/or calcium intake (retarded bone growth)	123
lowered carbohydrate consumption (low birth weight)	106
lack of calcium, phosphorus or vitamin D (retarded bone growth)	79
iodine deficiency in regions of the world in which the soils are deficient in iodine & where supplemental iodine not provided for pregnant mothers (endemic cretinism)	87
iron deficiency (infant anemia)	52,122
no effect on congenital defects	
poor quality diet	
poor diets in 483 Negro women (low birth weight)	28

maturity. They have succeeded in establishing a high degree of correlation between maternal physique, nutritional status, socioeconomic status, and reproductive efficiency (148). They demonstrated that women in poor physical condition are often shorter than those in better condition and, more recently, that shorter women on the average have poorer diets (Table 7.3) *(128)*. Although some differences seemed due to caloric intake, the reduced consumption of calcium and vitamin C could not be explained on this basis. Thus, their hypothesis that many short women have been poorly nourished during growth and have become stunted and generally unhealthy adults has received additional confirmation.

The incidence of fetal malformation in the women from the lower classes (0.72 per cent) was over twice that of a group from the upper classes (0.35 per cent) *(10)*. In a study of stillbirths and infant deaths due to congenital malformations, records of 37,585 single births in Aberdeen between 1938 and 1955 were examined. In 8,245 first pregnancies in Aberdeen in 1949-1955, there is clearly an excess of congenital absence of the brain (anencephaly) and, to a lesser extent, of malformations of the central nervous system in the lower social classes and in small women.

Data from the Registrar General for Scotland were analyzed in a similar fashion (Figure 7.2). It is clear that, as social status falls, there is a steady increase in the incidence of anencephalic stillbirths. There is a smaller, but similar, social-class trend in stillbirth rates due to other malformations of the central nervous system. Infant deaths due to "congenital malformation" also show an increase in rate as social class falls.

Table 7.3
mean nutritive values of daily diets
taken by tall, medium and short primigravidae

	tall (5 ft. 4 in. & over)	medium (5 ft. 1 in.- 5 ft. 3 in.)	short (Under 5 ft. 1 in.)
calories (kcal)	2595.00	2475.00	2229.00
protein (g)	80.00	75.10	69.20
calcium (g)	1.08	0.99	0.85
thiamine (mg)	1.24	1.18	1.08
riboflavin (mg)	1.95	1.86	1.67
nicotinic acid (mg)	12.10	11.70	11.00
ascorbic acid (mg)	76.50	63.80	56.90
number of subjects	133.00	239.00	117.00

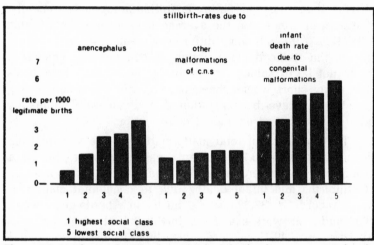

Figure 7.2. Incidence of stillbirths and infant deaths due to congenital malformations, according to social class (legitimate births, Scotland, 1950-55).

THERAPEUTIC FINDINGS

Lower Animal Observations: From Table 7.4 it is clear that a wide variety of dietary variables is teratogenic. However, it is equally evident that the investigations have been highly selective in at least two respects. First, attention has been focused almost exclusively on the vitamins, especially vitamins A and B complex. This is underscored by the fact that, in this survey of the literature, only eight of the almost ninety studies relate to nonvitamin fractions. Second, the studies have been equally restrictive in respect to the experimental animal species. At a recent large conference of scientists engaged in teratogenic testing, it was discovered that only rats, mice, and rabbits were being utilized (149).

The first reported study of inducing congenital malformations by dietary means involved a vitamin A deficiency in a Duroc-Jersey pig only thirty-odd years ago (54). Subsequently, malformations have been precipitated by a variety of other deficiency states, as well as by nutrient excesses and by the use of specific nutrient antagonists. More recently, interest has centered on the summating effect of several teratogens operating simultaneously.

Such an approach was utilized recently in one phase of a thalidomide study (43). One group of female rats was fed a complete diet. A second group was rendered deficient of one specific vitamin (either A, E, B12, folic acid, or nicotinic acid including tryptophan). This was done by feeding a basal diet containing all the vitamins except the one under study for a period of at least 18 days prior to the mating period and during the first 12 days of pregnancy.

Both groups were treated perorally with thalidomide (150 mg./kg. body weight) during the gestational period (days 3 to 12). The fecundated animals were sacrificed on day 19 and the following parameters evaluated: successful pregnancies, resorbed embryos and fetuses, litter size, fetal weight and viability, and dysmorphoses with particular attention to limbs, spine, and skull. The authors point out that, in rats, thalidomide is not ordinarily teratogenic and, in the strains used, does not customarily increase the incidence of fetal resorption.

Pantothenic acid deficiency enhanced the teratogenicity of thalidomide, causing an increase in both the incidence and the severity of appendicular skeletal deformations. It also resulted in a significant increase in fetal resorption. Fetal resorptions were also significantly increased in the vitamin E-deficient and riboflavin-poor groups of thalidomide-treated animals as compared with the thalidomide treated-normal diet animals. It was not possible to make an observation on a potential thalidomide-niacin deficiency synergism because the deficiency alone resulted in 100 per cent fetal resorption.

The fetus derived from the hypovitaminosed rat was consistently smaller, vitamin E and A deficiencies producing litters with the lowest weights. No difference in the number per litter was noted. The authors offer the hypothesis that thalidomide may act as an antimetabolite and they encourage additional investigation.

Although the exact mechanisms by which malformations are produced are still unknown, a number of important conclusions can be drawn from lower animal studies. The role of altered maternal nutrition as an important method of producing congenital malformations in lower animals is established. The teratogenic effect of a dietary variable must exert itself between the period of implantation and the completion of differentiation.

Table 7.4
diet and congenital defects
(lower animal therapeutic observations)

dietary variable (animal in parentheses) increased	reference
inanition (mouse)	65,114
large amounts of methionine derivatives (mouse)	99
sugar (chick)	59
various vitamin deficiencies plus thalidomide (rat)	43
hypervitaminosis A (rat)	9. 25. 26. 30. 47. 48. 49. 50. 51. 81. 82,135,140,150
hypervitaminosis A (mouse)	74
hypervitaminosis A. Trypan blue, cortisone acetate (rat)	3
vitamin A deficient (swine)	54. 55, 56
vitamin A deficient (cattle)	88
vitamin A deficient (rabbit)	83, 84.124
vitamin A deficient (rat)	4. 5. 61.111.138. 139,144,145,146
thiamine deficient (rat)	32
riboflavin & vitamin B12 deficient (rat)	53
riboflavin deficient (rat)	31, 44,100,136,137
riboflavin deficient & antagonist (rat)	93
riboflavin antagonist (mouse)	67
pantothenic acid deficient (rat)	12. 13
pantothenic acid deficient. niacin added (rat)	71
pantothenic acid antagonist (rat)	151
pantothenic acid deficient & antagonist (rat)	97
niacin antagonist (chick)	70
niacin antagonist (rat)	21
niacin antagonist (mouse)	107
choline deficient (swine)	40
folic acid & vitamin B12 deficiencies (rat)	102,110,141
folic acid deficient (rat)	62. 63. 64. 96. 98
folic acid deficient & antagonist (rat)	53.102
decreased folic acid synthesis (rat)	45
folic acid antagonists (rat)	92,116,125
folic acid antagonists (mouse)	113,130,131
vitamin D deficient (rat)	133
vitamin E deficient (rat)	19. 22. 23,117
manganese deficient (cattle)	35

no effect	
amino acid deficient (rat)	2,119
essential fatty acid deficient (rat)	72
choline deficient (mouse)	76
thiamine deficient (rat)	94
biotin deficient (mouse)	46
pyridoxine deficient (rat)	95
vitamin C deficient (guinea pig)	57
vitamin K deficient (rat)	89
copper (chick)	18

decreased	
vitamin A therapy of hydrocephalic offspring (rabbit)	80

The range within which a dietary variable produces malformations is narrow. Outside of this range the embryo either goes unharmed or is killed. The damage may be produced without any apparent harm to the mother. It is generally conceded that there are critical periods during which a particular tissue is especially susceptible to the action of a teratogen. This period of susceptibility is relatively short for any given tissue. As organ formation advances, vulnerability decreases, but increasing the severity of the dietary insult results in its prolongation. A host of different types has been produced by dietary variations. Folic acid deficiency has been called the "universal teratogen" *(106)* because of the wide variety of anomalies it can induce.

Human Observations: Despite the tremendous number of lower animal studies clearly demonstrating the ability of dietary disturbances to provoke the formation of congenital anomalies, very little has been done to explore the possible role of dietary defects in increasing the incidence of major congenital malformations in humans (Table 7.5).

Admittedly, such studies pose serious problems. The most critical period from the standpoint of congenital malformations is the first trimester. Relatively few women visit maternity clinics this early in gestation. The large number of pregnancies that would have to be followed in order to obtain enough information to provide statistically significant data is a second problem. For example, to collect findings on 100 cases of cleft lip, about 100,000 pregnancies would have to be studied *(42)*!

Peer and his associates *(104)* and others *(27,34,118)* have partially resolved the latter problem by selecting women who have previously given birth to a child with a cleft lip and/or cleft palate. In such a group, the likelihood of deformity is increased to about 5 per cent.

On the basis of lower animal studies performed in their laboratory *(103)* and the work of others, a study was begun to determine the effects of a prenatal vitamin capsule (containing vitamin B1, 10 mg.; vitamin B6, 2 mg.; vitamin B2, 10 mg.; vitamin B12, 4 mcg.; niacinamide, 100 mg.; calcium pantothenate, 20 mg.; and vitamin C, 300 mg.) supplemented with 5 mg. of folic acid and 10 mg. of B6 and taken daily

Table 7.5
diet and major congenital defects
(human therapeutic observations)

dietary variable	reference
increase in congenital defects	
administration of vitamin antagonists	
folic acid antagonist (aminopterin as an abortifacient)	126,127
4-aminopteroylglutamic acid as an abortifacient (case report)	78
ingestion of 12 mg. of aminopterin on day 55 and day 66 of pregnancy (case report)	134
decrease in congenital defects	
vitamin supplementation	
spouses of women who had previously produced anomalous infants given alpha-tocopherol prior to subsequent pregnancy	118
"compensatory nutrient" supplementation during the first trimester of women whose previous child had a congenital malformation	34
gravidas who had previously given birth to a cleft palate and/or lip child, given multivitamin supplement during first trimester	27
gravidas who had previously given birth to a cleft palate and/or lip child, given multivitamin supplement during first trimester	104

during the first trimester. One hundred seventy-six gravidas received the vitamin regime, and 418 women served as controls. Approximately 50 per cent reduction, not only in cleft lip and/or cleft palate deformities, but also in other defects as well, was observed (Figure 7.3). They concluded that their results were suggestive, but not statistically significant.

Thirty additional offspring were subsequently born to women in the group receiving first trimester vitamin therapy. These were not included in the original findings. None of these thirty additional infants had deformities. Obviously, if these offspring were added to the original series, the percentage difference in the two groups would be even more marked (Figure 7.3).

Shute (118) was the first to study the effects of dietotherapy in a group characterized by an increased incidence of anomalies. These were families in which grossly anomalous infants were born. In seventeen subsequent pregnancies from

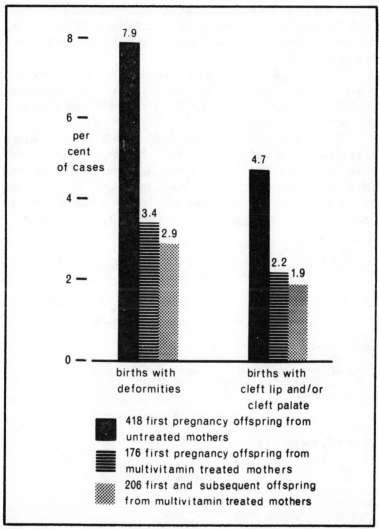

Figure 7.3. Incidence of malformed offspring from 418 untreated and 176 multivitamin treated mothers who had previously had a cleft lip and/or cleft palate child.

such families in which the sire took alpha-tocopherol immediately prior to conception, fifteen normal and two anomalous infants resulted. Of the seventeen couples represented by these seventeen pregnancies, four each had an additional infant without prior alpha-tocopherol supplementation of the father. Two of these four offspring were malformed. Other than this study, little consideration has been given to the nutritional status of the father as a possible contributor in congenital malformations.

The effect of diet on optimal development is summarized (Table 7.6). All save one study suggest a positive correlation of diet and physical condition but no parallelisms between diet and birth weight and/or length.

The details of the Toronto study *(36,37)* and the favorable influence of satisfactory diet on obstetrical complications have been described in the previous chapter (Chapter Six, Obstetrical Complications). Equally impressive is the effect on the offspring. The incidence of illness (pneumonia, bronchitis, frequent colds, otitis media, anemia, dystrophy, rickets,

Table 7.6
diet and minor congenital defects
(human therapeutic observations)

dietary variable	reference
decreased incidence of poor physical condition	
supplemental food and vitamins and/or diet instructions beginning fourth or fifth month	37
diet instructions and canned meat where necessary to assure consumption of 85 gms. protein daily in a subgroup	33
decreased incidence of hypovitaminosis A	
10,000 I.U. vitamin A for a few days in last trimester	52
no effect on incidence of low birth weight and/or length	
supplemental food and vitamins and/or diet instructions beginning fourth or fifth month	36
diet instructions and canned meat where necessary to assure consumption of 85 gms. protein daily in subgroup	33
diet instructions, also protein and vitamin supplements separately and in combination	108
no effect on incidence of physical condition	
diet instructions, also protein and vitamin supplements separately and in combination	68

and tetany) was markedly lower in the good diet groups; and in the words of the authors, "The difference in the appearance of the infants in the good diet groups was strikingly better than those born of mothers on a poor prenatal diet."

Two malformations occurred in the supplemental diet group and one each in the other two groups in this study. Of course, the number of malformations in such a study is too small from which to draw conclusions; nor would favorable results be expected since treatment was not initiated until the fourth or fifth month.

In the Philadelphia Lying-In Hospital study (68,108) the effects on the outcome of pregnancy of dietary counseling plus therapeutic amounts of a polyvitamin supplement and a commercial high protein preparation, each alone and in combination, were compared to the effects of dietary counseling alone. All fared well. This is consistent with the findings in the Toronto study in which the supplemented group and the group given only detailed dietary instructions both had significantly healthier offspring. Two-thirds of the babies were rated as good or excellent in health and less than 3 per cent as poor.

The study of vitamin antagonists in pregnancy has been almost exclusively confined to lower animals. However, it will be noted that, when they have been used in humans, the findings have been consistent with those observed in lower animals (78,126,127,134).

Although the number of clinical trials in humans is disappointingly small for an area of such vital importance, the preponderance of evidence seems to suggest that the diet and nutritional status during pregnancy may well be as important for the viable offspring as it is for the mother's health and her reproductive efficiency.

SUMMARY

As with most teratogens, the role of dietary disturbances remains vaguely defined. Yet a general association between diet and malformations seems to exist in the human. The role of diet in lower animal anomalies is more clearcut, and much light has been shed on the problem of when and where diet exerts its role. Nevertheless, the mechanisms by which the anomalies are produced are still unknown.

Obviously, thalidomide has left an indelible imprint on this field of study *(149)*.

Before thalidomide the amount spent in this country *(England)* annually on research into mammalian teratology was not quite sufficient to maintain two students at a university. Today I estimate the pharmaceutical industry to be spending on teratogenic experiments at least enough money each year to set up a new university in this country. Not surprisingly, the literature on teratology is now becoming swamped by a mass of information on the teratogenic effects of pharmaceutically interesting compounds.

Whether this rapidly accumulating "mass of information" will throw further light on the role of diet remains to be seen.

REFERENCES

1. Acosta-Sison, H. *Relation between the state of nutrition of the mother and the birthweight of the fetus.* J. Phillip.-Islands Med. Assn. 9: #5, 174-176, May 1929.

2. Albanese, A. A., Randall, R. M., and Holt, L. E. *The effect of tryptophane deficiency on reproduction.* Science 97: #2518, 312-313, April 2, 1943.

3. Amano, S. et al. *Congenital malformations in rats due to hypervitaminosis A in combination with trypan blue and cortisone acetate.* J. Osaka City Med. Cent. 12: #7, #9, 303-309, September 1963.

4. Andersen, D. H. *Incidence of congenital diaphragmatic hernia in the young of rats bred on a diet deficient in Vitamin A.* Amer. J. Dis. Child. 62: #4, 888-889, October 1941.

5. Andersen, D. H. *Effect of diet during pregnancy upon the incidence of congenital diaphragmatic hernia in the rat.* Amer. J. Path. 25: #1, 163-185, January 1949.

6. Anderson, W. J. R., Baird, D., and Thomson, A. M. *Epidemiology of stillbirths and infant deaths due to congenital malformations.* Lancet 1: #7034, 1304-1306, June 21, 1958.

7. Antonov, A. N. *Children born during Siege of Leningrad in 1942.* J. Pediat. 30: #3, 250-259, March 1947.

8. Aresin, N. and Sommer, K. H. *Missbildungen und Umweltfaktoren.* Zbl. Gynak. 72: #19, 1329-1336, 1950.

9. Baba, T. and Araki, E. *Morphogenesis of malformation due to excessive vitamin A. 1. Morphogenesis of exencephaly.* Osaka City Med. J. 5: 9, 1959.

10. Baird, D. *The influence of social and economic factors in stillbirths and neonatal deaths.* J. Obstet. Gynaec. Brit. Emp. 52: #3, #4, 217-234, 339-366, June & August 1945.

11. Berk, H. *Some factors concerned with the incidence of dental caries in children: multiple pregnancy and nutrition during prenatal, postnatal and childhood periods.* J. A. D. A. 30: #21, 1749-1754, November 1, 1943.

12. Boisselot, J. *Malformations congenitales provoquees chez le rat par une insuffisance en acide pantothenique du regime maternel.* C. R. Soc. Biol., Paris. 142: #13-14, 928-929, July 10, 1948.

13. Boisselot, J. *Malformations foetales par insuffisance en acide pantothenique.* Arch. Franc. Pediat. 6: 225-230, 1949.

14. Burke, B. S. *Study of the nutrition of groups of children select-

ed on the basis of no defective deciduous teeth. Child Develop. 11: 327-334, 1940.

15. Burke, B. S., Beal, V. A., Kirkwood, S. B., and Stuart, H. C. The influence of nutrition during pregnancy upon the condition of the infant at birth. J. Nutrit. 26: #6, 569-583, December 1943.

16. Burke, B. S., Stevenson, S. S., Worcester, J., and Stuart, H. C. Nutrition studies during pregnancy. V. Relation of maternal nutrition to condition of infant at birth: study of siblings. J. Nutrit. 38: #4, 453-467, August 1949.

17. Burke, B. S. and Stuart, H. C. Nutritional requirements during pregnancy and lactation. J. A. M. A. 137: #2, 119-128, May 8, 1948.

18. Butt, E. M., Pearson, H. E., and Simonsen, D. G. Production of meningoceles and cranioschisis in chick embryos with lead nitrate. Proc. Soc. Exper. Biol. and Med. 79: #2, 247-249, February 1952.

19. Callison, E. C. and Orent-Keiles, E. Abnormalities of the eye occurring in young vitamin E-deficient rats. Proc. Soc. Exper. Biol. and Med. 76: #2, 295-297, February 1951.

20. Carter, C. O. Congenital malformations. Eugen. Rev. 43: 83, 1951.

21. Chamberlain, J. G. and Nelson, M. M. Congenital abnormalities in the rat resulting from single injections of 6-aminonicotinamide during pregnancy. J. Exp. Zool. 153: #3, 285-299, August 1963.

22. Cheng, D. W. and Thomas, B. H. Relationship of time of therapy to teratogeny in maternal avitaminosis E. Proc. Iowa Acad. Sci. 60: 290, 1953.

23. Cheng, D. W. and Thomas, B. H. Histological changes in the abnormal rat fetuses induced by maternal vitamin E deficiency. Anat. Rec. 121: #2, 274, February 1955.

24. Coffey, V. P. and Jessop, W. J. E. A three year study anencephaly in Dublin. Irish J. Med. Sci. 6th Series: #393, 391-413, September 1958.

25. Cohlan, S. Q. Excessive intake of vitamin A as a cause of congenital anomalies in the rat. Science 117: #3046, 535-536, May 15, 1953.

26. Cohlan, S. Q. Congenital anomalies in the rat produced by excessive intake of vitamin A during pregnancy. Pediatrics 13: #6, 556-567, June 1954.

27. Conway, H. Effect of supplemental vitamin therapy on the limi-

tation of incidence of cleft lip and cleft palate in humans. Plast. and Reconstruct. Surg. 22: #5, 450-453, November 1958.

28. Crump, E. P., Horton, C. P., Masuoka, J., and Ryan, D. *Growth and development. 1. Relation of birth weight in Negro infants to sex, maternal age, parity, prenatal care, and socio-economic status.* J. Pediat. 51: #6, 678-697, December 1957.

29. Dean, R. F. A. *The effect of undernutrition on the size of the baby at birth and on the ability of the mother to lactate.* Proc. Roy. Soc. Med. 43: #4, 273-274, April 1950.

30. Deuschle, F. M., Geiger, J. F., and Warkany, J. *Analysis of an anomalous oculodentofacial pattern in newborn rats produced by maternal hypervitaminosis A.* J. Dent. Res. 38: #1, 149-155, January-February 1959.

31. Deuschle, F. M. and Warkany, J. *Congenital dentofacial malformations induced by maternal deficiency.* J. Dent. Res. 35: #5, 674-684, October 1956.

32. De Watteville, H., Jurgens, R., and Pfaltz, H. *Einfluss von Vitaminmangel auf Fruchtbarkeit, Schwangerschaft und Nachkommen.* Schweiz. Med. Wschr. 84: #30, 875-883, July 24, 1954.

33. Dieckmann, W. J., Turner, D. F., Meiller, E. J., Savage, L. J., Hill, A. J., Straube, M. T., Pottinger, R. E., and Rynkiewicz, L. M. *Observations on protein intake and the health of the mother and baby.* J. Amer. Dietet. Assn. 27: #12, 1046-1052, December 1951.

34. Douglas, B. *The role of environment factors in the etiology of "so-called" congenital malformations. II.* Plast. and Reconstruct. Surg. 22: #3, 214-229, September 1958.

35. Dyer, I. A., Cassatt, W. A., Jr., and Rao, R. R. *Manganese deficiency in the etiology of deformed calves.* Bioscience 14: #3, 31-32, March 1964.

36. Ebbs, J. H., Brown, A., Tisdall, F. F., Moyle, W. J., and Bell, M. *The influence of improved prenatal nutrition upon the infant.* J. Canad. Med. Assn. 46: #1, 6-8, January 1942.

37. Ebbs, J. H., Tisdall, F. F., and Scott, W. A. *The influence of prenatal diet on the mother and child.* J. Nutrit. 22: #5, 515-526, November 1941.

38. Edwards, J. H. *Congenital malformations of the central nervous system in Scotland.* Brit. J. Prev. and Soc. Med. 12: #3, 115-130, July 1958.

39. Eichmann, E. and Gasenius, H. *Die missgeburtenzunahme in*

Berlin und umgebung in den nachkriegsjahren. Arch. Gynak. 181: #2, 168-184, 1952.

40. Ensminger, M. E., Bowland, J. P., and Cunha, T. J. *Observations on the thiamine, riboflavin and choline needs of sows for reproduction.* J. Anim. Sci. 6: 409-423, 1947.

41. Ferrario, E. and Fortina, A. *Dati clinico-statistici sulle malformazioni fetali osservate nella Maternita e nel comune di Novara nell' ultimo ventennio.* Minerva ginec., Torino 2: #6, 248-251, June 1950.

42. Fraser, F. C. and Warburton, D. *No association of emotional stress or vitamin supplement during pregnancy to cleft lip or palate in man.* Plast. Reconstruct. Surg. 33: #4, 395-399, April 1964.

43. Fratta, I. D., Sigg, E. B., and Maiorana, K. *Teratogenic effects of thalidomide in rabbits, rats, hamsters, and mice.* Toxicol. and Appl. Pharmacol. 7: #2, 268-286, March 1965.

44. Giroud, A. and Boisselot, J. *Repercussions de l'avitaminose B2 sur l'embryon du rat.* Arch. Franc. Pediat. 4: #4, 317-327, 1947.

45. Giroud, A. and Lefebvres, J. *Anomalies provoquees chez le foetus en l'absence d'acide folique.* Arch. Franc. Pediat. 8: 648-656, 1951.

46. Giroud, A., Lefebvres, J., and Dupuis, R. *Carence en biotine et reproduction chez la ratte.* Compt. Rend. Soc. Biol., Paris 150: #12, 2066-2067, 1956.

47. Giroud, A. and Martinet, M. *Malformations diverses du foetus du rat suivant les stades d'administration de vitamine A en exces.* C. R. Soc. Biol., Paris 149: #11, #12, 1088-1090, June 1955.

48. Giroud, A. and Martinet, M. *Hydramnios et anencephalie.* Gynec. et Obstet. 54: #4, 391-399, 1955.

49. Giroud, A. and Martinet, M. *Hypovitaminose et hypervitaminose A chez le jeune et chez l'embryon.* Etud. Neo-nat. 5: #2, 55-68, June 1956.

50. Giroud, A. and Martinet, M. *Malformations de la face et hypervitaminose A.* Rev. Stomat., Paris 57: #7-8, 454-463, July-August 1956.

51. Giroud, A., Martinet, M., and Roux, C. *Ureterohydronephrose experimentale chez l'embryon par hypervitaminose A.* Arch. Franc. Pediat. 15: #3, 540-551, 1958.

52. Gopalan, C. *Effect of nutrition on pregnancy and lactation.* Bull. World Health Org. 26: 203-211, 1962.

53. Grainger, R. B., O'Dell, B. L., and Hogan, A. G. *Congenital mal-*

formations as related to deficiencies of riboflavin and vitamin B12, source of protein, calcium to phosphorus ratio and skeletal phosphorus metabolism. J. Nutrit. 54: #1, 33-48, September 1954.

54. Hale, F. Pigs born without eyeballs. J. Hered. 24: #3, 105-106, March 1933.

55. Hale, F. The relation of vitamin A deficiency to anophthalmia in pigs. Amer. J. Ophthal. 18: #12, 1087-1093, December 1935.

56. Hale, F. The relation of vitamin A deficiency to microphthalmia in pigs. Texas Med. J. 33: #7, 228-232, July 1937.

57. Harmon, M. T. and Gillum, I. Further observations on reproduction in guinea pigs fed vitamin C at different levels. Tr. Kansas Acad. Sc. 40: 369-376, 1937.

58. Houet, R. and Lecomte-Ramioul, S. Repercussions sur l'enfant des avitaminoses de la mere pendant la grossesse. Un cas de bec-delievre et xerophthalmie neonatale chez un enfant dont la mere presente une carence en vitamines A et B2. Ann. Paediat. 175: #5, 378-388, November 1950.

59. Hunt, E. L. Developmental abnormalities in chick embryos treated with sugar. Science 113: #2936, 386-387, April 6, 1951.

60. Ivanosky, A. Physical modifications of the population of Russia under famine. Amer. J. Phys. Anthrop. 6: #4, 331-353, October and December 1923.

61. Jackson, B. and Kinsey, V. E. Relation between vitamin-A intake, blood level, and ocular abnormalities in the offspring of the rat. Amer. J. Ophthal. 29: #10, 1234-1242, October 1946.

62. Johnson, E. M. Effects of maternal folic acid deficiency on cytologic phenomena in the rat embryo. Anat. Rec. 149: #1, 49-56, May 1964.

63. Johnson, E. M. Electrophoretic analysis of abnormal development. Proc. Soc. Exper. Biol. Med. 118: #1, 9-11, January 1965.

64. Johnson, E. M., Nelson, M. M., and Monie, I. W. Effects of transitory pteroylglutamic acid (PGA) deficiency on embryonic and placental development in the rat. Anat. Rec. 146: #3, 215-224, July 1963.

65. Kalter, H. Preliminary studies on metabolic factors involved in production of cleft palates in mice. Genetics 39: #6, 975, November 1954.

66. Kalter, H. and Warkany, J. Experimental production of congenital malformation in mammals by metabolic procedure. Physiol. Rev. 39: #1, 69-115, January 1959.

67. Kalter, H. and Warkany, J. Congenital malformations in inbred

strains of mice induced by riboflavin-deficient, galactoflavin-containing diets. J. Exper. Zool. 136: #3, 531-566, December 1957.

68. Kasius, R. V., Randall, A., Tompkins, W. T., Wiehl, D. G. *Maternal and newborn nutrition studies at Philadelphia Lying-In Hospital. Newborn studies. I. Size and growth of babies of mothers receiving nutrient supplements.* Milbank Mem. Fund Quart. 33: 230-245, July 1955.

69. Klebanow, D. *Die gefahrder keimschadigung bei ruckbildungsvorgangen in der weiblichen gonaden.* Deutsche Med. Wochenschr. 74: #23/24, 606-610, April 22, 1949.

70. Landauer, W. *Niacin antagonists and chick development.* J. Exper. Zool. 136: #3, 509-530, December 1957.

71. Lefebvres, J. *Role teratogene de la deficience en acide pantothenique chez le rat.* Ann. Med. 52: #3, 225-298, 1951.

72. Martinet, M. *Hemorragies embryonnaires par deficience en acide linoleique.* Ann. Med. 52: #3, 286-333, 1952.

73. Massler, M., Schour, I., and Poncher, H. G. *Developmental pattern of the child as reflected in the calcification pattern of the teeth.* Amer. J. Dis. Child. 62: #1, 33-67, July 1941.

74. Mauer, I. *Vitamin A-induced congenital defects in hairless mice.* Biol. Neonat. 6: #1, #2, 26-37, 1964.

75. McGanity, W. J., Bridgforth, E. B., Martin, M. P., Newbill, J. A., and Darby, W. J. *The Vanderbilt cooperative study of maternal and infant nutrition. VIII. Some nutritional implications.* J. Amer. Dietet. Assn. 31: #6, 582-588, June 1955.

76. Meader, R. D. and Williams, W. L. *Choline deficiency in the mouse.* Amer. J. Anat. 100: #2, 167-203, March 1957.

77. Mellanby, M. and Coumoulos, H. *The improved dentition of 5-year-old London school children: a comparison between 1943 and 1929.* Brit. Med. 1: #4355, 837-840, June 24, 1944.

78. Meltzer, H. J. *Congenital anomalies due to attempted abortion with 4-aminopteroylglutamic acid.* J. A. M. A. 161: #13, 1253, July 28, 1956.

79. M'Gonigle, G. C. M. and Kirby, J. *Poverty and public health.* 1936. London, Golancz.

80. Millen, J. W. and Dickson, A. D. *The effects of vitamin A upon the cerebrospinal-fluid pressures of young rabbits suffering from hydrocephalus due to maternal hypovitaminosis A.* Brit. J. Nutrit. 11: 440-445, May 24, 1957.

81. Millen, J. W. and Woollam, D. H. M. *Influence of cortisone on*

teratogenic effects of hypervitaminosis-A. Brit. Med. J. 2: #5038, 196-197, July 27, 1957.

82. Millen, J. W. and Woollam, D. H. M. (in press) 1961. Cited by Millen, J. W. The nutritional basis of reproduction. 1962. Springfield, Charles C. Thomas.

83. Millen, J. W. and Woollam, D. H. M. The effect of the duration of vitamin A deficiency in female rabbits upon the incidence of hydrocephalus in their young. J. Neurol. Psychiat. 19: #1, 17-20, February 1956.

84. Millen, J. W., Woollam, D. H. M. and Lamming, G. E. Congenital hydrocephalus associated with deficiency of vitamin A. Lancet 2: #14, 679-683, 2 October 1954.

85. Millis, J. A study of the effect of nutrition on fertility and the outcome of pregnancy in Singapore in 1947 and 1950. Med. J. Malaya 6: 157-179, March 1952.

86. Mitani. S. Malformations of the newborn and fetus. In Int. Congress Gynaec. Obstet. Exposition scientifique. Documents de recherches cliniques et experimentales. Bale, Sandoz. 1954.

87. Montagu, M. F. A. Prenatal influences. 1962. Springfield, Charles C. Thomas.

88. Moore, L. A. and Sykes, J. F. Terminal cerebrospinal fluid pressure values in vitamin A deficiency. Amer. J. Physiol. 134: #2, 436-439, September 1941.

89. Moore, R. A., Bittenger, I., Miller, M. L. and Hellman, L. M. Abortion in rabbits fed a vitamin K deficient diet. Amer. J. Obstet. Gynec. 43: #6, 1007-1012, June 1942.

90. Murphy, D. P. Congenital malformations. 2nd Edition. 1947. Philadelphia, Lippincott, University Press.

91. National Center for Health Statistics, Series 3, Number 1, The change in mortality trend in the United States. U. S. Dept. of Health, Education and Welfare, Washington, D. C., March 1964.

92. Nelson, M. M., Asling, C. W. and Evans, H. M. Production of multiple congenital abnormalities in young by maternal pteroylglutamic acid deficiency during gestation. J. Nutrit. 48: #1, 61-80, September 1952.

93. Nelson, M. M., Baird, C. D. C., Wright, H. V. and Evans, H. M. Multiple congenital abnormalities in the rat resulting from riboflavin deficiency induced by the antimetabolite galatoflavin. J. Nutrit. 58: #1, 125-134, January 1956.

94. Nelson, M. M. and Evans, H. M. Relation of thiamine to reproduction in the rat. J. Nutrit. 55: #1, 151-163, 10 January 1955.

95. Nelson, M. M. and Evans, H. M. *Effect of pyridoxine deficiency on reproduction in the rat.* J. Nutrit. 43: #2, 281-294, 10 February 1951.

96. Nelson, M. M., Wright, H. V., Asling, C. W. and Evans, H. M. *Multiple congenital abnormalities resulting from transitory deficiency of pteroylglutamic acid during gestation in the rat.* J. Nutrit. 56: #3, 349-369, 11 July 1955.

97. Nelson, M. M., Wright, H. V., Baird, C. D. C. and Evans, H. M. *Teratogenic effects of pantothenic acid deficiency in the rat.* J. Nutrit. 62: #4, 395-406, 10 August 1957.

98. Nelson, M. M., Wright, H. V., Baird, C. D. C. and Evans, H. M. *Effect of a 36 hour period of pteroylglutamic acid deficiency on fetal development in the rat.* Proc. Soc. Exp. Biol., New York, 92: #3, 554-556, July 1956.

99. Nishimura, H., Kageyama, M. and Hayashi, K. *Teratogenic effect of the methionine derivatives upon the mouse embryos.* Acta. Schalre Med. Univ. Kirto. 38: 193-197, 1962.

100. Noback, C. R. and Kupperman, H. S. *Anomalous offspring and growth of Wistar rats maintained on a deficient diet.* Proc. Soc. Exp. Biol., New York, 57: #2, 183-185, November 1944.

101. Nowak, J. *Haufigkeit der missgeburten in den nachkriegsjahren 1945-1949.* Zenbralbl. Gynak. 72: #19, 1313-1328, 1950.

102. O'Dell, B. L., Whitley, J. R. and Hogan, A. G. *Vitamin B12, a factor in prevention of hydrocephalus in infant rats.* Proc. Soc. Exp. Biol. Med. 76: #2, 349-353, February 1951.

103. Peer, L. A., Bryan, W. H., Strean, L. P., Walker, J. C., Bernhard, W. G., and Peck, G. C. *Induction of cleft palate in mice by cortisone and its reduction by vitamins.* J. Internat. Coll. Surgeons 30: #2, 249-254, August 1958.

104. Peer, L. A., Gordon, A. W., Bernhard, W. G. *Effect of vitamins on human teratology.* Plastic and Reconstruct. Surg. 34: #4, 358-362, October 1964.

105. Peller, S. *Growth, heredity, and environment.* Growth. 4: #3, 277-289, November 1940.

106. Perlstein, M. A. and Levinson, A. *Birth weight. Its statistical correlation with various factors.* Amer. J. Dis. Child. 53: #6, 1645-1646, June 1937.

107. Pinsky, L. and Fraser, F. C. *Production of skeletal malformations in the offspring of pregnant mice treated with 6-aminonicotinamide.* Bio. Neonat. 1: #2, 106-112, April 1959.

108. Randall, A., Randall, J. P., Kasius, R. V., Tompkins, W. T. and

Wiehl, D. G. *Maternal and newborn nutrition studies at Philadelphia Lying-In Hospital. Newborn studies, IV. Clinical findings at birth and one month for babies of mothers receiving nutrient supplements.* The Milbank Memorial Fund Quarterly 24: 321-353, October 1956.

109. Record, R. G. and McKeown, T. *Congenital malformation of the central nervous system.* Brit. J. Soc. Med. 3: #4, 183-219, October 1949.

110. Richardson, L. R. and Hogan, A. G. *Diet of mother and hydrocephalus in infant rats.* J. Nutrit. 32: #4, 459-465, 10 October 1946.

111. Rokkones, T. *Experimental hydrocephalus in young rats.* Int. Z. Vitaminforsch. 26: #1, #2, 1-9, 1955.

112. Roszkowski, I. and Kietlinska, Z. *Indirect causes of congenital malformations. An analysis of 212 cases.* Gynaecologia (Basel) 159: #1, 47-53, 1965.

113. Runner, M. N. *Inheritance of susceptibility to congenital deformity - embryonic instability.* J. Nat. Cancer Inst. 15: #3, 637-647, December 1954.

114. Runner, M. N. and Miller, J. R. *Congenital deformity in the mouse as a consequence of fasting.* Anat. Rec. 124: #2, 437-438, February 1956.

115. Sanders, B. S. *Environment and growth.* 1934. Baltimore, Warrick and York.

116. Sansone, G. and Zunin, C. *Embriopatie spermentale de somministrazioni di antifolici.* Acta vitamin Milano. 8: 73, 1954.

117. Shute, E. V. *The relation of deficiency of vitamin E to the antiproteolytic factor found in the serum of aborting women.* J. Obstet. Gynaec. Brit. Emp. 43: #1, 74-86, February 1936.

118. Shute, E. V. *The prevention of congenital anomalies in the human: experiences with alpha-tocopherol as a prophylactic measure.* J. Obstet. Gynaec. Brit. Emp. 64: #3, 390-395, June 1957.

119. Sims, F. H. *Methionine and choline deficiency in the rat with special reference to the pregnant state.* Brit. J. Exp. Path. 32: #6, 481-492, December 1951.

120. Smith, C. A. *The effect of wartime starvation in Holland upon pregnancy and its product.* Amer. J. Obstet. Gynec. 53: #4, 599-608, April 1947.

121. Sontag, L. W. and Harris, L. M. *Evidence of disturbed prenatal and neonatal growth in bones of infants aged one month.* Am. J. Dis. Child. 56: #6, 1248-1255, December 1938.

122. Strauss, M. B. Anemia of infancy from maternal iron deficiency in pregnancy. J. Clin. Invest. 12: #2, 345-353, March 1933.

123. Stuart, H. C. Effects of protein deficiency on the pregnant woman and fetus and on the infant and child. New England J. Med. 236: #14, #15, 507-513, 537-541, 3 April, 10 April 1947.

124. Tennyson, V. M. An electron microscopic study of newborn choroid plexus from normal and hydrocephalic rabbits. Anat. Rec. 136: #2, 290, February 1960.

125. Thiersch, J. B. Effect of certain 2, 4-Diaminopyridine antagonists of folic acid on pregnancy and rat fetus. Proc. Soc. Exp. Biol., New York. 87: #3, 571-577, December 1954.

126. Thiersch, J. B. Therapeutic abortions with a folic acid antagonist 4-aminopteroylglutamic acid (4-amino P. G. A.) administered by the oral route. Amer. J. Obstet. Gynec. 63: #6, 1298-1304, June 1952.

127. Thiersch, J. B. Discussion, in Ciba Foundation symposium on congenital malformations. eds. Wolstenholme, G. E. W. and O'Conner, C. M. 1960. London, Churchill.

128. Thomson, A. M. and Billewicz, W. Z. Nutritional states, maternal physique and reproductive efficiency. Proc. Nutrit. Soc. 22: #1, 55-60, 1963.

129. Toverud, K. U. and Toverud, G. Studies on the mineral metabolism during pregnancy and lactation and its special bearing on the disposition to rickets and dental caries. Acta Paediat. (Suppl. 2) Vol. 12, 1-116, 1931.

130. Trasler, D. G. Genetic and other factors influencing the pathogenesis of cleft palate in mice. Ph. D. Thesis, McGill Univ. Montreal. 1958.

131. Tuchmann-Duplesis, H. and Mercier-Parot, L. Sur l'action teratogene de l'acide x-methylfolique chez la Souris. C. R. Acad. Sci. 245: Part Two, 1963-1965, 25 November 1957.

132. Warkany, J. Prenatal effects of nutrition on the development of the nervous system. Proceedings Assoc. Res. Nerv. and Ment. Disease. 33: Part I, 76-83, 1954.

133. Warkany, J. Effect of maternal rachitogenic diet on skeletal development of young rat. Amer. J. Dis. Child. 66: #5, 511-516, November 1943.

134. Warkany, J., Beaudry, P. H. and Hornstein, S. Attempted abortion with aminopterin (4-aminopteroylglutamic acid); malformations of the child. Amer. J. Dis. Child. 97: #2, 274-281, February 1959.

135. Warkany, J., Kalter, H. and Geiger, J. F. *Experimental teratology.* Pediat. Clin. N. Amer. 983-994, November 1957.

136. Warkany, J. and Nelson, R. C. *Skeletal abnormalities in the offspring of rats reared on deficient diets.* Anat. Rec. 79: #1, 83-94, January 1941.

137. Warkany, J. and Nelson, R. C. *Congenital malformations induced in rats by maternal nutritional deficiency.* J. Nutrit. 23: #4, 321-334, April 1942.

138. Warkany, J. and Roth, C. B. *Congenital malformations induced in rats by maternal vitamin A deficiency. II. Effect of varying the preparatory diet upon the yield of abnormal young.* J. Nutrit. 35: #1, 1-11, 10 January 1948.

139. Warkany, J. and Schraffenberger, E. *Congenital malformations of the eyes induced in rats by maternal vitamin A deficiency.* Proc. Soc. Exp. Biol., New York, 57: #1, 49-52, October 1944.

140. Warkany, J., Wilson, J. G. and Geiger, J. *Myeloschisis and myelomeningocoele produced experimentally in the rat.* J. Comp. Neurol. 109: #1, 35-64, February 1958.

141. Whitley, J. R., O'Dell, B. L. and Hogan, A. G. *Effect of diet on maze learning in second-generation rats. Folic acid deficiency.* J. Nutrit. 45: #1, 153-160, 10 September 1951.

142. Wilson, J. G. *Experimental teratology.* Am. J. Obst. and Gynec. 90: #7, Part 2, 1181-1192, 1 December 1964.

143. Wilson, J. G. *Experimental studies on congenital malformations.* J. Chron. Dis. 10: #2, 111-129, August 1959.

144. Wilson, J. G., Roth, C. B. and Warkany, J. *An analysis of the syndrome of malformations induced by maternal vitamin A deficiency. Effects of restoration of vitamin A at various times during gestation.* Amer. J. Anat. 92: #2, 189-217, March 1953.

145. Wilson, J. G. and Warkany, J. *Aortic arch and cardiac anomalies in the offspring of vitamin A deficient rats.* Amer. J. Anat. 85: #1, 113-155, July 1949.

146. Wilson, J. G. and Warkany, J. *Cardiac and aortic arch anomalies in the offspring of vitamin A deficient rats correlated with similar human anomalies.* Pediatrics 5: #4, 708-725, April 1950.

147. Wilson, J. L. *Congenital malformations.* Compiled, edited, and published by the International Medical Congress, Ltd. New York. 1964.

148. Wolff, H. (editor) *Mechanisms of congenital malformation.* New York City, Association for the Aid of Crippled Children. 1954.

149. Woollam, D. H. M. *Principles of teratogenesis: mode of action of thalidomide.* Proc. Roy. Soc. Med. 58: #7, 497-501, July 1965.

150. Woollam, D. H. M. and Millen, J. W. *Effect of cortisone on the incidence of cleft palate induced by experimental hypervita-minosis-A.* Brit. Med. J., 2: #5038, 197-198, 27 July 1957.

151. Zunin, C. and Borrone, C. *Embriopatie da carenza di acido pan-totenico.* Acta vitamin., Milano. 8: 263, 1954.

8. MENTAL RETARDATION

DOCTOR GEORGE TARJAN (SUPERINTENDENT AND MEDICAL DIRECTOR, Pacific State Hospital, Pomona, California, and Associate Professor, Department of Psychiatry, University of California School of Medicine at Los Angeles) set the stage for the multifactorial concept of mental retardation and identifies its two major performance parameters *(59):*

> There is general agreement that mental retardation is a syndrome which can be caused by many factors acting singly or in combination....In practice we use significant impairments in two aspects of behavior - intelligence and general adaptation - as the guideposts of diagnosis.

In most instances, the term mental retardation refers to a significant, subaverage intellectual functioning that is manifested during the developmental period and is characterized by inadequacy in adaptative behavior.

Doctor Tarjan, in a presidential address to the Eighty-Third Annual Meeting of the American Association on Mental Deficiency (Milwaukee, 22 May 1959), discussed at length the multicausality of deficient mentality *(58):*

> We know that mental deficiency is not a singular entity; it represents a group of complex processes....a primary causative agent - be it a trauma, a virus, a gene, any other noxa, or a combination of these - has been identified in only a few types of mental deficiencies....causation is so complex that there is a tendency toward artificial over-simplification.

In their current textbook on mental retardation, the late Doctor Abraham Levinson (Professor of Pediatrics, Northwestern University Medical School; Chief of Pediatric Neuropsychiatry Service and Chief of Staff, Children's Division, Cook County Hospital) and Doctor John A. Bigler (Professor and Head of Department of Pediatrics, Northwestern Uni-

versity Medical School; Chief of Staff, Children's Memorial
Hospital, Chicago) quote appalling figures on the incidence
of mental subnormality *(30)*:

In 1946, the American Association on Mental Deficiency estimated
that 7% of the population is mentally or intellectually deficient.
Of 13,000,000 men examined for Selective Service up to 1944,
4.3% were rejected because of mental deficiency....The figures
given for the incidence of mental retardation in children vary.
Dr. Charlotte Grave states that there is an estimated 10 million
exceptional children in the United States or 25% of the child
population under 18 years of age. Other authorities believe that
there are 5,000,000 retarded children in the United States, or
12.5% of the child population.

The conservative estimate of mental retardation in the
United States approaches 3 per cent *(62)*. Thus, there are
approximately five million intellectually deficient people in
this country. In another frame of reference, 126,000 babies
born each year will be retarded *(45)*.

Epidemiologic data show that mental deficiency is more
common among males, and that in this civilization it is found
more frequently in the culturally, socially, and economically
deprived groups. The detection of mental retardation increases
progressively with age up to about 15 years *(58)*. H. A. Stevens
and R. Heber *(55)* have demonstrated the effects of these
socioeconomic factors upon the reported incidence of mental
subnormality very effectively in their excellent monograph
which was prepared for the American Association on Mental
Deficiency. In the lower economic sections of Syracuse, New
York, the number of cases of mental retardation per 1000
population in 10-14 year old whites is significantly higher than
in the remainder of the city (152 versus approximately 90). For
the 10-14 year old nonwhites (318 cases per 1000 population)
from these poorer sections of Syracuse, however, the
incidence of subnormal mentality was more than double and
tripled the figure for the remainder of the city *(55)*.

The late President Kennedy, in calling together a panel of distinguished experts in October 1961 to formulate a national plan to
combat mental retardation, stated....'we as a nation have for too
long postponed an intensive search for solutions to the problems
of the mentally retarded....Our goal should be to prevent retardation *(22)*.'

Helen M. Hille (Institutional Nutritional Consultant, Children's Bureau, United States Department of Health, Education and Welfare) and Mary Reeves (Regional Nutritional Consultant, Children's Bureau, United States Department of Health, Education and Welfare), as well as others (44), insist that (22):

> To prevent mental retardation the accent must be on prevention - prevention of the physical conditions in mothers and infants that lead to mental retardation and prevention of the social and emotional conditions that block the development of whatever potential retarded children have.

According to the American Association on Mental Deficiency, a biochemical approach to mental subnormality should be initiated (55).

> ...if mental retardation is to be prevented rather than treated, then one must look to the biochemical investigations to provide the necessary information...
> The biochemical approach must take at least three directions. The first is that basic work on the role of lipids, carbohydrates, and amino acids in the brain needs to be examined....The second approach is the biochemical investigation of the mentally retarded child....A third need is...pursuing the study of experimentally produced mental retardation in animals.

Doctor Joaquin Cravioto (Associate Director, Institute of Nutrition of Central America and Panama, Guatemala City, Guatemala) in a presentation before the Association Symposium of the American Public Health Association at its Ninetieth Annual Meeting (Miami Beach, Florida, 19 October 1962) affirmed that, of the biochemical parameters that may be investigated, diet and nutrition should certainly be considered (12):

> In an increasingly complicated world of sophisticated technology in which even a mild reduction in mental performance may be a serious handicap, the possible effect of early malnutrition on mental capacity and personality development should be a major consideration.

In their synopsis of investigations in the area of diet and mental performance, Helen M. Hille and Mary Reeves (22) note that:

> Research over the past quarter century has clearly shown that the nutrition of the mother is one of the important environmental

factors that influences the health of the expectant mother and the well being of the infant....

Efforts to reduce the incidence of mental retardation caused by premature birth and complications associated with childbearing include programs geared to improving the dietary habits of all women of childbearing age and to providing nutritional supervision early in pregnancy.

CORRELATIVE FINDINGS

Lower Animal Observations: It is comprehensible because of the nature of the subject that the medical literature reviews do not cite lower animal studies of a correlative nature.

Human Observations: Even though an infant receives enough food there appears to be a significant correlation between artificial feeding methods and mental inferiority *(23)*. Doctor Mattie Crumpton Hardy and her associate (Carolyn Hoefer) from Elizabeth McCormick Memorial Fund have observed (Table 8.1) a definitely superior mentality in breast-fed children. *(23)*. These results were based on a comparison of intelligence, educational, and performance quotients, and the age at which talking began. From their observations of exceptionally bright children it is interesting that none was artificially fed during infancy (Table 8.1). It may be noted in Table 8.2 that dietary inadequacy has been reported as a problem factor in the etiology of subnormal mentality.

The lower division of Table 8.2 points out the correlation between various body nutrient levels and mental deficiency. Although the concentration of these blood and salivary nutrients is a resultant of many operating factors, dietary intake is most certainly playing an important role *(15,26,48)*. Not only is the consumption of a nutrient a determining factor in its body fluid level, but the complex dietary nutrient interrelationships (Chapter Four, Dietary Interrelationships) are equally important.

Particular emphasis was placed in Chapter One (The American Diet) upon the dietary alterations during the past century. It was pointed out that the major significant change has been a replacement of starch by the simple carbohydrates. The ingestion of these sugars causes wide fluctuations in the blood sugar and glucose levels *(7,9,10)*. Thus, the two items

Table 8.1
method of infant feeding in children
of superior intelligence

| | per cent of each group with intelligence quotients of | |
	120 or above	130 and above
artificially fed	5.2	0.0
breast fed	14.2	4.9
3 months or less	15.4	5.1
4-9 months	20.8	9.1
10-15 months	12.4	3.3
16 months or more	8.1	2.7

Table 8.2
diet and mental retardation
(human correlative observations)

dietary variable	type or degree of mental retardation	reference
chronic malutrition	significantly low behavior and central nervous system capacity scores	11,40
protein-calorie malnutrition	lowered intelligence quotient	41
bottle feeding	lowered intelligence quotient	23

body nutrient level		
increased salivary sodium and calcium	mongoloid	64
lowered serum calcium	mongoloid	51,53
increased serum inorganic phosphate	mongoloid	53
hypermagnesemia	mongoloid; other mentally retarded	54
decreased serum albumin	mongoloid	51,52
increased serum gamma globulin	mongoloid	51,52
decreased absorption of vitamin A	mongoloid	51,1
elevated serum cholesterol	mongoloid; undifferentiated mental deficiency	49
decreased glucose tolerance	mongoloid	47
neonatal hypoglycemia	mental subnormality	43
decreased plasma ascorbic acid	lowered I.Q. in normal students	28

in Table 8.2 concerned with abnormal carbohydrate metabolism and mental deficiency may be a much more important factor than previously recognized *(43,47)*.

Doctors Reisner, Forbes, and Cornblath *(43)* from the Department of Pediatrics, University of Illinois College of Medicine, and Research and Education Hospitals of Chicago have proposed hypoglycemia as a possible etiologic factor for the mental subnormality and slow development seen in the smaller twin as compared with his larger sibling. The smaller twin is thought to be an example of intrauterine malnutrition, with the larger twin as a natural control during the gestational period.

Workers in the field of mental retardation have postulated that mongolism may be of metabolic origin and may actually progress with aging *(1,25,43,47,49,51-54,64)*. One may note in Table 8.2 a variety of biochemical abnormalities reported in mongoloids. Doctor Gretchen H. Runge *(47)* of the Austin State School in Austin, Texas, has observed not only a high incidence of decreased glucose tolerance in mongoloids but a dramatic increase in the percentage of abnormal tolerance curves with age (Table 8.3). The normal curve was defined as one in which the blood sugar did not reach a level higher than 250 mg. per cent following intravenous glucose, showed a striking drop by 30 minutes, and returned to the fasting level within 60 minutes.

A very interesting correlation has been noted between season of birth and intelligence *(27,38)*. In a paper presented before the Mental Health Section of the American Public Health Association (Eighty-Fifth Annual Meeting, Cleveland, Ohio, 12 November 1957), Doctor Hilda Knobloch (Director, Clinic of Child Development; Associate Professor of Pediatrics, Ohio State University, College of Medicine) and Doctor Benjamin Pasamanick (Director of Psychiatry, Ohio State University, College of Medicine) reported that significantly more mentally defective children (Columbus State School, 1913-1948) had been born in the winter months *(27)*.

Since the third month after conception is known to be the period during pregnancy when the cerebral cortex of the unborn child is becoming organized, any damage which occurred at that time could affect intellectual functioning. The months when this might happen would be June, July and August, the hot summer months, when pregnant women might decrease their food intake, particularly protein, to dangerously low levels and consequently damage their developing babies. If this were so, one would expect that hotter summers would result in significantly more mental defectives born than following cooler summers. This was exactly what was found to a highly significant degree.

According to Doctors Knobloch and Pasamanick, there is a growing body of knowledge which indicates that it is quite necessary for the women in the child-bearing age to consume a good diet to produce a healthy, normally developing child *(27)*.

Inadequate dietary intake during pregnancy, because of heat as well as substandard economic conditions, may be an important link in the vicious cycle that results in poor physical and mental growth.

Table 8.3
abnormal glucose tolerance curves
in mongoloids according to age

age in years	number mongoloids	per cent abnormal curves
0-10	41	30
10-20	50	34
20-30	15	73
30-40	10	60
40-56	11	99

THERAPEUTIC FINDINGS

Lower Animal Observations: Table 8.4 provides a summary of lower animal research concerning the effect of diet upon mental achievement. These studies of dietary deficiency and supplementation have almost exclusively utilized rats. In most instances the evaluation of mental performance or learning ability has been through the use of the maze or some similar device designed to evaluate an animal's choice-making ability and/or efficiency.

The data in Table 8.4 demonstrate a therapeutic relationship between diet and mental retardation in the rat. It is concluded that the B complex group of vitamins must be

Table 8.4
diet and mental retardation
(lower animal therapeutic observations)

dietary variable	clinical effect	reference
phosphorus deficiency	slight decrease in maze performance (rat)	5
iron deficiency	adverse effect on maze performance (rat)	5
protein deficiency	reduced learning performance (rat)	4
B complex deficiency	reduced maze learning ability (rat)	6,32,33,39
B1 deficiency	reduced maze learning ability (rat)	34,37
B1 excess	improved maze performance above normal (rat)	37
B2 deficiency	reduced maze performance (rat)	35
B6 deficiency	reduced learning performance (rat)	50
folic acid deficiency	inferior maze learning ability (rat)	63
glutamic acid supplement	enhanced learning ability (rat)	14

present in liberal quantities for the normal functional development of a rapidly growing nervous system. Furthermore, should a deficiency exist, the earlier its onset, the more damaging is it to reducing learning ability. Thus, a deficiency during gestation or before weaning and followed by a normal diet exerts a more profound effect on learning efficiency than at some later period in the animal's life. The loss of weight or stunting of growth in the deficient groups is apparently not the factor in the production of mental subnormality. This is confirmed by the fact that pair-fed controls maintained at the same weight and growth status with a normal diet prove mentally superior to the deficient animals but no different from controls fed a normal diet ad libitum.

Not only has the cause-and-effect relationship between B complex components and subnormal mentality been demonstrated by complete withdrawal of these nutrients but the effects of graded dietary intake have also been noted *(34,37)*. In rats subjected to dietary regimes differing in thiamine content, the watermaze learning ability was quite different (Table 8.5). The author (Philip H. O'Neill, S. J., Department of Psychology, Fordham University) was able to demonstrate evidence for the following conclusions (37):

1. The amount of thiamine in the diet of the very young rats affected their ability to learn a watermaze. Larger amounts of thiamine led to better maze performance.

2. A daily allowance of less that 3 gamma of thiamine diminished maze learning below normal; more than 100 gamma a day improved maze performance above normal. The amount of improvement and impairment was statistically significant and reliable above the one per cent level of confidence.

3. Variations in the thiamine content of the diet between 3 gamma and 100 gamma a day did not produce any significant effect on maze learning ability.

4. When rats received an excess of thiamine, they did not make any further improvement in maze learning ability when large amounts of riboflavin (B2), pyridoxine (B6), and calcium pantothenate were added to the diet.

Table 8.5
thiamine deficiency and the
average maze learning scores
of rats (36 rats per group)

dietary regime*	total time (minutes)	number of trials	number of errors
B complex deficient diet + 20 gamma B2 and B6, 40 gamma calcium pantothenate and 2 or 3 gamma B1 daily	19.0	18.2	77.2
B complex deficient diet + 20 gamma B2 and B6, 40 gamma calcium pantothenate and 4 or 6 gamma B1 daily	14.0	14.9	57.8
B complex deficient diet + 20 gamma B2 and B6, 40 gamma calcium pantothenate and 10 gamma B1 daily- or normal diet	14.0	13.9	56.9
normal diet + 5 gamma B1 per cc. water or B complex deficient diet + 5 gamma B1, B2, B6 and 10 gamma calcium pantothenate per cc. water (100-200 gamma B1 daily)	9.8	11.4	36.1

*this diet fed for first eight weeks of life, followed by normal
diet for one week prior to tests and during test trials

Animal research demonstrates, therefore, that even *marginal* malnutrition during early life may lead to permanent stunting of mental capacity. These observations, as will become evident, have far-reaching implications regarding the health and welfare of mankind.

Human Observations: One of the most revealing developments in the field of nutrition, according to Doctor Richard H. Barnes *(3)*, Dean, Graduate School of Nutrition, Cornell University, has been the demonstration that malnutrition during early life may retard the rate of mental development in man. In this increasingly technologic society even a *slight* reduction in mental performance may be a very serious handicap, said Doctor Joaquin Cravioto *(12)* of the Institute of Nutrition of Central America and Panama in a presentation before the American Public Health Association (Ninetieth Annual Meeting, Miami Beach, Florida, 19 October 1962).

It is recognized that mental deficiency frequently results from abnormal nutrient metabolism in early life. However, the so-called genetic errors of metabolism will not be considered in the review. Here, the primary concern is with the congenital and postnatal effects of dietary nutrients upon mental achievement.

A review of the literature reveals a plethora of data concerning the nutritional aspects of mental retardation. Table 8.6 is a summary of reports demonstrating the effects of dietary deficiency and supplementation upon various parameters of intelligence in human beings. From a study of Table 8.6, four characteristics are noteworthy. First, the majority of publications deal with dietary supplementation rather than deficiency. It is obvious that, in human research, improvement of mental status is the only therapeutic avenue open for investigation. Second, a rather wide variety of nutrients has been utilized, both singly and in combination, for improvement of mentation. Third, these reports have not only dealt with a broad age distribution in both males and females, but significant improvement was achieved in individuals of so-called normal mentality as well as with different gradations of retardation. Finally, from a perusal of Table 8.6, it becomes apparent that most of the researchers employed controls, and, in four instances, the studies were double-blind with a

Table 8.6
diet and mental retardation
(human therapeutic observations)

dietary variable	effect on mental status	reference
deficiency		
malnutrition during infancy	significantly lowered I.Q. (children)	56*
omission of breakfast	increased simple & choice reaction time (normal young women)	60*
	detrimental effect on attitude & scholastic attainment (boys)	61*
nicotinic acid	loss of memory; mental retardation (all ages)	13
supplementation		
correction of protein-calorie malnutrition	progressive decrease in mental retardation (children)	46
provision of good diet	significant increase in I.Q. (normal & retarded children)	29*
orange juice	significant gain in I.Q. when plasma ascorbic acid was >1.1 mg. %	28*
coffee	significant increased power to form associative bonds (various ages)	42*
C; B1 + B2 + niacin + iron	significant I.Q. increases (3 & 4 year old children of supplemented mothers)	21**
B complex	significant improvement in each of a battery of mental tests (normal children)	2
monosodium glutamate + B complex (L-Glutavite)	mental improvement of mongoloids & non-mongoloid retardates (children)	18*
	improvement in alertness, comprehension & intelligence in various types of mental subnormality (children & adults)	19
glutamic acid	I.Q. increases (all aged retardates)	14
lecithin + B1	significant increased arithmetic performance & graphomotor expansion (normal high school seniors)	36**
nicotinic acid	improvement in memory & retardation (all ages)	13
thiamine (B1)	significantly improved mental performance (children)	20**
vitamin E	improvement of subnormal mentality (children)	16,17, 24*
	mental improvement of mongoloids (children)	57
ribonucleic acid	improvement of memory (aged)	8**

* untreated controls
**double-blind with placebo-treated controls

placebo-treated control group.

A team of investigators (Ruth F. Harrell, Ella R. Woodyard, and Arthur I. Gates) *(21)*, from the Department of Psychology and Education at the College of William and Mary in Williamsburg, Virginia, and the Teachers College of Columbia University, has demonstrated the prenatal effect of vitamin supplementation upon the intelligence of the offspring at three and four years of age (Table 8.7). Significant differences were noted in the frequency distribution of intelligence quotients between placebo and vitamin (2 mg. thiamine, 4 mg. riboflavin, 20 mg. niacinamide, and 15 mg. iron) treated pregnancies. Actually, the mean I.Q. scores of the children are significantly different at the one per cent level of confidence. This is particularly noteworthy in view of the fact that maternal therapy was not administered until relatively late in gestation. Second, the supplement was modest in both quantity and quality. Finally, the offspring, themselves, received no treatment. This is in contrast to other observations in the same report with women consuming presumably adequate diets. In this latter group there were no differences in I.Q. with vitamin versus placebo supplementation.

The effect of diet upon intellectual capacity is not limited to therapy during the gestation period. Stoch and Smythe *(56)*, from the Department of Child Health, Red Cross War Memorial Children's Hospital and University of Cape Town, South Africa, have noted significantly less brain growth and a significantly lower intelligence quotient in Cape Colored children who were grossly undernourished during the first year of life when compared to a matched control group. They reported no improvement in the retarded mentality during the seven year follow-up period. At the final testing, the mean I.Q. of the undernourished group (70.86) differed from that of the control group (93.48) by 22.62 points. The difference of the means was highly significant (P < 0.01).

The far-reaching effects of diet upon intellect have even been demonstrated in the presumably normal child. In a controlled study of dietary improvement upon child mentality, Doctor I. Newton Kugelmass, Doctor Louise E. Poull, and Emma L. Samuel *(29)* noted an increase in the intelligence quotient of both retarded and mentally normal children (Table

Table 8.7
frequency distribution of intelligence quotients
for four year old children of women receiving a
placebo or vitamin (2 mg. B1, 4 mg. B2, 20 mg.
niacin and 15 mg. iron) supplement during pregnancy

intelligence quotient	vitamin (one pill daily)	placebo (one pill daily)
66		1
69		1
72		1
75	1	3
78	1	4
81	4	4
84	2	10
87	8	11
90	4	6
93	8	15
96	7	6
99	15	18
102	8	4
105	10	8
108	2	1
111	10	3
114	2	1
117	1	1
120	1	
123	3	
126	1	
129	2	
150	1	
total children	91	98
mean	101.7	93.6
P	< 0.01	

8.8). The group of children, malnourished at the time of the
first mental test and well nourished at the second, showed a
rise of 10 points for the retarded and 18 points for the mentally
normal. In contrast, there was relatively no change (-0.3 and
-0.9) for the well nourished retarded and normal groups,
respectively, on both occasions.

Doctor Ruth F. Harrell (20) of the Department of
Educational Psychology, Teachers College, Columbia University, found that in closely matched (age, sex, weight, education
status, and mentality) groups of presumably normal orphanage
children, the double-blind daily administration of a placebo
versus 2 mg. thiamine tablet for one year produced a superior

Table 8.8
effect of dietary improvement
upon child mentality

malnourished

	retarded (n=41)		normal (n=50)	
	range	mean	range	mean
age (years)	2- 8	3.8	2- 10	4.7
I.Q. (initial)	20-90	45	95-145	110
I.Q. (change)	-8 to + 44	+ 10	-12 to + 55	+ 18

well-nourished

	retarded (n=41)		normal (n=50)	
	range	mean	range	mean
age (years)	2- 8	4.8	2- 10	5.0
I.Q. (initial)	20-90	52	95-140	110
I.Q. (change)	-20 to + 11	-0.3	-25 to + 20	-0.9

Table 8.9
mental response to placebo and thiamine
(2 mg. daily) supplementation for
one year in orphanage children
9 to 19 years of age

evaluation activity	per cent relative mean gains		
	placebo* group	thiamine group	P
remembering: word-number pairs	100	175	.002
code substitution	100	400	.003
memorizing new material	100	530	.007
remembering: Morse code	100	230	.020
intelligence: power type test	100	215	.040
reaction time	100	120	.050

*placebo gain equals 100%

mental response in the vitamin group. The thiamine supplemented group not only excelled but the improvement was regarded as statistically significant (Table 8.9). The percentage of improvement over the controls ranged from approximately 25 to 3200. Thus, it appears that mental achievement in children of presumably normal mentality consuming a presumably normal diet can be remarkably increased through the employment of dietary supplements.

That mental advancement may even be extended into the late teens has been vividly demonstrated by Hans Muecher and Gerhard Gruenwalt *(36)* of the Psychiatric Clinic of the Medizinischen Akademic Duesseldorf. The double-blind daily administration of a placebo or supplement (lecithin, .65 mg., vitamin B1, 2 mg.) to high school seniors significantly improved (P < 0.001) arithmetic mental performance in the subjects receiving the nutrient supplement. The supplement effectiveness was noted by the end of the first day of the six days of therapy. Placebo supplementation to both groups before and after this period revealed no differences in performance.

SUMMARY

Although not mentioned in Table 8.6, the ingestion of various chemical substances (which may or may not be regarded as dietary) produces neurologic intoxication. Many of the individuals who do not die become mental retardates. As illustrative, lead encephalopathy is not an infrequent cause of subnormal mentality *(31)*.

A significant volume of evidence from both lower animal and human studies has been presented to support the relationship between diet and mental retardation. Since the incidence of subnormal intelligence is of great magnitude, every avenue of prevention should be investigated.

In a presidential address before the American Association on Mental Deficiency at its Eighty-Third Annual Meeting (22 May 1959), Doctor George Tarjan *(58)* urged the initiation of preventive programs in the following words:

> In closing, may I underscore a few points. The present imperfection of our knowledge should not delay the initiation of preventive programs. We have already identified, on an experimental or

empirical basis, sufficient facts which can be put to good preventive use.

Doctor Hilda Knobloch and Doctor Benjamin Pasamanick *(27)* underscore the role of diet and other environment influences versus genetics as the logical avenues for such preventive programs.

...Except for a comparatively few and rare hereditary disorders, life experiences, rather than inherited characteristics, may be the primary factors making one individual significantly different from the next...It does not appear necessary, however, to wait until the last iota of evidence is in proving the association of diet and disability. Present knowledge...would appear sufficient to demand that public health workers turn their attention more directly to this problem. We are well beyond the stage of paying lip service to the importance of the chronic diseases; possible avenues of prevention should be seized upon--and action taken. In a field as complex as behavioral functioning prevention of dysfunction is often the only method of demonstrating etiology.

REFERENCES

1. Auld, R. M., Pommer, A. M., Houck, J. C. and Burke, F. G. *Vitamin H absorption in mongoloid children.* Am. J. Ment. Defic. 63: #5, 1010-1013, March 1959.

2. Balken, E. R. and Maurer, S. *Variations in psychological measurements associated with increased vitamin B complex feeding in young children.* J. Exp. Psychol. 17: #1, 85-92, February 1934.

3. Barnes, R. H. *Malnutrition in early life and mental development.* N. Y. State J. Med. 65: #22, 2816-2817, 15 November 1965.

4. Bernhardt, K. S. *Protein deficiency and learning in rats.* J. Comp. Psychol. 22: #2, 269-272, October 1936.

5. Bernhardt, K. S. *Phosphorus and iron deficiencies and learning in the rat.* J. Comp. Psychol. 22: #2, 273-376, October 1936.

6. Bernhardt, K. S. and Herbert, R. *A further study of vitamin B deficiency and learning with rats.* J. Comp. Psychol. 24: #2, 263-267, October 1937.

7. Burns, T. W., Bregant, R., Van Peenan, H. J. and Hood, T. E. *Observations on blood glucose concentration of human subjects during continuous sampling.* Diabetes 14: #4, 186-193, April 1965.

8. Cameron, D. E. and Solyom, L. *Effects of ribonucleic acid on memory.* Geriatrics 16: #2, 74-81, February 1961.

9. Cheraskin, E. and Ringsdorf, W. M., Jr., *Homeostasis: a study in carbohydrate metabolism.* J. Med. Assn. Ala. 35: #3, 173-182, September 1965.

10. Conn, J. W. and Newburgh, L. H. *The glycemic response to iso-glucogenic quantities of protein and carbohydrate.* J. Clin. Invest. 15: #6, 665-671, November 1936.

11. Coursin, D. B. *Effects of undernutrition on central nervous system function.* Nutrition Rev. 23: #3, 65-68, March 1965.

12. Cravioto, J. *Application of newer knowledge of nutrition on physical and mental growth and development.* Am. J. Pub. Health 53: #11, 1803-1809, November 1963.

13. Eiduson, S., Geller, E., Yuwiler, A. and Eiduson, B. T. *Biochemistry and behavior.* 1964. Princeton, New Jersey, D. Van Nostrand Company. pp. 20-26.

14. Eiduson, S., Geller, E., Yuwiler, A. and Eiduson, B. T. *Biochemistry and behavior.* 1964. Princeton, New Jersey, D. Van Nostrand Company. pp. 122-128.

15. *Expert committee on medical assessment of nutritional status: Report.* World Health Organization Technical Report Series #258. Geneva World Health Organization, 1963.

16. Giudice, D. A. *Large doses of vitamin E as a factor in the mental improvement of subnormal children.* The Summary 12: #1, 21-22, June 1960.

17. Giudice, D. A. *Vitamin E for mental defect.* The Summary 13: #1, 1-4, June 1961.

18. Goldstein, H. *L-Glutavite as a therapeutic aid in mentally retarded children.* Med. Times 89: #8, 848-851, August 1961.

19. Goven, J. W. and Lade, A. *Mental subnormality helped with L-Glutavite.* Psychosomatics 3: #6, 480-483, November-December 1962.

20. Harrell, R. F. *Mental response to added thiamine.* J. Nutrit. 31: #3, 283-298, March 11, 1946.

21. Harrell, R. F., Woodyard, E. R. and Gates, A. I. *The influence of vitamin supplementation of the diets of pregnant and lactating women on the intelligence of their offspring.* Metabolism 5: #5, 555-562, September 1956.

22. Hille, H. M. and Reeves, M. *The battle against mental retardation; the dietitian's share.* Hospitals 38: #22, 101-106, 16 November 1964.

23. Hoefer, C. and Hardy, M. C. *Later development of breast fed and artificially fed infants.* J. A. M. A. 92: #8, 615-619, 23 February 1929.

24. Houze, M., Wilson, H. D. and Goodfellow, H. D. L. *Treatment of mental deficiency with alpha tocopherol.* Am. J. Ment. Defic. 69: #3, 328-329, November 1964.

25. Ingalls, T. H. *The problem of mongolism.* Ann. N. Y. Acad. Sci. 57: #5, 551-557, 15 January 1954.

26. Jonas, L., Miller, T. G. and Teller, T. *All day blood sugar curves in nondiabetic individuals and in diabetic patients with and without insulin.* Arch. Int. Med. 35: #3, 289-314, March 1925.

27. Knobloch, H. and Pasamanick, B. *Seasonal variation in the births of the mentally deficient.* Am. J. Public Health 48: #9, 1201-1208, September 1958.

28. Kubala, A. L. and Katz, M. M. *Nutritional factors in psychological test behavior.* J. Genetic Psychol. 96: #2, 343-352, June 1960.

29. Kugelmass, I. N., Poull, L. E. and Samuel, E. L. *Nutritional improvement of child mentality.* Am. J. Med. Sc. 208: #5, 631-633, November 1944.

30. Levinson, A. and Bigler, J. A. *Mental retardation in infants and children.* 1960. Chicago, The Year Book Publishers. p. 29.

31. Levinson, A. and Bigler, J. A. *Mental retardation in infants and children.* 1960. Chicago, The Year Book Publishers. pp. 278-281.

32. Maurer, S. and Tsai, L. S. *Vitamin B deficiency in nursing young rats and learning ability.* Science 70: #1819, 456-458, 8 November 1929.

33. Maurer, S. and Tsai, L. S. *Vitamin B deficiency and learning ability.* J. Comp. Psychol. 11: #1, 51-62, October 1930.

34. Maurer, S. *III. The effect of partial depletion of vitamin B (B1) upon performance in rats.* J. Comp. Psychol. 20: #2, 309-317, October 1935.

35. Maurer, S. *IV. The effect of early depletion of vitamin B2 upon performance in rats.* J. Comp. Psychol. 20: #2, 385-387, October 1935.

36. Muecher, H. and Gruenwald, G. *Pharmacologic stimulation of arithmetic performance and graphomotor expansion.* Perceptual and Motor Skills 15, 101-102, August-December, 1962.

37. O'Neill, P. H. *The effect on subsequent maze learning ability of graded amounts of vitamin B1 in the diet of very young rats.* J. Genetic Psychol. 74: First Quarter, 85-95, March 1949.

38. Orme, J. E. *Intelligence and season of birth.* Brit. J. Med. Psychol. 35, 233-234, 1962.

39. Poe, E., Poe, C. and Muenzinger, K. F. *The effect of vitamin deficiency on the acquisition and retention of the maze habit in the white rat: IV. Vitamin B complex, B1 and B2 (G).* J. Comp. Psychol. 27: #2, 211-214, April 1939.

40. Ramos-Galvan, R., Perez-Navarr, etc., J. L. and Cravioto-Nunoz, J. *Various aspects of growth and development of Mexican children.* Bol. Med. Hosp. Infantil de Mexico 17, 455-474, 1960.

41. Ramos-Galvan, R. cited by Cravioto, J. *Application of newer knowledge of nutrition on physical and mental growth and development.* Am. J. Pub. Health 53: #11, 1803-1809, November 1963.

42. Reiman, G. *The influence of coffee on the association constant.* J. Exp. Psychol. 17: #1, 93-104, February 1934.

43. Reisner, S. H., Forbes, A. E. and Cornblath, M. *The smaller of twins and hypoglycemia.* Lancet 1: #7384, 524-526, 6 March 1965.

44. Richmond, J. B., Tarjan, G. and Gardner, G. E. *Mental retardation; a handbook for the primary physician.* J. A. M. A. 191: #3, 183-222, 18 January 1965.

45. Richmond, J. B. *Mental retardation.* J. A. M. A. 191: #3, 243, 18 January 1965.

46. Robles, B., Ramos-Galvan, R. and Cravioto, J. cited by Cravioto, J. *Application of newer knowledge of nutrition on physical and mental growth and development.* Am. J. Public Health 53: #11, 1803-1809, November 1963.

47. Runge, G. H. *Glucose tolerance in mongolism.* Am. J. Ment. Defic. 63: #5, 822-828, March 1959.

48. Seelig, M. S. *The requirement of magnesium by the normal adult; summary and analysis of published data.* Am. J. Clin. Nutrit. 14: #6, 342-390, June 1964.

49. Simon, A., Ludwig, C., Gofinan, J. W. and Croak, G. H. *Metabolic studies in mongolism.* Am. J. Psychiatry 111: #2, 139-145, August 1954.

50. Sloane, H. N., Jr. and Chow, B. F. *Vitamin B6 deficiency and the initial acquisition of behavior.* J. Nutrit. 83: #4, 379-384, August 1964.

51. Sobel, A., Strazzulla, M., Sherman, B. S., Elkan, B., Morgenstern, S. W., Marius, N. and Meisel, A. *Vitamin A absorption and other blood composition studies in mongolism.* Am. J. Ment. Defic. 62: #4, 642-656, January 1958.

52. Stern, J. and Lewis, W. H. P. *Serum proteins in mongolism.* J. Ment. Sc. 103: #430, 222-226, January 1957.

53. Stern, J. and Lewis, W. H. P. *Calcium, phosphate and phosphatase in mongolism.* J. Ment. Sc. 104: #436, 880-883, July 1958.

54. Stern, J. and Lewis, W. H. P. *Blood magnesium in children with mongolism and other mentally retarded children.* Am. J. Ment. Defic. 64: #6, 972-977, May 1960.

55. Stevens, H. A. and Heber, R. *Mental retardation.* 1964. Chicago, University of Chicago Press. pp. 279-280.

56. Stoch, M. B. and Smythe, P. M. *Does undernutrition during infancy inhibit brain growth and subsequent intellectual development?* Arch. Dis. Child. 38: #202, 546-552, December 1963.

57. Szasz, H. *Vitamin E in the treatment of mongolian idiocy. Influence on the organism of vitamin E given from birth onward until puberty.* The Summary 11: #2, 49-51, December 1959.

58. Tarjan, G. *Prevention, a program goal in mental deficiency.* Am. J. Ment. Defic. 64: #1, 4-11, July 1959.

59. Tarjan, G. *The next decade: Expectations from the biological sciences.* J. A. M. A. 191: #3, 160-163, 18 January 1965.

60. Tuttle, W. W., Wilson, M. and Daum, K. *Effect of altered breakfast habits on physiologic response.* J. Appl. Physiol. 1: #8, 545-559, February 1949.

61. Tuttle, W. W., Daum, K., Larse, R., Salzano, J. and Roloff, L. *Effect on school boys of omitting breakfast.* J. Am. Dietet. Ass. 30: #7, 674-677, July 1954.

62. Warren, S. L. *Implementation of the president's program on mental retardation.* Am. J. Psychiatry 121: #6, 549-554, December 1964.

9. PSYCHOLOGIC DISORDERS

THERE IS AMPLE REASON TO BELIEVE THAT MENTAL ILLNESS AND ITS impact on health care resources will be one of the major future public health issues *(68)*. In nonfederal hospitals, listed by the American Hospital Association in 1959, there were 1,434,000 beds and 440,515,000 days of hospital care. Almost half (48 per cent) of the beds and more than half (53 per cent) of the days were classified for psychiatric care. Phrased another way, the 234,000,000 days of psychiatric hospital care per annum for a population of 180,000,000 persons means approximately 1.3 psychiatric hospital days per capita per year. These shocking figures were presented at a national symposium (Health Care Issues of the 1960's, October 1961) by Doctor William H. Stewart *(68)*, formerly Chief, Division of Public Health Methods, United States Public Health Service.

Current research is looking critically for a biochemical basis of mental illness. Because of their conviction that any behavioral phenomenon is preceded by biochemical change, Doctors Eiduson, Geller, Yuwiler (University of California, Los Angeles) and Eiduson (Reiss-Davis Clinic for Child Guidance) have written a text entitled *Biochemistry and Behavior*. They expressed, in their introductory remarks, the belief that behavior must be mediated like all other body functions, via biochemical pathways *(15)*:

> Whatever behavioral process takes place, whether feeling or overt action, it is our belief that there necessarily must be concomitant or correlative biochemical reactions....We cannot conceive of even a thought occurring without its counterpart of biochemical and physiological events....

> ...Different organs of the body subserve different functions, and it is reasonable to expect, therefore, that each organ will carry

out specific and unique biochemical processes....Underlying these individual peculiarities, however, may be found general metabolic pathways common to all systems regardless of their specific function. Thus, for example, the myriad of biochemical reactions required to utilize carbohydrate as a fuel and convert it to needed stored chemical energy is essentially common to all metabolizing cells and organs whether they are found in plants, bacteria, or any other living organism. It should, therefore, be clear that general biochemical principles which are applicable to the liver and lungs are found equally applicable to the brain.

Doctor T. L. Sourkes (Senior Research Biochemist, Allen Memorial Institute of Psychiatry and Associate Professor of Psychiatry, McGill University) in his *Biochemistry of Mental Disease* underscores two aims for the chemical approach to the study of mental disorders *(52)*.

...the search for causative factors of a chemical nature; and the investigation of chemical parameters whereby the disease may be characterized, its severity quantified, or its course indicated.

Further, he quotes Doctor Derek Richter of the Medical Research Council, Neuropsychiatric Research Unit in Carshalton, Surrey, who is keenly aware of the need for more investigation in this area:

...biochemical research is especially urgent since the knowledge of biochemical defects can lead quite directly to the suggestion of remedies. Thus the discovery of specific biochemical deficiencies in rickets, diabetes, and pernicious anemia led rapidly to successful treatment by rational methods and replacement therapy. Faulty working of the brain due to an imbalance of enzyme systems or to a biochemical deficiency might also be rectified by similar methods.

As a warning to those who cling to the Freudian concepts of mental diseases, Doctor D. W. Woolley of the Rockefeller Institute concluded his text, *The Biochemical Bases of Psychoses*, with this statement:

It really seems that the biochemical aspects of various features of the mind have become clear enough that formal philosophy must take official recognition of them if it wishes to protray a comprehensive and true picture of men and the world. Formal philosophers cannot continue to remain aloof from the laboratory. If they do, the full nature of consciousness may escape them.

It is possible that the biochemical bases for psychologic

disorders may be in part related to diet and nutrient metabolism. Realizing the complex interrelationships between nutrients (Chapter Four) and the average American's eating habits (Chapter One), one should suspect that not all mental patients are well nourished. Doctors Ian Gregory and R. H. Paul *(28)* of the Department of Psychiatry, University of Western Ontario, published blood nutrient analyses in mental hospital patients. According to their figures (Table 9.1) from 4 to 37 per cent of the patients in different diagnostic groups revealed relative nutritional deficiencies of one or several nutrients. Thus, dietary inadequacies do apparently exist in psychologically disoriented individuals.

Investigations dealing with the dietary and neuropathology are not to be considered in this chapter. This survey is limited to a review of diet and behavioral disorders.

CORRELATIVE FINDINGS

Lower Animal Observations: The investigations of relationships between diet and behavioral disorders in animals have been primarily those of a cause and effect variety. A number of nutrient deficiencies have been observed to affect, significantly, experimental animal behavior. These are reported under *Therapeutic Findings.*

Human Observations: Considerable research effort on the biochemical patterns of abnormal behavior has been expended. There is some degree of correlation between chemical es-

Table 9.1
percentages of selected diagnostic groups
showing relative nutritional deficiencies

	thiamine	ribo-flavin	niacin	ascorbic acid	vitamin A	caro-tene	pro-tein
schizophrenia	15.5	25.8	16.5	27.9	15.5	7.2	18.6
affective psychoses	7.7	13.5	11.5	17.3	19.3	9.6	17.3
organic psychoses or senility	16.7	16.7	14.3	16.7	11.9	19.1	28.6
psychoneuroses and pathologic personality	15.7	37.4	13.7	27.5	7.8	3.9	7.8
alcoholism and alcoholic psychoses	9.1	31.8	9.1	22.7	18.2	9.1	9.1
other diagnoses	12.5	25.0	20.9	33.4	10.4	4.2	16.7

timates of various body nutrients and the dietary intake *(2,32)*. Doctor D. W. Woolley, while discussing the origin of the chemical hypothesis of mental disease, underlined the historic role of dietary deficiency in man *(73)*.

The cure of the mental defect of pellagra by nicotinic acid assumes considerable historical importance because it was one of the first demonstrations that a chemical cause could be ascribed to an obscure mental disease....when it became possible, as it did in 1937, to treat patients in mental hospitals in the southern United States with nicotinic acid, and to find that a few of them became well (that is, the ones who owed their mental defect to unrecognized pellagra), a powerful argument was presented to some minds that other mental diseases of obscure causation might have a biochemical basis.

Research data demonstrating a relationship between certain biochemical patterns and mental disorders is just now beginning to make some small cracks in the psychoanalytic ice. The Freudian view has, until recently, dominated the ideas concerning mental disease causation.

Table 9.2 presents a summary of known associations between nutrients and psychologic disorders. The upper division demonstrates the association of abnormal behavior with certain flaws in the metabolism of nutrients. The lower part notes some biochemical correlates with mental disorders. These correlations are, for the most part, observations of metabolic flaws in individuals with behavioral disturbances. Even though many of the biochemical correlates with disorders of behavior were noted in the absence of any dietary consideration, some have definite dietary implications. For instance, the relationships observed between carbohydrate metabolism and the disorders listed followed the administration of an oral glucose supplement. Others, such as the observations of altered blood amino acid, serum cholesterol, or mineral levels, may well be, in part, a function of dietary intake.

In some cases, an increased nutrient requirement may render the dietary intake inadequate. For example, the increased oxidation of nicotinamide observed in schizophrenics may make the intake very insufficient. The elevation of ceruloplasmin levels noted in schizophrenics is thought to increase the need for ascorbic acid by enhancing its destruction in the body.

Not all investigations in this area confirm these correlations. However, the preponderance of evidence favors such
a correlation.

Three reports in the very recent literature show well
tabulated correlations between nutrients and behavioral
disorders. These may be noted in Tables 9.3, 9.4, and 9.5.
Table 9.3 (5) demonstrates that normal subjects, other hos-

Table 9.2
diet and psychologic disorders
(human correlative observations)

nutrient variable	behavioral disorder	reference
nutrient metabolism		
subnutrition	depressive psychoses	25
increased nicotinamide oxidation	schizophrenia	30
low absorption of vitamin B12	confusion, paranoia, affective disorders	62
abnormal N-K metabolism	affective illnesses	4
sodium retention	psychotic depression	3, 9
abnormal sodium distribution	melancholia	12
abnormal trytophane metabolism	schizophrenia	22,55,72
abnormal ascorbic acid metabolism	schizophrenia	5
low glucose tolerance	schizophrenia, depressive psychosis	21,56
	catatonic, endogenous depression	56
high glucose tolerance	manic psychosis	21,56
hypoglycemia	anxiety, irritability, fatigue, mental confusion, uncontrolled emotional outbursts	49,70
nutrient levels		
elevated blood lactic and pyruvic acid	psychoses	21
increased serum arginine, glutamine	catatonia	27
decreased glycine reserves	schizophrenia	53
reduced plasma glutamic acid	schizophrenia	47,54
elevated plasma ceruloplasmin	schizophrenia	5,22,65
hypercholesterolemia	manic depression	57
hypomagnesemia	disoriented, delirious	63
hypermagnesemia	psychotic depression, schizophrenia	9
hypokalemia	mania	9

Table 9.3
urinary ascorbate metabolites in schizophrenia

subjects type	number	mean ratio*
schizophrenia	20	43
other patients	32	69
normal subjects	20	73

*ascorbic acid x 100

dehydroascorbic acid + diketogulonic acid + ascorbic acid

Table 9.4
relationship between subnutrition
and psychiatric status in elderly patients

group	number	depressive psychosis	organic psychosis with depressive symptoms
subnutrition without contributing physical disease	48	15 (31%)	8 (16%)
average nutrition without contributing physical disease	27	2 (7%)	4 (14%)

Table 9.5
nicotinamide oxidation in schizophrenics,
drug addicts and normal individuals

subjects	urine N-methyl-2-pyridone-5-carboxamide (mg. per gm. creatinine)
female schizophrenics	624
female normals	477
male schizophrenics	404
male normals	345
male drug addicts	340

pitalized patients, and schizophrenics had remarkably different ascorbate excretion patterns even though all received the same diet. The schizophrenic excretes more ascorbic metabolites in the form of dehydroascorbic acid and diketogulonic acid than nonschizophrenic persons. This is reflected in Table 9.3 by a lower ratio number of ascorbic acid to its metabolites.

The correlation between subnutrition and psychiatric state in elderly patients is presented in Table 9.4 *(25)*. From these data, subnutrition appears to be over fourfold more common in subjects with depressive psychosis.

Schizophrenics, drug addicts, and normal individuals fed the same diet and receiving supplements of nicotinamide have been shown to oxidize the vitamin at different rates. Table 9.5 *(30)* indicates that schizophrenics metabolize the vitamin considerably faster.

Thus, the accumulating scientific data strongly suggest that some of the relationships noted between various nutritional parameters and psychologic disorders suggest an abnormal biochemical profile in the mental patient.

THERAPEUTIC FINDINGS

Research efforts in this section are directed only at the biochemical patterns of behavior. While dietary and biochemical analyses are different estimates of nutritional status, there is a reasonable degree of agreement between them *(2,32)*.

Lower Animal Observations: Table 9.6 lists several dietary variables which have been noted to produce abnormal behavior in lower animals. Additionally, it may be pointed out that a deficiency of blood glucose (hypoglycemia) has been found to initiate psychopathy *(14)*. These and other nutrient or dietary alterations frequently give rise to neurologic changes, disorders and lesions of the central and peripheral nervous systems, without producing a psychologic disturbance.

Doctor Josef Brozek *(7)*, Professor and Chairman of the Department of Psychology at Lehigh University, recently published a review of Soviet studies on nutrition and higher nervous system activity. The Russian publications in this field are, for the most part, investigations of the effect of dietary deficiencies

Table 9.6
diet and psychologic disorders
(lower animal therapeutic observations)

nutrient variable	reference
semistarvation	6
dietary thiamine deficiency	18
dietary riboflavin deficiency	59
dietary magnesium deficiency	59
dietary antimetabolites of nicotinic acid	73
low protein dietary	13
dietary pyridoxine deficiency	35

with conditioned-reflex methods. Soviet researchers regard conditioned reflex activity as the sole adequate criterion for an objective evaluation of the effects of dietary deficiency on the higher functions of the central nervous system. They have reported that conditioned responses were disturbed by deficiencies of thiamine, riboflavin, niacin, pyridoxine, protein and certain amino acids.

Recently, investigators from the Department of Psychology at the University of Pittsburgh *(23)* were able to demonstrate behavioral disruption in primates following intraperitoneal injections of blood substances from schizophrenic or stressed normal donors. Although the biochemical nature of the active blood substance or substances is not known, it may conceivably be a nutritional flaw of dietary origin.

Human Observations: A review of the literature reveals a considerable volume of data concerning the nutritional aspects of behavioral disorders summarized as the effects of dietary deficiencies (Table 9.7), nutrient supplementation (Table 9.8), and flaws in nutrient metabolism (Table 9.9) upon the psychologic status of human beings.

Of the listed deficiencies, thiamine and nicotinic acid produce the most definitive behavioral disorders (Table 9.7). A number of oral or parenteral supplements (Table 9.8) have been shown to produce significant clinical improvement in a variety of abnormal behavioral patterns. On the other hand, a deterioration of behavior may follow the use of an antimetabolite or an excess of manganese or bromide (Table 9.8). Disturbances in carbohydrate metabolism have been observed to be directly related to the psychic state (Table 9.9). Hypoglycemia has been observed to mimic many psychiatric, somatic and neurologic disorders (Table 9.10) *(51)*. The restoration of normal blood sugar levels through dietary alteration

Table 9.7
diet deficiencies and psychologic disorders
(human therapeutic observations)

nutrient variable	psychologic assessment	references
fasting (4 to 6 days)	irritability & depression	34
semistarvation	increase in "psycho-neurotic scales" of MMPI	6
dietary riboflavin deficiency	depression	17
dietary pyridoxine deficiency	extreme nervousness or confusion	61
dietary nicotinic acid deficiency	confusion, depression, psychosis	16,60,73
dietary thiamine deficiency	agitation, confusion, depression, anxiety increase of "psycho-neurotic scales" of MMPI	18,58 6
dietary pantothenic acid deficiency	depression, sullenness	19
dietary iodine deficiency	dullness, apathy in adult	6

usually results in a behavioral recovery *(51)*. Such restitution was noted in elderly subjects with marked cerebral arteriosclerosis. The decreased blood glucose supply to the brain was compensated for by intravenous glucose infusion (Table 9.8).

Three recent publications of controlled studies demonstrate that dietary supplementation may become an important therapeutic adjunct in the treatment of abnormal behavior. In a double-blind study of 42 long-term hospitalized, elderly, schizophrenic patients, dietary fortification with a supplement (monosodium l-glutamate, nicotinic acid, pyridoxine, thiamine, riboflavin, ascorbic acid, ferrous sulfate, and dicalcium phosphate) resulted in significant behavioral improvement *(24)*. Actually, 19 out of 22 supplemented subjects improved while only 5 out of the 20 controls improved (87 per cent versus 25 per cent). A number of different aspects of their behavior was analyzed, and the patients receiving the supplement demon-

Table 9.8
diet supplementation
and psychologic disorders
(human therapeutic observations)

nutrient variable	psychological assessment	references
nutrient supplementation		
food sensitivity	behavior disorders & mental illness	39
low carbohydrate, adequate protein & fat diet	recovery from depression violent temper, fatigue, & irritability	10,50
dietary L-Glutavite (mono-sodium l-glutamate + vitamins + minerals) supplement	behavior improvement in elderly deteriorated schizophrenics	24
dietary sodium glutamate supplement	behavior improvement in elderly patients with psychiatric disorders	31
dietary l-methionine or l-tryptophane supplement	clinical improvement in schizophrenics	43
dietary ascorbic acid supplement	improvement in depression, & paranoid symptom complexes & overall personality functioning	41,42
dietary sitosterol supplement	beneficial effect in elderly on mental ability & alertness	46
dietary antimetabolite (6-aminonicotinamide) supplement	psychotic episodes, confusion, depression	16,73
intramuscular B12 supplement	complete recovery from severe depression, anxiety & paranoia	69
intramuscular pyridoxine supplement	disappearance of neurasthenia symptoms	36
intravenous glucose infusion	improvement in senile confusion	29
manganese poisoning	dullness, apathy, incoherent speech, euphoria, aggressiveness	64
high bromide intake	apathy, paranoia, delirium, memory loss	66

strated superior progress in each parameter (Table 9.11) *(24)*. This study by Doctor Louis P. Fincle and Doctor L. J. Reyna of the Veterans Administration Hospital in Bedford, Massachusetts, and Boston University, Department of Psychology, extended over a one-year period.

Doctor Ralph M. Reitan and Doctor Robert E. Shipley *(46)* (Department of Neurology, Indiana University Medical

Table 9.9
nutrient metabolism and psychologic disorders
(human therapeutic observations)

nutrient metabolism	psychologic assessment	references
low glucose tolerance	schizophrenia	45
improvement in glucose tolerance	improvements in various mental disorders	38,45,56
hypoglycemia	depression, anxiety, neuroses, any aspect of entire range of psychiatric disorders	11,37,40 1,10
increase in plasma potassium	recovery from mania	8

Center), using a battery of eleven standardized psychologic tests, found that dietary sitosterol (principal sterols of plant oils) supplementation for twelve months produced a beneficial effect on mental ability and alertness. These results were only noted in older men whose serum cholesterol levels were reduced by 10 per cent or more. Figure 9.1 *(46)* clearly portrays this beneficial effect of lowering the serum cholesterol on the psychologic test performance.

A controlled double-blind trial of dietary ascorbic acid versus placebo supplementation in 40 male, chronic, psychiatric patients was published by Doctor G. Milner *(41)*, Registrar in Psychiatry at the Towers Hospital in Leicester, England. A clinical state of subscurvy was found in these patients and, when it was corrected by dietary supplementation, a statistically significant improvement in behavior followed. The six days required for ascorbic acid saturation in these patients was at least three times that for normal subjects and approached the seven to ten day requirement for scorbutics. Depressive, manic, and paranoid symptom complexes, together with overall personality function, improved (Table 9.12) *(41)*. Doctor Milner suggested that states of depression and anxiety associated with psychiatric disorders are probably accentuated by an inadequate intake of ascorbic acid.

ALCOHOLISM

In commenting on the psychiatric aspects of alcoholism, Doctor Ruth Fox *(26)* (Medical Director, National Council on

Table 9.10

major symptoms in 300 cases
of relative hypoglycemia

symptoms	per cent of patients reporting symptoms
psychiatric	
depression	60
insomnia	50
anxiety	50
irritability	45
crying spells	32
phobias	31
lack of concentration	30
forgetfulness or confusion	26
unsocial or antisocial behavior	22
restlessness	20
previous psychosis	12
suicidal	10
somatic	
exhaustion or fatigue	67
sweating	41
tachycardia	37
anorexia	32
chronic indigestion or bloating	29
cold hands or feet	26
joint pains	23
obesity	19
abdominal spasm	16
neurologic	
headache	45
dizziness	42
tremor (inward or external)	38
muscle pains and backache	33
numbness	29
blurred vision	24
muscular twitching or cramps	23
staggering	18
fainting or blackouts	14
convulsions	4

Table 9.11
percentage of improved elderly
schizophrenics receiving placebo
and nutritional supplements for one year

behavior	experimental group (22 patients)	placebo group (20 patients)
eating habits	86	20
toilet habits	82	25
interests	77	25
aggression	77	15
verbal interaction	77	0
bizarre behavior	77	0
appearance	73	20
productiveness	68	20
initiative	68	15

Alcoholism, Inc.) points out that this disorder is a chronic behavioral disturbance. She further states that alcoholism causes a regression in the patients to infantile states. Psychologic characteristics found with a battery of tests on 300 consecutive private patients showed the following character traits, many of which disappeared when the alcoholic became consistently abstinent *(26)*:

...inner battle between passivity and aggression, low frustration tolerance; inability to endure anxiety or tension; feelings of isolation, devaluated self-esteem, sometimes with overcompensation; undue sensitiveness; impulsive; repetitive acting out of conflicts; masochistics; self-punitive behavior and extreme narcissism or exhibitionism; strong sense of guilt; hostility, either overt or covert; strong dependent needs; marked rebellion; repressed grandiose ambitions with little ability to persevere; and sexual maladjustment.

Doctor Roger J. Williams *(71)*, Director of the Clayton Foundation for Research, has repeatedly noted that nutritional support reduces the physiologic craving for alcohol. He recommends a high-protein diet supplemented with therapeutic amounts of the available vitamins and minerals. Doctor Williams, in commenting on his dietary regime, made the following assertion *(71)*:

It is our opinion that in the great majority of individual alcoholics, the practical elimination of alcoholic craving can be assured, provided the recommendations which we have made are followed.

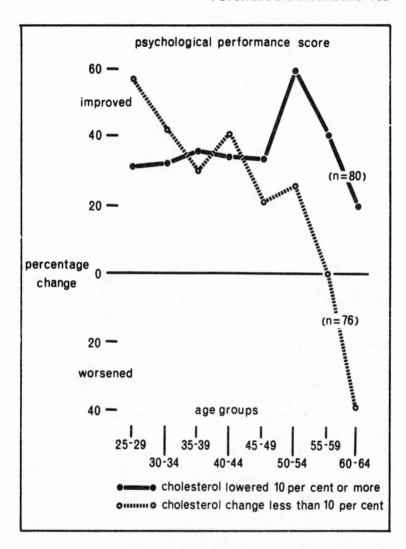

Figure 9.1
mean change in psychologic test performance (between a first and second examination) in healthy males with (n = 80) or without (n = 76) reductions of 10 per cent or more in serum cholesterol.

Table 9.12
effect of ascorbic acid and placebo
supplementation on psychologic test
scores in 40 chronic
psychiatric male patients

		before	after	P
MMPI results				
depression	active	72.8	64.8	< 0.01
	placebo	71.3	72.8	*
Wittenborn results				
depressed state	active	117	89	< 0.01
	placebo	124	116	< 0.05
manic state	active	66	50	< 0.02
	placebo	49	42	*
paranoid state	active	53	46	< 0.05
	placebo	45	45	*
schizophrenic	active	96	85	*
excitement	placebo	95	95	*
paranoid	active	87	82	*
schizophrenia	placebo	77	78	*
hebephrenic	active	112	102	*
schizophrenia	placebo	104	108	*

*statistically not significant

Whether they are followed is a question which must be answered separately in each individual case.

More evidence that alcoholism is, in part, a nutritional disorder comes from an experimental group at the Harlem Hospital Center, Department of Surgery, Division of Surgical Research. Doctor Aaron Prigot and co-workers (44) have found that, compared to 51 controls, intravenous amino acid supplements consistently reduce the duration of morbidity, severity of seizures and the necessity for ancillary sedation in patients with delirium tremens. These investigators pointed out that:

...amino acid preparations were employed prophylactically with a high degree of success to forestall delirium in patients whose clinical status or low amino acid levels indicated their susceptibility.

Assay of serum from these patients, by two-dimensional paper chromatography, revealed that depletion of amino acids was characteristic of delirium tremens. The values for the amino acids reverted to higher levels as the clinical manifestations of delirium abated following the administration of amino acid medication.

...Determinations before, during, and at the end of therapy showed no variation in total protein or albumin globulin ratios.

Doctor Herbert E. Karolus *(33)* of the Keelsy Institute in Dwight, Illinois, believes that the alcoholic is peculiarly sensitive to certain beverages. In 442 patients, skin tests for various foods revealed an average of seven allergic reactions per patient. The most frequently positive tests were for rye (308) and for wheat (239). Desensitization through weekly injections of allergenic extracts of offending substances appears "to be offering both physiologic and psychologic therapy" according to Doctor Karolus.

SUMMARY

In discussing the biochemical aspects of schizophrenia, Doctor Derek Richter *(48)* noted that the three primary etiologic factors are heredity, stress, and constitutional defense mechanisms. According to Doctor Richter, these defense factors include all the normal mechanisms that combat infection and deal with other forms of stress. He *(75)* commented further that:

It is hardly likely that every case can be explained on any one hypothesis and that a single 'cause of schizophrenia' will be found. On the other hand, there is evidence that the schizophrenias include a considerable group characterized by an impairment of the homeostatic control mechanisms situated in the hypothalamus.

Evidence of an abnormal biochemical profile in individuals with psychologic disorders has been presented. Many of these parameters are either directly or indirectly related to the dietary intake. Controlled studies employing dietary deficiencies and supplements have demonstrated, in part, cause-and-effect relationships.

Although not mentioned in the text, hormonal imbalances can lead to gross behavioral distortions *(20,67)*. The direct influence of diet upon the endocrines is well known.

The influence of diet upon homeostatic mechanisms such as glucose tolerance (Chapter Three, Nature of Health and Disease) and the ultimate role of abnormal carbohydrate metabolism in various disease manifestations is repeatedly asserted in this book. As pointed out in Chapter Three, disease is essentially a breakdown in the body's homeostatic metabolic control. The evidence cited in this chapter indicates that abnormal behavior may be a metabolic disorder, in part, related to diet and nutrition.

REFERENCES

1. Abrahamson, E. M. and Pezet, A. W. *Body, mind and sugar.* 1951. New York, Henry Holt and Company.
2. Albanese, A. A. *Protein and amino acid nutrition.* 1959. New York, Academic Press. p.309.
3. Anderson, W. McC. and Dawson, J. *Verbally retarded depression and sodium metabolism.* Brit. J. Psychiat. 109: #459, 225-230, March 1963.
4. Anderson, W. McC., Dawson, J. and Margerison, J. H. *Serial biochemical, clinical and electroencephalographic studies in affective illness.* Clinic. Sc. 26: #2, 323-336, April 1964.
5. Briggs, M. H. *Possible relations of ascorbic acid, ceruloplasmin and toxic aromatic metabolites in schizophrenia.* New Zealand Med. J. 61: #356, 229-236, April 1962.
6. Brozek, J. *Experimental studies on the impact of deficient diet on behavior.* Borden's Rev. Nutrit. Res. 20: #6, November-December 1959.
7. Brozek, J. *Soviet studies on nutrition and higher nervous activity.* Ann. New York Acad. Sc. 93: #15, 665-714, September 12, 1962.
8. Cade, J. F. J. *The relation between recovery and plasma potassium levels in manic states.* Med. J. Australia 2: #23, 911-913, December 8, 1962.
9. Cade, J. F. J. *The biochemistry of schizophrenics and affective psychoses.* Med. J. Australia 1: #23, 878-881, June 6, 1964.
10. Cerkez, C. T. and Ferguson, K. G. *Diabetes mellitus with secondary reactive hypoglycemia simulating a neuropsychiatric disorder.* Canad. Med. Assn. J. 92: #24, 1270-1273, June 12, 1965.
11. Conn, J. W. and Seltzer, H. S. *Spontaneous hypoglycemia.* Amer. J. Med. 19: #3, 460-478, September 1955.
12. Coppen, A. and Shaw, D. M. *Mineral metabolism in melancholia.* Brit. Med. J. 2: #5370, 1439-1444, December 7, 1963.
13. Cowley, J. J. and Griesel, R. D. *Low protein diet and emotionality in the albino rat.* J. Genet. Psychol. 104: #1, 89-98, 1964. Abstract in Psycholog. Abst. 39: #2, 462, April 1965.
14. Cumings, J. N. and Kremer, M. *Biochemical aspects of neurological disorders.* In Richter, D. *Biochemical aspects of anoxic and hyperglycemic states.* 1959. Oxford, England, Blackwell Scientific Publications. pp. 135-146.

15. Eiduson, S., Geller, E., Yuwiler, A. and Eiduson, B. T. *Biochemistry and behavior.* 1964. Princeton, D. Van Nostrand Company. pp. 4-5.

16. Eiduson, S., Geller, E., Yuwiler, A. and Eiduson, B. T. *Biochemistry and behavior.* 1964. Princeton, D. Van Nostrand Company. pp. 20-26.

17. Eiduson, S., Geller, E., Yuwiler, A. and Eiduson, B. T. *Biochemistry and behavior.* 1964. Princeton, D. Van Nostrand Company. pp. 26-29.

18. Eiduson, S., Geller, E., Yuwiler, A. and Eiduson, B. T. *Biochemistry and behavior.* 1964. Princeton, D. Van Nostrand Company. pp. 29-37.

19. Eiduson, G., Geller, E., Yuwiler, A. and Eiduson, B. T. *Biochemistry and behavior.* 1964. Princeton, D. Van Nostrand Company. pp. 37-39.

20. Eiduson, S., Geller, E., Yuwiler, A. and Eiduson, B. T. *Biochemistry and behavior.* 1964. Princeton, D. Van Nostrand Company. pp. 175-250.

21. Eiduson, S., Geller, E., Yuwiler, A. and Eiduson, B. T. *Biochemistry and behavior.* 1964. Princeton, D. Van Nostrand Company. pp. 261-270.

22. Eiduson, S., Geller, E., Yuwiler, A. and Eiduson, B. T. *Biochemistry and behavior.* 1964. Princeton, D. Van Nostrand Company. pp. 272-274.

23. Ferguson, D. C. and Fisher, A. E. *Behavior disruption in Cebus monkeys as a function of injected substances.* Science 139: #3561, 1281-1282, March 29, 1963.

24. Fincle, L. P. and Reyna, L. J. *A one year study of L-Glutavite on long term hospitalized, elderly, schizophrenic patients.* J. Clin. & Exper. Psychopath. 19: #1, 7-18, March 1958.

25. Fowlie, H. C., Cohen, C. and Anand, M. P. *Depression in elderly patients with subnutrition.* Geront. Clin. 5: 215-225, 1963.

26. Fox, R. *Psychiatric aspects of alcoholism.* Amer. J. Psychotherapy 19: #3, 408-416, July 1965.

27. Gjessing, L., Bernhardsen, A. and Froshaug, H. *Investigation of amino acids in a periodic catatonic patient.* J. Ment. Sc. 104: #434, 188-200, January 1958.

28. Gregory, I. and Paul, R. H. *Nutritional deficiencies in patients admitted to mental hospital.* Canad. M. A. J. 80: #3, 186-189, February 1, 1959.

29. Helps, E. P. W. *Senile confusion and the blood sugar level.* Lancet 1: #6960, 138-139, January 19, 1957.

30. Heyman, J. J. *Nicotinamide metabolism in schizophrenics, drug addicts and normals: the effect of psychotropic drugs and hormones.* Trans. New York Acad. Sc. 26: #3, 354-360, January 1964.

31. Himwich, H. E., Wolff, K., Hunsicker, A. L. and Himwich, W. A. *Some behavioral effects associated with feeding sodium glutamate to patients with psychiatric disorders.* J. Nerv. & Ment. Dis. 121: #1, 40-49, January 1955.

32. Interdepartmental Committee on Nutrition for National Defense. *Suggested guide for intepreting dietary and biochemical data.* Public Health Rep. 75: #8, 687-698, August 1960.

33. Karolus, H. E. *Alcoholism and food allergy.* Illinois Med. J. 119: #3, 151-152, March 1962.

34. Kollar, E. J., Slater, G. R., Palmer, J. O., Doctor, R. F. and Mandell, A. J. *Measurement of stress in fasting man.* Arch. Gen. Psychiat. 11: #2, 113-125, August 1964.

35. Kosenko, S. A. *The significance of vitamin B6 in normal activity of the cerebral cortex.* Zh. vipsh. nervn. Deiatel. 10: 291-296, 1960. Abstract in Psycholog. Abst. 35: #1, 55-56, February 1961.

36. Krjukova, N. A. *Pyridoxine (vitamin B6) in the treatment of deficiency disorders.* Klin. Med. Moscow 42: #9, 123-127, 1964, Abstract 2720 in Nutrit. Abst. & Rev. 35: #2, 477, April 1965.

37. Lortie, G. and Laird, D. M. *Hypoglycemia simulating psychoses.* New Eng. J. Med. 256: #25, 1190-1191, June 20, 1957.

38. Mann, S. A. *Blood sugar studies in mental disorders.* J. Ment. Sc. 71: #294, 443-473, July 1925.

39. Medical Tribune-World Wide Report. *Food sensitivity implicated in cases of mental disorder.* Med. Tribune 5: #101, September 23, 1964.

40. Medical Tribune-World Wide Report. *Diet corrects hypoglycemia mimicking psychopathology.* Med. Tribune & Med. News 6: #102, August 25, 1965.

41. Milner, G. *Malnutrition and mental disease.* Brit. Med. J. 1: #5272, 191, January 20, 1962.

42. Milner, G. *Ascorbic acid in chronic psychiatric patients—a controlled trial.* Brit. J. Psychiat. 109: #459, 294-299, March 1963.

43. Pollin, W., Cardon, P. V., Jr. and Kety, S. S. *Effects of amino acid feedings in schizophrenic patients treated with Iproniazid.* Science 133: #3446, 104-105, January 13, 1961.

44. Prigot, A., Corbin, E. E., Maynard, A. deL., Roden, T. P. and Hjelt-Harvey, I. *The treatment of delerium tremens with amino acids.* Quart. J. Studies Alcohol 23: #3, 390-410, September 1962.

45. Procter, L. M., Dewan, J. G. and McNeel, B. H. *Variations in the glucose tolerance observations in schizophrenics before and after shock treatment.* Amer. J. Psychiat. 100: 652-658, March 1944.

46. Reitan, R. M. and Shipley, R. E. *The relationship of serum cholesterol changes to psychological abilities.* J. Gerontol. 18: #4, 350-357, October 1963.

47. Richter, D. *Schizophrenia; somatic aspects.* 1957. New York, Permagon Press. pp. 56-59.

48. Richter, D. *Schizophrenia; somatic aspects.* 1957. New York, Permagon Press. pp. 68-72.

49. Richter, D. *Biochemical aspects of anoxic and hypoglycemic states.* In Cummings, J. N. and Kremer, M. *Biochemical aspects of neurological disorders.* 1959. Oxford, England, Blackwell Scientific Publications. pp. 144-146.

50. Rosenfeld, C. *Nutritional guidance can forestall broken marriages.* New Med. Materia 51: #8, 51-52, August 1962.

51. Salzer, H. M. *Relative hypoglycemia as a cause of neuropsychiatric illness.* J. National Med. Assn. 58: #1, 12-17, January 1966.

52. Sourkes, T. L. *Biochemistry of mental disease.* 1962. New York, Hoeber Medical Division, Harper and Row. p. 10.

53. Sourkes, T. L. *Biochemistry of mental disease.* 1962. New York, Hoeber Medical Division, Harper and Row. pp. 32-36.

54. Sourkes, T. L. *Biochemistry of mental disease.* 1962. New York, Hoeber Medical Division, Harper and Row, pp. 49-53.

55. Sourkes, T. L. *Biochemistry of mental disease.* 1962. New York, Hoeber Medical Division, Harper and Row. pp. 80-81.

56. Sourkes, T. L. *Biochemistry of mental disease.* 1962. New York, Hoeber Medical Division, Harper and Row. p. 156.

57. Sourkes, T. L. *Biochemistry of mental disease.* 1962. New York, Hoeber Medical Division, Harper and Row. pp. 171-172.

58. Sourkes, T. L. *Biochemistry of mental disease.* 1962. New York, Hoeber Medical Division, Harper and Row. pp. 206-208.

59. Sourkes, T. L. *Biochemistry of mental disease.* 1962. New York, Hoeber Medical Division, Harper and Row. pp. 216, 251-252.

60. Sourkes, T. L. *Biochemistry of mental disease.* 1962. New York, Hoeber Medical Division, Harper and Row. pp. 220-223.

61. Sourkes, T. L. *Biochemistry of mental disease.* 1962. New York, Hoeber Medical Division, Harper and Row. pp. 228-230.

62. Sourkes, T. L. *Biochemistry of mental disease.* 1962. New York, Hoeber Medical Division, Harper and Row. pp. 239-241.

63. Sourkes, T. L. *Biochemistry of mental disease.* 1962. New York, Hoeber Medical Division, Harper and Row. pp. 251-252.

64. Sourkes, T. L. *Biochemistry of mental disease.* 1962. New York, Hoeber Medical Division, Harper and Row. pp. 252-254.

65. Sourkes, T. L. *Biochemistry of mental disease.* 1962. New York, Hoeber Medical Division, Harper and Row. pp. 259-261.

66. Sourkes, T. L. *Biochemistry of mental disease.* 1962. New York, Hoeber Medical Division, Harper and Row. pp. 265-266.

67. Sourkes, T. L. *Biochemistry of mental disease.* 1962. New York, Hoeber Medical Division, Harper and Row. pp. 296-350.

68. Stewart, W. H. *Who gets what care and how?* In *The health care issues of the 1960's.* 1963. New York, Group Health Insurance, Inc. pp. 22-23.

69. Wiener, J. S. and Hope, J. M. *Cerebral manifestations of vitamin B12 deficiency.* J. A. M. A. 170: #9, 1038-1041, June 27, 1959.

70. Williams, D. *Clinical aspects of anoxic and hypoglycemic states.* In Cummings, J. N. and Kremer, M. *Biochemical aspects of neurological disorders.* 1959. Oxford, England, Blackwell Scientific Publications. pp. 147-155.

71. Williams, R. J. *Alcoholism, the nutritional approach.* 1959. Austin, Texas, University of Texas Press.

72. Woolley, D. W. *The biochemical bases of psychoses.* 1962. New York, John Wiley and Sons. pp. 170-171.

73. Woolley, D. W. *The biochemical bases of psychoses.* 1962. New York, John Wiley and Sons. pp. 268-276.

74. Woolley, D. W. *The biochemical bases of psychoses.* 1962. New York, John Wiley and Sons. p. 310.

10. CANCER

CANCER IS THE SECOND LEADING CAUSE OF MORTALITY, ACCOUNTING for approximately one in every seven deaths in the United States. The following figures reflect the changing dimensions of the oncologic problem *(143)*:

> In 1900, only 3.7 per cent of the deaths in the United States were attributed to cancer, whereas in 1962, this figure had risen to 15.9 per cent. The proportion of overall mortality attributed to cancer...indicates one peak for the age interval 5 - 10 and another during the interval 46 - 65. The American Cancer Society recently estimated 295,000 cancer deaths for 1965....

Important as they are, death statistics by themselves cannot adequately define the problem. Obviously, everyone who develops cancer does not necessarily die from cancer. Its true impact can be better visualized in Table 10.1 which shows the actual projected figures for new cases and cases under treatment, as well as cancer deaths, for 1940 through 1975. That the estimates in this table are conservative is suggested by the projected figure for cancer deaths in 1965 (282,000). This is actually less by 13,000 than occurred according to the previously cited American Cancer Society estimate of 295,000. Under conditions existing in 1954, it was estimated that 32 of every 100 newborn children could be expected to develop cancer at some time during their life and that approximately 50,000,000 people then alive could also anticipate cancer *(34)*.

A little known fact is that the incidence of cancer in children under fourteen has almost doubled in little more than a decade, and that of leukemia has increased almost sixfold in the fifty-year period ending in 1951 *(80)*. Although carcinoma of the colon and rectum have not received wide-

Table 10.1
estimates of cancer incidence, prevalence,
and mortality, United States, 1940-1975

year	new cases	cases under treatment	cancer deaths
1940	380,000	528,000	165,255*
1950	497,000	668,000	210,733*
1953	530,000	711,000	225,000
1960	605,000	811,000	259,000
1965	656,000	879,000	282,000
1970	706,000	945,000	304,000
1975	753,000	1,008,000	326,000

*actual number reported by the National Office
of Vital Statistics, Public Health Service

spread publicity, they account for 29 per cent of the cancer deaths in this country. This is more than for any other organ site. Death rates from prostatic cancer since 1930 have almost doubled for the white and have tripled for the nonwhite groups. Among men, the most substantial increases in both death rate and frequency of occurrence for the period 1930-1960 have been leukemia and cancers of the lung, pancreas, and prostate. For women in the same period the increases have been most marked for leukemia and cancers of the lung, pancreas, colon (excluding rectum), and ovary. The increases for women are not as pronounced as those for men (143). While part of the increment is due to improved reporting and medical diagnosis, there has unquestionably been a true increase in incidence and mortality.

Faced with a problem of this magnitude, it is not surprising that a tremendous multidisciplinary force of investigators has been mobilized in every civilized nation to combat cancer. Although this mighty effort was initiated well over a half century ago and pursued with dedication, there is evidence that the results have been disappointing. Doctor E. Grunberg, addressing the Division of Microbiology of the New York Academy of Sciences in 1963, reflects this point of view:

In retrospect our experimental approach to the therapy of inoperable malignancies has, more or less, been a failure....For many years now the experimental chemotherapist has been searching for a cytotoxic agent. Unfortunately, experience has shown that an agent toxic for malignant cells is usually toxic for the normal cell. Might it not be worthwhile now to reconsider...that a process within the body is responsible for the development of neoplastic cells....This might mean not treating the tumor cell but rather the host.

Expressing his concern for the lack of progress during the last fifty years of research, Sir Charles Dodds (Professor of Biochemistry, University of London, England) made this perceptive analogy in 1949 *(37)*:

A hundred years ago one of the great menaces to life was suppuration....One can well imagine a group of philanthropic people banding together to form an organization to investigate the fatal malady. Having collected the money, they would be faced with how to proceed to spend it. One way would be to form institutions for the study of suppuration, and those would correspond to the purely cancer research institutions.

Here one can imagine the workers collecting purulent discharges, analyzing, investigating them microscopically, and so forth. We know today that they could have gone on doing this to the present time without getting any nearer to the solution. Before the mystery of suppuration could be solved, Pasteur had to found the science of bacteriology....we then had to have Lister with his development of antiseptic surgery....

We should take this lesson to heart and realize that everyone who is working in the biological sciences is a potential cancer research worker and actually may be paving the way to the knowledge that will discover a cure of this disease.

With a concept of the ecologic nature of cancer in mind, the following conclusion reached by Doctor Thomas A. McCoy in an extensive 1959 review in the first edition of the *World Review of Nutrition and Dietetics* takes on added significance *(114)*:

Nutrition is the process by which living matter can absorb and utilize exogenous substances for maintenance and/or growth. Since the neoplasm in the body is dependent upon the host for a supply of amino acids, carbohydrates, fats, vitamins, minerals, and a number of cofactors, it is only reasonable that the critical period of tumor development, as well as tumor growth, can be influenced by the dietary regime and the nutritional status of the host.

CORRELATIVE FINDINGS

Lower Animal Observations: The paucity of this type of observation in cancer etiology research and some of the probable reasons for it has recently been discussed *(80)*.

At a California border station, hepatic carcinoma in epidemic proportions was discovered during routine inspection of a shipment of rainbow trout from an Idaho hatchery *(213)*. It subsequently became clear that hepatomas or hepatocarcinomas are almost endemic in hatched trout all over the world, but they seldom, if ever affect wild trout. The intensive investigations that followed and the subsequent findings have been thoroughly reviewed *(92,212)*. It appears well established now that the outbreak was brought about by a change from an unprocessed, largely meat diet to a processed, dry pelleted ration consisting of steam or flame dried animal meal and vegetable meal, vitamins, minerals, antioxidants, antibiotics, antifungicides, and other substances. Since not all commercial rations produced hepatomas, it was concluded that processing, storage, or source of ration component had something to do with the carcinogenicity of the "hot" rations. Subsequently, investigation *(66)* suggested that the lipid fraction alone extracted from the total ration contains the carcinogen(s). A still later study based on the component parts of the ration indicated that cottonseed meal was the one essential for carcinogenesis *(212)*. Prior to the implication of cottonseed meal, processing degradation products (largely concentrated in fish meal) were the prime suspect. The carcinogenic process is thought to be initiated through absence of vitamin E or antioxidants and presence of lipid peroxides or polymers which hasten lipoid degeneration of the liver and ultimate development of liver cancer *(58)*. Other factors being investigated are pesticides, defoliants and fungal metabolites found in the rations.

In the south and east of England over 100,000 turkey poults died, victims of a mysterious disease. On postmortem examination, the turkeys were found to have acute hepatic necrosis with generalized bile duct proliferation *(15)*. The mystery of the turkey deaths was more rapidly resolved. "Turkey X disease," as it was called, has been found to be related to peanut meal contaminated with a toxic mold known to cause hepatic carcinoma in rats *(15)*. A poison called afla-toxin, produced by the fungus *Aspergillus flavus*, was identified as the culprit. It is but one of a series of fungal contaminants which may occur in cereal products and other foods. Ramifi-cations of this finding will be considered subsequently.

These two incidents in 1960, widely separated geographi-cally, focused major attention on possible parallelisms between diet and cancer in lower animals.

Human Observations: In Table 10.2 it will be noted that some thirty-odd reports of relationships between neoplasia and diet are listed. The target organs most frequently impli-cated are the digestive tract, liver and genitals. Most of the studies can be broadly grouped into four categories: those relating to obesity and generalized overeating; those associated with generalized undernutrition; those identified with the consumption of a specific food item, beverage, or food con-taminant; and those concerned with relatively "immune" cancer groups.

In view of the frequency of overnutrition and obesity in this country (Chapter One, The American Diet), the findings relating these dietary problems to cancer carry added signi-ficance. The rather extensive study of dietary habits of cancer patients and the surveys of life insurance statistics suggest that individuals who overeat and are overweight when past middle-age are more likely to die of cancer than are persons of average weight or less *(168, 169)*. In the few instances where neoplasms were classified according to site, obesity seemed to correlate most closely with malignancies of the intestines, liver and gallbladder, and genitourinary organs.

The most convincing findings relating overnutrition to carcinomatosis have emerged from investigations of patients with endometrial cancer *(56,70,124,215)*. These patients are frequently characterized by obesity, decreased glucose tolerance, nulliparity, and a history of numerous spontaneous abortions. Of equal interest are the five-year survival rates after irradiation of patients with cancer of the uterine cervix *(73)*. A survival rate of only 38 per cent was noted among patients weighing over 170 pounds as compared with 55 per cent of those less than 170 pounds.

The reports of generalized malnutrition in Western coun-

Table 10.2
diet and cancer
(human correlative observations)

dietary variable	site	references

reported to inhibit incidence of cancer

dietary variable	site	references
undernutrition during	not specified	74*
World War I	stomach	130,132
certain primitive diets	not specified	8, 35, 108, 145, 153
	breast	98
certain oriental diets	stomach	17
	liver	122

reported to favor incidence of cancer

dietary variable	site	references
generalized malnutrition	not specified	12, 55
	upper alimentary tract	2, 214
high fat and obesity	genitourinary tract	78
	upper alimentary tract, stomach, intestines, liver and gall bladder, genitourinary tract	169
	genitourinary tract	56, 70, 73, 124, 215
	skin	44
protein deficiency	genitourinary	1
	liver and gall bladder	11, 12
alcohol	mouth	216
	stomach	146
sugar	intestine, genitourinary tract	166
vitamin A deficiency	upper alimentary tract	193
mineral excesses (sodium chloride, lead, arsenic, nitrate, boron, manganese, chromium, titanium)	not specified	30, 197
	stomach	75
mineral deficiencies (strontium, calcium, trace minerals, iodine)	not specified	30
	stomach	75, 185
	thyroid gland	167, 201
food cooking & processing methods, contaminants, seasoning agents, coffee, tea	upper alimentary tract	62
	stomach	39, 146, 194
	liver and gall bladder	148
	genitourinary tract	166
	hemopoietic tissues	102

*mortality rather than incidence of cancer

tries seem chiefly related to malignancies of the upper alimentary tract *(2,214)*. Those reports emanating from the non-western countries *(1,11,12,55,78)* are concerned primarily with hepatic and genitourinary cancer. This includes nutritional disturbances classed as protein lack. Parenthetic mention should be made that, clinically, protein deficiency without an accompanying lack of vitamins and/or minerals is rarely encountered.

Excessive consumption of several specific food and beverage items has been implicated as a possible cause of cancer, usually of specific target organs. Items of particular interest because of their high rate of consumption in this country are animal fats, alcohol, sugar, and coffee.

A much higher incidence of various types of skin cancer in New Zealand than in England, France or the United States has been reported. This, in turn, has been related to New Zealand's higher animal fat consumption *(44)*. In this country a high correlation between oral cancer and alcohol consumption has been described *(216)*. This may be associated with the generalized malnutrition which so frequently accompanies excessive alcohol use.

Recently *(166)*, statistical relationships between coffee and sugar consumption of twenty-two countries and the age-adjusted death rate from cancer of urogenital and digestive organs were analyzed (Table 10.3). Both coffee and sugar consumption correlated with prostatic cancer. Sugar consumption also correlated with breast, ovarian, bladder, intestinal, and rectal malignancy. Although the roasting procedure of coffee is emphasized as a possible etiologic factor, at the International Union Against Cancer (Rome, 1956), Doctor D. G. Steyn *(154)*, Professor of Pharmacology, Medical Faculty, University of Pretoria, South Africa, focused attention on caffeine in carbonated soft drinks and coffee as a possible carcinogen.

Heat, various condiments, table salt, and smoked meat and fish have been strongly implicated in malignancies of the mouth, pharynx, esophagus, and stomach. Japan has the highest incidence of gastric cancer in the world. An excellent investigation *(75)* of stomach cancer in Japan suggested that an extremely high intake of salty food and, to a lesser extent,

Table 10.3
correlation coefficients between estimated
national average consumption of coffee and
sugar with age-adjusted death rate from cancer
of urogenital and digestive organs in 20 countries

age-adjusted death rate from	coffee		sugar	
	male	female	male	female
prostate cancer	0.700***		0.771***	
breast cancer		0.420		0.833***
ovary cancer (13 countries)		0.403		0.828***
uterus cancer		− 0.158		0.097
bladder cancer (13 countries)	0.039	0.144	0.500	0.649*
esophagus cancer	0.058	0.196	− 0.047	0.198
stomach cancer	0.201	− 0.146	− 0.165	− 0.187
intestine cancer	0.315	0.344	0.697**	0.709***
rectum cancer	0.258	0.125	0.680**	0.656**

* $P < 0.05$
** $P < 0.01$
***$P < 0.001$

a low intake of milk were the major factors.

The previously mentioned discovery of the carcinogenic effects of aflatoxin in moldy products, such as peanuts, rice, and corn, has world-wide significance in both the human and animal (92) and is intimately related to dietary habits. The high incidence of malignant hepatoma and liver cirrhosis among Orientals and some natives of Central Africa has been attributed to protein deficiency and generalized malnutrition (11). It is obvious that the effects of moldy diet components also must be considered, and this is presently being studied (92). The problem is not just one for the underdeveloped nations. Aflatoxin (0.2 to 0.3 p.p.m.) has been found in Dutch peanut butter samples. It has also been isolated from the milk (but not from the liver or blood) of cows fed toxic peanut meal. Fungal contamination could involve many cereal products and protein sources utilized by man, such as soybeans, corn, oats, wheat, milk powders, cheese, and bread (92).

Another food contaminant has been indicted as a possible carcinogen. The high incidence of leukemia in Nebraska, and especially among the farmers whose leukemic incidence is twice what would be predicted for them, has led to speculation that milk-borne and egg-borne viruses may be responsible (102).

It should be noted that calcium in milk and iodine and strontium in the soil and plants have been associated with a decreased incidence of neoplasia; whereas the reverse has been true in the case of arsenic, nitrate, boron, manganese, chromium, titanium, and lead in soil and plant samples. Certainly this is an area deserving of more definitive investigation.

Relatively little attention has been directed toward cancer-free or relatively free groups. Diets reported to be associated with a low incidence of cancer vary markedly as to content, but they are surprisingly similiar in a number of aspects if the wartime diets are disregarded. First, they are nutritionally balanced and adequate. Second, prolonged cooking is generally avoided. Finally, excessive amounts of salt, condiments and nutritionally empty foods such as alcohol and sugar are seldom used. Wartime diets have been discussed in Chapter Six (Obstetrical Complications). Except in time of outright famine, these seem to be not undesirable in that they emphasize simple, wholesome foods in moderate amounts rather than nutritionally undesirable luxury items.

The famous Arctic explorer, Vilhjalmur Stefansson, has written about the diets of primitive peoples who seemed remarkably healthy, long-lived and free of cancer (153). Doctor Philip R. White, with the Roscoe B. Jackson Memorial Laboratory in Bar Harbor, Maine, made the following comments in the preface of Stefansson's book, *Cancer: Disease of Civilization* (210):

> Here is the sort of thing we call *basic research*, just as much so as if it were being conducted in the latest of laboratories. Here are the data from a series of experiments which Nature has performed for us - in the Arctic northland, in the tropic forests of Gabon, and in the temperate valley of Hunzaland. She has varied a series of environmental factors yet come up with a like result in the three places, and a result which she has produced, so far as we know, *only* in those three special combinations of environments....

THERAPEUTIC FINDINGS

Lower Animal Observations: A wide variety of nutrients has been studied in lower animals in terms of possible relationships to neoplasia. A lack or an excess of calories per se, fats, proteins, carbohydrates, and to a lesser extent, vitamins and even minerals, has been implicated in the inhibition or prevention (Table 10.4), and encouragement (Table 10.5) of malignant growths. Some nutrients are reported to have no effect (Table 10.6) upon neoplasia. As with teratogeny investigations, an extremely limited number of animal species has been utilized, chiefly rats and mice.

A number of writers *(10,114,168)* have cited the problems in experimental design. Paired feeding, caloric restriction, and forced feeding are each conceded to have limitations. Because of the active nutritional parasitism of malignancies and their consequent priority on the utilization of dietary components, the manner of feeding of the experimental and control animals may be of critical importance. What cannot be exactly equated in the control animal by any of the above mentioned alternatives is the extraction of nutrients from the host that occurs when the malignancy outstrips the dietary supply. Studies have been concerned with the incidence (genesis), rate of growth, time of appearance, and metastatic variabilities of neoplasms. Most attention has been focused on the first two characteristics. It is quite apparent that a factor affecting the origin of a tumor in one way may influence its growth in quite a different manner or not at all.

On the basis of the lower animal experimental studies, it appears that dietary variations seem to exert more influence on the initiation of neoplasms than on their growth. Reducing total food consumption without changing the ratio of the nutrients or reduction in the amounts of carbohydrate, fat or proteins singly and in various combinations have all resulted in a reduced incidence of tumor formation *(167)*.

As might be expected, this inhibiting effect varies considerably *(131)*. The kind of tumor, the nature and potency of the carcinogen(s), the degree of caloric restriction, and the composition of the restricted diet are factors of special importance. Halving the caloric intake may reduce the incidence of certain tumors to zero and exert little or no effect upon

Table 10.4
diet and cancer
(lower animal therapeutic observations
reported to inhibit or prevent neoplasia)

dietary variable	species used	sites	references
caloric restriction			
underfeeding all nutrients, fat & carbohydrates, & carbohydrates alone; reduction of induced obesity	mouse rat	intestines, liver & gall bladder, breast, skin, subcutaneous & fibrous tissues, hemopoietic tissues, lung	13, 14, 18, 23, 29, 42, 52, 81, 109, 110, 111, 112, 113, 120, 136, 137, 138, 141, 142, 157, 171, 172, 173, 174, 175, 176, 177, 180, 181, 188, 199, 204, 205
fat intake			
linolenic acid, cholesterol, heptaldehyde supplements	mouse, rat & dog	liver & gall bladder	144, 155, 156
protein & amino intake			
low protein, high protein, low amino acid, high amino acid	mouse rat	liver & gall bladder, breast, skin, subcutaneous & fibrous tissues, hemopoietic tissues, kidney	9, 36, 41, 51, 59, 61, 64, 67, 76, 84 117, 121, 123, 126, 127, 139, 151, 161, 162, 163, 179, 180, 189, 190, 191, 192, 202, 205, 206, 209, 211
carbohydrate intake			
qualitative changes	mouse	liver & gall bladder	122, 151
vitamin & mineral intake			
riboflavin, thiamine, B complex, biotin, B12, vitamin C & hesperidin, copper salts & allinase supplements; riboflavin antagonist, pyridoxine deficient-high riboflavin & vitamin C deficient	mouse, rat & guinea pig	liver & gall bladder, breast, subcutaneous & fibrous tissue, lung	5, 28, 49, 50, 84, 86, 90, 95, 116, 117, 119, 125, 133, 134, 151, 158

Table 10.5
diet and cancer
(lower animal therapeutic observations
reported to favor neoplasia)

dietary variable	species used	sites	references
caloric restriction			
induced overeating & high calorie diets	mouse & rat	liver & gall bladder, breast, skin	9, 19, 22, 27, 47, 51, 53, 71, 72, 100, 118, 128, 137, 138, 163, 164, 165, 172, 200, 207, 218
fat intake			
low fat (one study), high fat with high or low calorie, high fat-low choline, lard and/or cholesterol, cotton-seed & sesame oil, egg lipids, corn oil, & cod-liver oil supplements	mouse, rat & chicken	liver & gall bladder, breast, subcutaneous & fibrous tissue, skin, genitourinary tract, ear, eye, lung, mesentery, lym-phatic tissue	9, 19, 22, 27, 47, 51, 53, 71, 72, 118 128, 137, 138, 163, 164, 165, 172, 218
protein & amino acid intake			
low protein-variable fat & carbohydrate, high protein (liver, casein, lactalbumin, peanut meal, lysophilyzed tumor tissue), low cystine, high amino acid (methi-onine, tryptophane)	mouse & rat	liver & gall bladder, genitourinary tract, breast, subcutaneous & fibrous tissue, ear, lung, kidney, lym-phatic tissues	4, 9, 28, 40, 41, 51, 57, 77, 115, 138, 139, 140, 147, 151, 164, 204, 208
carbohydrate intake			
sugar injections, rice in place of sugar, polished rice	mouse & rat	stomach, liver & gall bladder, subcutaneous & fibrous tissue	6, 128, 159
vitamin & mineral intake			
low vitamins A or ribo-flavin; maintenance level of synthetic B vitamin supplement; biotin or B12 added; low iodine; iron-dextran, lead, or sodium fluoride added	rat, mouse, sheep, fly	stomach, thyroid gland, liver & gall bladder, genitourinary tract, breast, skin, subcu-taneous & fibrous tissue, kidney	26, 43, 54, 60, 69, 106, 107, 119, 133, 184, 187, 219, 220
cooking or processing methods & contaminants			
milk-borne virus, toxic peanut meal & cotton-seed meal	mouse, rat, trout	liver & gall bladder, hemopoietic tissues	66, 94, 96, 212

Table 10.6
diet and cancer
(lower animal therapeutic observations
reported to have no effect on neoplasia)

dietary variable	species used	sites	references
caloric restriction			
underfeeding all nutrients, restricted calorie-variable protein, carbohydrate	mouse, rat	liver & gall bladder, breast, skin, subcutaneous & fibrous tissues, lung, adrenal gland	29, 32, 42, 87, 103, 135, 136, 137, 157, 170, 174, 178
fat intake			
cottonseed oil & sesame seed oil or cholesterol supplement	mouse, rat	breast, skin	9, 22, 165
protein & amino acid intake			
high to low protein with & without cystine & riboflavin supplements; low tryptophane, lysine, cystine intake	mouse, rat	liver & gall bladder, breast, skin, subcutaneous tissues, hemopoietic tissues	4, 41, 91, 97, 121, 160, 179, 202, 203, 209
carbohydrate intake			
sugar injections	rat	subcutaneous & fibrous tissues	71
vitamin, mineral & enzyme intake			
multivitamin, yeast, or vitamin E supplements, low biotin, mineral supplement, allinase supplement	mouse, rat	liver & gall bladder, breast, skin, hemopoietic tissues	28, 85, 95, 158, 180
food processing			
heating of fats	mouse, rat	stomach, subcutaneous & fibrous tissues	88, 89, 100

others. Again, even a small reduction in food intake may be beneficial in the suppression of tumor formation in still another situation. The duration of the period of dietary restriction also appears to be an important determinant in some instances. In the mouse, mammary tumors and hepatomas are most susceptible, and skin tumors and sarcomas least sensitive to caloric restriction.

Several theories have been advanced to explain the inhibitory effect of dietary restriction on neoplasia: a generalized inhibitory effect on mitotic activity including that of the latent cancer cell *(24)*, the limited ability of the tumor cells to compete with normal ones in the critical period when there is a nidus of relatively few cells with no independent blood supply *(99)*, and the lack of oil on the skin which increases the penetration of rays in the case of ultraviolet radiation *(137)*. Doctor A. Tannenbaum (Director, Department of Cancer Research, Medical Research Institute, Michael Reese Hospital, Chicago, Illinois) believes that an excessive fat intake, regardless of the total caloric consumption, enhances tumor formation *(173)*. Certainly the evidence, Table 10.5, would seem to substantiate this opinion. He suggests two mechanisms. Acting as a solvent, fat concentrates the carcinogen in the skin; as a co-carcinogen, fat causes a metabolic stimulation of carcinogenesis.

More recent studies (163-165) suggest a relationship between the types of malignancies and the composition of the lipids ingested by the animals. For example, a strain of mice maintained on a cholesterol supplemented diet developed a high incidence of lung adenocarcinoma but minimal mammary cancer. When lard was added to the diet, there was a high incidence of both *(165)*.

The response of neoplasms to changes in protein intake parallels changes in the host itself. Incidence, rate of appearance, and growth vary little with protein intakes suitable for good general health, i.e., 9 to 45 per cent milk protein (casein) *(179)*. No doubt, varying the experimental conditions would influence the latitude within which no influence on neoplasia would be exerted. Evaluation of individually added amino acids in respect to their effect on carcinogenesis is difficult. The problem is one of discerning whether the effect is due to the specific role of the amino acid or simply to the fact that the protein is more complete.

The literature relating vitamin intake to cancer is rather limited (Tables 10.4, 10.5 and 10.6). An inhibitory effect on neoplasia has been noted in instances of various vitamin deficiency states. However, with few exceptions as with protein, this has been achieved only at levels that markedly impair the growth and well-being of the host.

The most notable exception to the foregoing has been the

favorable effect of protein and some B vitamins on azo dye-induced hepatomas. The favorable effect of both casein and methionine on azo dye-induced hepatomas has been attributed to an improvement in the liver's ability to retain riboflavin.

The recent findings regarding the role of food contaminants as carcinogens will necessitate a reappraisal of many earlier studies upon which such conclusions are based. The original work of Engel, Copeland, and Salmon (48) suggesting that choline-deficient diets potentiate hepatomagenesis has been cited as an example (92). Recent work (140) now ascribes the contributing role in this hepatomagenesis to the fungal metabolites in peanut meal, the protein source in the diet. It is now clear that no dietary component or food should be labeled carcinogenic until all associated entities have been defined.

Biotin has been reported to increase the incidence of hepatoma. However, eggwhite protein, regardless of its content of avidin (biotin-antagonist) or the biotin supply of the animal, also inhibits liver neoplasia (90). Pyridoxine deficiency under certain circumstances has been reported to retard azo dye-induced hepatomas (116,119). Folic acid antagonists have generally been reported to inhibit certain kinds of transmissible mouse leukemia and a few other types. An inhibitory effect of ascorbic acid deficiency on the growth of transplanted sarcomas in guinea pigs has been recognized (134).

Generally speaking, modification of the proportion of dietary mineral salts within the limits supporting good body growth has had no noteworthy effect on carcinogenesis (180). An exception has been the reported inhibitory effect of added copper salts on azo dye carcinogenesis (86). A more recent report credits 0.5 per cent cupric oxyacetate with providing a better degree of protection than riboflavin (in the form of two extracts—yeast autolysate or a bovine tissue mixture) against one of the most potent of the azo dye carcinogens (50).

Today there is an increased awareness of the extent and severity of the metabolic lesion in the tumor-bearing animal. However, knowledge as to why malignant cells can synthesize protein, for example, at the expense of the host is still limited. Doctor G. B. Mider, Director in charge of Research at the National Cancer Institute, and his associates established that lyophilized tumor tissue used as a source of nitrogen in the diet can stimulate food intake and weight gain in tumor-bearing rats that have reached a weight plateau on a 20 per cent casein diet (115,208). Subsequent investigation suggests that this activity is due primarily to the sodium ion content (207).

The role of diet and its influence on metastasis has recently come under scrutiny for the first time (51). The intraportal injection of carcinoma cells into rats was done to evaluate the effect of diet (protein intake and high fat, choline-free and choline-supplemented diets) on the development of hepatic metastases. This site was selected because the liver is the organ most frequently affected by metastases regardless of the source of the primary carcinoma. The effect of varying both fat and protein dietary components prior and subsequent to tumor cell injection was evaluated. It was observed that, when the amount of protein consumed in the diet was decreased without altering caloric intake, the number of animals demonstrating hepatic metastases two weeks after injecting the tumor cells was also reduced. Reversing the protein-free and high-protein diets after tumor inoculation reversed the incidence of metastases also. It was concluded that the inhibitory effect involved tumor growth rather than neoplastic initiation. Also it was concluded that variations in the amount of dietary fat, per se, do not influence metastatic growth. Only when a fatty liver develops, as happened on a high fat, choline-free diet, was metastatic incidence increased.

An Italian study (28), employing the same technique, noted the inhibitory effect of a low protein diet on liver and pulmonary metastases. Administration of an ascorbic acid-bioflavonoid-benzoylcarbinol preparation produced an inhibition of pulmonary lesions. No effect was observed with high protein, vitamin E supplemented, or vitamin deficient diets.

The significance of these studies is underscored by the finding that, in intestinal cancer, operative technique plays a minor role in the degree of dissemination of tumor cells in the blood. Tumor cells were found in the blood of 51 per cent of a series of such cancer patients at the time of operation who survived five to nine years (46).

Human Observations: An examination of Table 10.7 reveals that the very modest number of attempts to apply cancer dietotherapy can be divided into two general categories: those involving preventive measures in populations and those concerned with the treatment of individual cancer patients.

In the former group only two attempts have been recorded. One relates to an inherent iodine deficiency of the plants and the soil in which they are grown (195). The second has to do with dietary deficiencies brought about by food processing procedures and/or improper food selection in the Arctic Circle (217).

Iodized salt has been used successfully to reduce goiter formation in areas where iodine deficiency is endemic. Since goiter formation was thought to be a frequent cancer precursor, a reduction in thyroid cancer was also expected. Although there is some indication that the more severe forms are seen less frequently, the overall incidence appears unchanged according to a Swiss study (195,196).

Wynder (Division of Cancerigenesis, Sloan-Kettering Institute of Cancer Research, New York City) and his associates (217) continued the earlier investigations (2) of the Swedish women living in the Arctic Circle. It was felt that the initial steps taken by the Swedish Public Health Service in 1938, the addition of iron and vitamins to flour and a general dietary improvement, might be responsible for the reduction observed in some types of cancer related to Plummer-Vinson syndrome. The diets of the victims of this syndrome were almost totally lacking in vitamin C, as well as being low in other vitamins and protein. It was thought that this might have been an important factor in reducing the absorption of an already marginal intake of iron, thus leading to anemia, atrophic changes, and the precancerous stages.

Specific nutrients or nutrient-antagonists have been used therapeutically in a few instances on individual patients to inhibit or destroy neoplasms. The nutrients have not been used so much to correct a suspected deficit, but rather as pharmacologic entities. The best controlled and most extensive studies of this type have been those involving the treatment, with massive doses of vitamin A, of oral leukoplakia, a frequently precancerous lesion similar to that seen in Plummer-Vinson disease. This therapy has been repeatedly demonstrated to be effective *(82,149,150,152)*. Symptoms of overdosage may occur, however, but remissions will result with discontinuation of therapy. In a study of 40 subjects with leukoplakia conducted under double-blind conditions *(82)*, 400,000 I. U. of

Table 10.7
diet and cancer
(human therapeutic observations)

dietary variable	lesion studied	references
reported to inhibit neoplasia		
general dietary improvement		
high calorie, protein, vitamin & mineral diet tube-fed	cachexia from advanced cancer	129
general dietary improvement in subjects with malnutrition & Plummer-Vinson's disease	upper alimentary tract cancer	217
protein intake		
addition of amino acids to create amino acid imbalance	leukemia	3
low protein, purine-free diet	leukemia	65
vitamin and mineral intake		
massive doses of vitamin A	leukoplakia	82, 149, 150, 152
massive doses of vitamin B12	neuroblastoma	16
doses of folic acid antagonist	leukemia	25
	choriocarcinoma	105
iodized salt in endemic goiter areas	goiter formation	195
food decomposition product		
rancid fat component (heptaldehyde) injection	breast cancer	101
reported to favor neoplasia		
caloric increase		
force feeding patients in a metabolic ward	cachexia and cancer growth rate	104, 182, 186, 198
mineral intake		
dextran-iron IM in one patient with uterine cancer (stage II) developed	metastasis at injection site	183
reported to have no effect on neoplasia		
mineral intake		
use of iodized salt in endemic goiter areas	thyroid cancer	195, 196
dextran-iron complex IM, 40 million injections in 3 million patients	no malignancy at injection site	183

vitamin A were administered daily to one-half of the subjects for 21 days. A reduction in size, favorable qualitative change in the lesions, and histologic evidence of improvement in a substantial sample of the vitamin A supplemented group resulted.

Vitamin antagonists have been used in the treatment of tumors of embryonal origin. This approach to therapy is based on the observed ability of these agents to precipitate miscarriage and teratogenesis. Metastatic uterine choriocarcinoma usually causes death within a year, and testicular choriocarcinoma has nearly 100 per cent mortality in two years, regardless of the therapeutic approach. Using amethopterin, a folic acid antagonist, Doctor Min C. Li (Sloan-Kettering Institute, New York City) obtained temporary or sustained remissions for two years or more (105). Temporary remissions have also been reported with folic acid antagonists in acute leukemias in children (25).

Tentative success of a limited nature in the use of dietotherapy for the treatment of cancer in children has been reported by others. The use of massive dosages of vitamin B12 in the treatment of neuroblastoma is suggested (16). Acute leukemia has been treated with a low protein, purine-free diet (65) and by the addition of two amino acids to the diets to create an amino acid imbalance at the cellular level (3).

A chemical factor in rancid fat, heptaldehyde, was used in the treatment of two patients with inoperable metastatic breast cancer with apparent limited success according to a preliminary report (101). Its use was based on the low incidence of breast cancer in Eskimo women, who consume large amounts of rancid fat in cooking, and the reported regression of mammary tumors produced in mice and dogs with heptaldehyde (155,156).

It has been pointed out that the devastation brought about by cancer utilizes two basic mechanisms (33). One is mechanical interference with strategic organs. Second, tumors can usurp the host's food intake and, when their needs outgrow this supply, feed on the host itself "until the neoplasm literally eats itself out of its home" (68). It is estimated that as much as 30 per cent of all cancer deaths are due to the latter metabolic mechanism (33).

In an attempt to ameliorate this neoplastic parasitism, sixty-four terminal cancer patients were selected to evaluate the effects of continuous or frequent tube feeding (129). The standard daily ration contained 3500 calories, 210 gm. of protein, and vitamins and minerals at levels recommended as therapeutic by the National Research Council. All other indicated forms of therapy had been used. The patients were cachectic, mostly bedfast, and had been hospitalized for terminal, nonspecific care. The results were truly remarkable (Table 10.8) (129) as described by Doctor Morton D. Pareira, Associate Professor, Department of Surgery, Washington University School of Medicine, St. Louis, Missouri.

> While most of the advanced-cancer patients were actually near death when admitted, as would be expected in a city institution, many who were thought to be terminal and had been bedfast because of "cachexia" were rehabilitated for a period of many months.
>
> Practically all...showed some increase in general strength and a majority became at least partially ambulatory, more comfortable, and able to care for themselves and hence happier and less of a nursing problem. Many who were bedfast in the hospital were temporarily restored to family living without special care.... Tumors...seemed to increase in size pari passu with gain in body weight.

There are other reports of cancer patients who have been force-fed diets that varied in regard to protein (40 gms. to 80 gms./day) and calories under metabolic ward conditions (104,182,186,193). Rapid weight loss upon discontinuation of the forced feeding, accumulation of large quantities of intercellular fluid, and possible acceleration of the malignancy were reported. These studies seem to differ in several respects from those of Pareira et al (129). The patients were fed by mouth, usually diets of their own choosing, except that at times they were supplemented as needed with protein and calories to establish the desired levels of intake. They apparently were not in as severely a cachectic state. Thus it would appear that there were important variations in frequency of feeding, protein content, possible micronutrient intake, as well as degree of cachexia. Because of the differences in experimental design, it would seem that the results obtained by Pareira and co-workers warrant further investigation.

SUMMARY

The information at hand clearly implies that, although much remains to be learned, diet does play an important role in neoplasia, especially in carcinogenesis. Most of the present knowledge of these relationships is derived from lower animal observations.

For example, findings in the hatched rainbow trout in California and the turkey poults in England in 1960 have demonstrated man's ability to precipitate tumor formation in epidemic proportions by dietary manipulation. Other important oncologic-dietary relationships have been elicited by a host of lower animal experimental studies which have been carried on since almost the turn of the century.

The restriction of calories has the most striking inhibitory effect on the genesis of almost all experimental tumors. The formation of spontaneous mammary carcinomas, some induced skin tumors and, possibly, some hepatomas is encouraged by fat-supplemented diets. A low protein intake involving an amino acid deficiency may inhibit spontaneous hepatoma formation but favors the genesis of induced hepatomas. Riboflavin may play a special protective role in azo-dye induced hepatomas.

Tumor growth, in contrast to tumor genesis, reflects less response to dietary variations. A tumor appears capable of feeding on the host if its own nutrient supply is outstripped. Caloric restriction and severe protein or vitamin lack may inhibit neoplastic growth but only at levels that markedly impair the growth and well-being of the host.

Another area of investigation that appears promising is the influence of diet on metastases. Low protein intake, an ascorbic acid-bioflavonoid-benzoylcarbinol supplement and a high fat-choline free diet exert an inhibitory effect on metastatic growth.

The cancer sites which account for the most deaths and some of the organ sites experiencing the greatest increases in cancer deaths in the United States are among those mentioned most frequently in diet-carcinomatosis relationships. Human

Table 10.8
rehabilitation by tube feeding of completely
invalided patients with advanced cancer

age and sex	primary site	body weight (per cent loss)	duration invalid-ism (days)	eventuality
71 F	cervix	35	56	discharged, eating well; employed 6 months thereafter
37 F	cervix	8	21	discharged, eating well, active
68 M	stomach	25	14	discharged, eating well, active
70 M	pharynx	59	56	activity & normal appetite retained until 1 week prior to death 3 months later
46 F	cervix	21	14	discharged, actively engaged in housework, eating well
59 M	pancreas	34	42	discharged, eating well, active
47 M	pancreas	34	175	discharged, eating well, active
47 F	breast	31	42	discharged, eating well, active
34 F	cervix	23	56	discharged, eating well, active
56 F	cervix	29	21	became ambulatory; able to return home

reports relate oncosis especially to obesity, generalized malnutrition, sugar consumption, alcohol intake, deficiencies of vitamin A and of various minerals, seasonings, food processing, and contaminants. A few cancer-free primitive peoples have been studied from a dietary standpoint.

Qualified success has been reported in the two instances where the effect of diet improvement on the incidence of neoplasia has been recorded, iodine supplementation in one instance and correction of generalized deficiencies in the other. Limited success in the pharmacologic use of individual nutrients and nutrient-antagonists has been reported, primarily in embryonal tissue malignancies.

Within the last decade, Nutrition Reviews echoed the conclusion reached over a quarter of a century ago by Tannenbaum (45):

Certainly a recommendation can be drawn both from the statistical data in man and the experimental work in animals; the avoidance of overweight is probably one way to prevent, or delay, the appearance of some malignant processes.

The implication of sugar in malignancies also acquires heightened significance when considered against the background of the studies relating carcinomatosis to disturbed carbohydrate metabolism. A recent paper reporting a positive correlation between cervical carcinoma and increased blood glucose levels indicates well over one hundred such reports *(31)*. For example, hyperglycemia was even noted in three consecutive cases of the rare disease, solitary metastatic carcinoma of the mandible, at the Mayo Clinic *(21)*.

In the case of endometrial cancer, whose amazingly detailed proneness profile includes obesity and decreased glucose tolerance, discussions of prevention for the prone individual have not included development of dietary habits that would discourage lipogenesis and hyperglycemia. Since there have been no great advances in therapeutic techniques in the past ten years *(83)*, evaluation of such preventive measures would seem to be doubly warranted.

The reported effects of forced tube-feeding of terminal cancer patients are impressive but have not been pursued in the interim period of over fifteen years. Another important

Table 10.9
natural and man-made agents regarded
as established lower animal carcinogens

agent	established or suspected tumor site
estrogens (natural or synthetic) as a dietary additive	cutaneous lymph nodes (rat)
DDT as a food contaminant	liver (rat)
tannic acid as an ingredient of fruit, wine, coffee, and tea	liver (rat)
thiourea and derivatives as citrus fruit preservatives	liver (rat) thyroid (rat)
p-Phanetylurea (Dulcin) as artificial sweetening agent	liver (rat)
8-Hydroxyquinoline as a food preservative or as an adhesive ingredient for paraffin-ized food containers	bladder (mouse) uterus (rat)
vegetable oils (polymerized and oxidized) used as a margarine emulsifier	subcutaneous tissue (rat)
safrol as a flavoring agent	liver (rat)
oil orange E as a food dye	liver (mouse)
oil yellow HA as a food dye	liver (mouse)
oil orange TX as a food dye	subcutaneous tissue and colon (mouse)
carboxymethylcellulose as a food additive	subcutaneous tissue (rat)

Table 10.10
natural and man-made agents regarded
as established human carcinogens

agent and its dietary significance	reported tumor sites
aromatic amines in production of colored margarine, butter, baked goods, cheese crackers	bladder ureter renal pelvis
Dulcin as an artificial sweetener	intestine? lung? liver? prostate?
soot from smoking and roasting foodstuffs (meats, fish, coffee, etc.); charcoal broiling of meats and fish, hard liquor aged in charred wood caskets	skin scrotum lung alimentary system
drinking water polluted with mineral oils (naturally or artificially), foodstuffs sprayed with insecticides	skin scrotum larynx? lung?
paraffin and petroleum waxes as coating (fruit and vegetable preserves, eggs, beer can lining, bottle cap liner, cheese, paper milk bottles, fruit and vegetables, and soda straws), chewing gum ingredient, dehydrated food packages, drinking cup impregnation, egg preservatives, field ration package, feather remover of fowl, tank tar treatment for wine, etc.	skin lung? stomach?
ionizing radiations in sterilization of foods, radiography of chicken eggs, foodstuffs contaminated with radioactive fallout, and drinking water contaminated with radioactive fallout	skin subcutaneous tissue bones hematopoietic tissues lung liver larynx thyroid kidney breast? uterus?

observation pertinent to supportive therapy was recently made. It was noted that radiation injury in the guinea pig increased the capacity for ascorbic acid absorption by the blood proteins, thus causing a vitamin C improverishment of a number of organs *(38)*.

Again, mention needs to be made of a problem that has only been alluded to because it occupies a gray zone between food technology and dietotherapy. The preparation of a food can change it from a nutrient into a carcinogen. Food may

Table 10.11
natural and man-made agents regarded
as potential human carcinogens

agent and its dietary significance	reported tumor sites
urethan (ethyl carbamate) as a latent flavor developer in packaged food	lung hemapoietic organs
DDT as residue on foodstuffs	liver lung skin
estrogens (natural and synthetic) as animal feeds and implants in fowl (to stimulate production of eggs and to induce chemical caponization)	uterus breast prostate, bladder blood-forming tissues
8-Hydroxyquinoline in adhesive of paraffinized milk containers and food preservatives	uterus rectum bladder brain
surfactants-detergents as additive to foodstuffs (emulsifiers, fat substitutes, or stabilizers)	skin lung alimentary tract bladder
tannic acid as clarification agent of fruit juices, precipitant of gelatin, ingredient of red wine, tea, nuts, fruits, hops, etc.	liver
thiourea as fungicide; thioacetamide as solubilizer of riboflavin; foodstuffs contaminated with these substances	liver thyroid
thermic and oxidation products of oils and fats of vegetables and animal derivation such as lard, vegetable oils and fats, shortenings, margarine emulsifier, fish oils, polymerized and oxidized fatty acid emulsifiers and contaminants of heated fats and oils	lung alimentary system bladder
carbon polymers in impregnation of food containers, bottles, tubes, boxes, sausage skins	site of mucosal contact
products with contact to hydrophilic carbon polymers: sodium carboxymethyl cellulose as emulsifier and stabilizer of ice cream, cheese, thickener of foodstuffs; polyvinyl pyrrolidone as suspending agent of foodstuffs, clearing agent of beer and fruit juices; polyvinyl alcohol as emulsifier and gelatin substitute in foodstuffs (ice cream, coating of candies and confectionery, sausage casings)	lung mucosal contact areas organs and tissue of retention and deposition
cobalt in vitamin B12 supplements	connective tissue lung
selenium in foodstuffs naturally contaminated (seleniferous plants grown in seleniferous soil (grain) and meat from food animals eating such plants) and as an additive for insect repelling and poisoning in greenhouses and citrus fruit	liver thyroid

serve as a carrier or breeding ground for a carcinogenic contaminant. An additive designed to enhance food appearance or taste may eventuate as a cancer-inducing agent. Doctor Hueper has outlined a host of such substances. Some of these are listed in Tables 10.9, 10.10 and 10.11. This distinguished investigator from the National Cancer Institute has described the origins of the problem and has ably expressed the philosophy upon which its management should be based *(80)*:

...During the last 150 years, man has fundamentally changed and revolutionized the natural environment in which he and animals are living by the effects of a rapidly increasing industrialization of the human activities and by the alarmingly growing chemicalization of environment of man and animals, including their food supply, with synthetic substances many of which never existed before....While it is not possible to avoid all risks to man and animals from human efforts for progress and improvements, whereas it will be necessary sometimes to balance risks for obtaining the maximal general benefits, the taking of avoidable, unnecessary and foolish risks entailing possible or even probable cancer hazards for young and old, man and animals, is foolhardy and irresponsible....

REFERENCES

1. Acosta-Sison, H. *Studies in choriocarcinoma from 88 patients admitted to the Philippine General Hospital from 1950-1961.* Philippine J. Cancer 4: 197-203, July-September 1962.

2. Ahlbom, H. E. *Simple Achlorhydric Anaemia, Plummer-Vinson syndrome, and carcinoma of the mouth, pharynx, and oesophagus in women.* Brit. Med. J. 2: #3945, 331-333, 15 August 1936.

3. Allen, S. D., Ireland, J. T., Milner, J. and Moss, A. D. *Treatment of leukemia by amino acid imbalance.* Lancet 1: #7380, 302-303, 6 February 1965.

4. Allison, J. B., Wannemacher, R. W. J., Hilf, R. and Hetzel, C. A. *The effect of methionine supplementation upon the tumor-host relationship in the rat.* J. Nutrit. 59: #1, 27-38, 10 May 1956.

5. Antopol, W. and Unna, K. *The effect of riboflavin on the liver changes produced in rats by p-dimethylaminoazobenzene.* Cancer Res. 2: #10, 694-696, October 1942.

6. Arakawa, S. *Experimental production of sarcoma of mice with the subcutaneous high concentrated sugar solutions, especially lactose, and mixture of laevulose and glucose.* Gann 46: #2 & 3, 363-364, September 1955.

7. Armstrong, D. B., Dublin, L. I., Wheatly, G. M. and Marks, H. H. *Obesity and its relation to health and disease.* J. A. M. A. 147: #11, 1007-1014, 10 November 1951.

8. Banik, A. E. and Taylor, R. *Hunza land.* 1960. Long Beach, California, Whitehorn Publishing Company.

9. Baumann, C. A., Jacobi, H. P. and Rusch, H. P. *Effect of diet on experimental tumor production.* Am. J. Hyg. 30: #1, 1-6, July 1939.

10. Begg, R. W. *Tumor-host relations.* Advances in Cancer Res. 5, 1-54, 1958.

11. Berman, C. *Etiology of primary carcinoma of the liver with special reference to the Bantu races of South Africa.* South Africa J. M. Sc. 6: #1 & 2, 11-26, April 1941.

12. Berman, C. *Primary carcinoma of the liver. A Study in incidence, clinical manifestations, pathology and aetiology.* 1951. London, H. K. Lewis.

13. Bischoff, F. and Long, M. L. *The influence of calories per se upon the growth of sarcoma 180.* Amer. J. Cancer 32: #3, 418-421, March 1938.

14. Bischoff, F., Long, M. L. and Maxwell, L. C. *Influence of caloric intake upon the growth of sarcoma 180.* Amer. J. Cancer 24: #3, 549-554, July 1935.

15. Blount, W. P. *Turkeys* 9: 52, 55-58, 61-71, 1961.

16. Bodian, M. *Neuroblastoma: an evaluation of its natural history and the effects of therapy, with particular reference to treatment by massive doses of vitamin B12.* Arch. Dis. Child. 38: #202, 606-619, December 1963.

17. Bonne, C. *Cancer and human races.* Am. J. Cancer 30: #3, 435-454, July 1937.

18. Boutwell, R. K., Brush, M. K. and Rusch, H. P. *Some physiological effects associated with chronic caloric restriction.* Amer. J. Phys. 154: #3, 517-524, September 1948.

19. Boutwell, R. K., Brush, M. K. and Rusch, H. P. *The stimulating effect of dietary fat on carcinogenesis.* Cancer Res. 9: #12, 741-746, December 1949.

20. Boyland (1960) Chester Beatty Research Institute, cited by Warren, H. V. *Trace elements and epidemiology.* J. College Gen. Practit. 6: #4, 517-531, November 1963.

21. Brown, W. F. *Solitary metastatic cancer of the mandible: three cases with associated hyperglycemia.* Mayo Clin. Proc. 40: #5, 392-396, May 1965.

22. Bryson, G. and Bischoff, F. *Tumors in Evans rats fed vegetable oils.* Proc. Am. Assn. Cancer Res. 5: #1, 8 March 1964.

23. Bullough, W. S. *Mitotic activity and carcinogenesis.* Brit. J. Cancer 4: #3, 329-336, September 1950.

24. Bullough, W. S. and Eise, E. A. *Effects of graded series of restricted diets on epidermal mitotic activity in the mouse.* Brit. J. Cancer 4: #3, 321, September 1950.

25. Burchenal, J. H., Karnofsky, D. A., Kingsley-Pillers, E. M., Southam, C. M., Myers, W. P. L., Escher, G. C., Craver, L. F., Dargeon, H. W. and Rhoads, C. P. *The effects of folic acid antagonists and 2,6-diaminopurine on neoplastic disease with special reference to acute leukemia.* Cancer 4: #3, 549-569, May 1951.

26. Burk, D., Spangler, J. M., DuVigneaud, V., Kensler, C. J., Sugiura, K. and Rhoads, C. P. *Biotin-avidin balance in p-dimethylaminoazobenzene tumor formation.* Cancer Res. 3: #2, 130-131, February 1943.

27. Bykorez, A. I. *The diet of rats during liver-tumor induction with N-dimethylaminoazobenzene.* Vop. Onkol. 9: #11, 15-18, 1963.

28. Cagliani, P. and Sforza, M. *Effect of various nutritional conditions on the hematogenic distribution of metastases.* Biol. Lat. (Milano) 15: #2, 177-182, April-June 1962.

29. Carlson, A. J. and Hoelzel, F. *Apparent prolongation of the life span of rats by intermittent fasting.* J. Nutrit. 31: #3, 363-375, 11 March 1946.

30. Cannon, H. L. and Fidler, D. A. Cited in *Environmental variables in disease.* Science 146: #3646, 954-955, 13 November 1964.

31. Cheraskin, E., Ringsdorf, W. M., Jr., Hutchins, K., Setyaadmadja, A. T. S. H. and Wideman, G. L. *Carbohydrate metabolism and cervical (uterine) carcinoma.* 1967. Am. J. Obstet. Gynecol. 97, #6, 817-820, 15 March 1967.

32. Clayton, C. C. and Baumann, C. A. *Diet and azo dye tumors: effect of diet during a period when the dye is not fed.* Cancer Res. 9: #10, 575-582, October 1949.

33. Costa, G. and Weathers, A. P. *Cancer and the nutrition of the host.* J. Am. Diet. Assn. 44: #1, 15-17, January 1964.

34. Cutler, S. J. and Haenszel, W. M. *The magnitude of the cancer problem.* Pub. Health Rep. 69: #4, 333-339, April 1954.

35. Dahl-Iversen (personal communication) cited by Lawson. R. N.. Saunders, A. L. and Cowen, R. D. *Breast cancer and heptalde-hyde.* Canad. Med. Assn. J. 75: #5. 486-488, 1 September 1956.

36. Devik, F., Elson, L. A., Koller, P. C. and Lamerton, L. F. *The influence of diet on the Walker rat carcinoma and its response to x-radiation, cytological and histological investigations.* Brit. J. Cancer 4: #3, 298-314, September 1950.

37. Dodds, C. *The problem of cancer.* Science News 13: 26-42, October 1949. Harmondsworth, England, Penguin Books, Ltd.

38. Dolgova, Z. Y. *Ascorbic acid exchange during the action of x-rays on the organism.* Fed. Proc. 22: #1, Part II, T130-T131, January-February 1963.

39. Dungal, N. *The special problem of stomach cancer in Iceland.* J. A. M. A. 178: #8, 789-798, 25 November 1961.

40. Dunning, W. F. and Curtis, M. R. *The role of dietary tryptophane in the incidence of 2-acetylaminofluorene-induced bladder cancer in rats.* Acta Unio. Int. Contra Cancrum 11: #6, 654-657, 1955.

41. Dunning, W. F., Curtis, M. R. and Maun, M. E. *The effect of added dietary tryptophane on the occurrence of diethylstilbestrol-induced mammary cancer in rats.* Cancer Res. 10: #5, 319-323, May 1950.

42. Dunning, W. F., Curtis, M. R. and Maun, M. E. *The effect of dietary fat and carbohydrate on diethylstilbestrol-induced mammary cancer in rats.* Cancer Res. 9: 354-361, June 1949.

43. DuVigneaud, V., Spangler, J. M., Burk, D., Kensler, C. J., Sugiura,

K. and Rhoads, C. P. *The procarcinogenic effect of biotin in butter yellow tumor formation.* Science 95: #2459, 174-176, 13 February 1942.

44. Eastcott, D. F. *Epidemiology of skin cancer in New Zealand.* Nat. Cancer Inst. Mongr. 10: 141-151, February 1963.

45. Editorial. *Nutrition and cancer.* Nutrition Reviews 15: #6, 178-179, June 1957.

46. Engell, H. C. *Cancer cells in the blood.* Ann. Surg. 149: #4, 457-461, April 1959.

47. Engel, R. W. *Influence of 2-acetylaminofluorene on the metabolism of fat and protein by the rat.* Cancer Res. 11: #4, 246-247, April 1951.

48. Engel, R. W., Copeland, D. H. and Salmon, W. D. *Carcinogenic effects associated with diets deficient in choline and related nutrients.* Ann. New York Acad. Sc. 49: Part I, 49-67, 7 September 1947.

49. Eversole, W. J. and Biancifiori, C. *Some dietary factors in experimental liver cancer.* Lavori Inst. Anat. V. Perugia 22: #3, 197-202, 1962.

50. Fare, G. *Protective effects of beef and yeast extracts and copper acetate in the diet against rat liver carcinogenesis by 4-dimethylaminoazobenzene.* Brit. J. Cancer 18: #4, 782-791, December 1964.

51. Fisher, B. and Fisher, E. R. *Experimental studies of factors influencing hepatic metastases: VI. Effect of nutrition.* Cancer 14: #3, 547-554, May-June 1961.

52. Flory, C. M., Furth, J., Saxton, J. A. and Reiner, L. *Chemotherapeutic studies of transmitted mouse leukemia.* Cancer Res. 3: #11, 729-743, November 1943.

53. Fredrickson, T. N. *Cod liver oil and lymphocytoma in the chicken.* Dissertation. Abstr. 24: #1, 255, July 1963.

54. Fujimaki, Y. *Formation of gastric carcinoma in albino rats fed on deficient diets.* J. Cancer Res. 10: #4, 469-477, December 1926.

55. Gangadharan, D. and Reddy, D. B. *Carcinoma of the stomach.* Indian J. Path. Bact. 5: #2, 80-92, April 1962.

56. Garnet, J. D. *Constitutional stigmas associated with endometrial carcinoma.* Am. J. Obstet. & Gynecol. 76: #1, 11-19, July 1958.

57. Ghadially, F. N. and Wiseman, G. *The effect of excess dietary methionine on the rate of growth of RD3 Sarcoma.* Brit. J. Cancer 10: #3, 570-574, September 1956.

58. Ghittino, P. and Ceretto, F. *The etiopathogenesis of hepatoma in*

hatchery rainbow trout. Turmoi 48: #6, 393-409, November-December 1962.

59. Green, J. W. and Lushbaugh, C. C. *Histopathologic study of the mode of inhibition of cellular proliferation: effect of 4-dimethylaminostilbene on the growth of Walker rat carcinoma 256.* Cancer Res. 9: #11, 692-700, November 1949.

60. Griffin, A. C. and Baumann, C. A. *Hepatic riboflavin and tumor formation in rats fed azo dyes in various diets.* Cancer Res. 8: #6, 279-284, June 1948.

61. Griffin, A. C., Clayton, C. C. and Baumann, C. A. *The effects of casein and methionine on the retention of hepatic riboflavin and on the development of liver tumors in rats fed certain azo dyes.* Cancer Res. 9: #2, 82-87, February 1949.

62. Grishin, E. N. *Etiology and incidence of cancer of the esophagus in Aktiubinsk Oblast.* Tr. Inst. Klin. i Eksp. Khir., Akad. Nauk Kaz SSR 8: 23-27, 1962.

63. Grunberg, E. *Aspects of cancer research.* Trans. New York Acad. Sc. 25: #4, 433-443, February 1963.

64. Gyorgy, P., Poling, E. C. and Goldblatt, H. *Necrosis, cirrhosis and cancer of liver in rats fed a diet containing dimethylaminoazobenzene.* Proc. Soc. Exp. Biol. Med. 47: #1, 41-44, May 1941.

65. Halikowski, B., Armata, J. and Garwicz, S. *Low protein purine-free diet in treatment of acute leukaemia in children: preliminary communication.* Brit. Med. J. 1: #5486, 519-521, 26 February 1966.

66. Halver, J. E. Natl. Inst. Health Rep., April 11-12, 1962.

67. Harris, P. N. *The effect of diet containing dried egg albumen upon p-dimethylaminoazobenzene carcinogenesis.* Cancer Res. 7: #3, 178-179, March 1947.

68. Henderson, J. F. and LePage, G. A. *The nutrition of tumors: a review.* Cancer Res. 19: #9, 887-902, October 1959.

69. Herskowitz, I. H. and Norton, I. L. *Increased incidence of melanotic tumors in two strains of Drosophila Melanogaster following treatment with solium fluoride.* Genetics 48: #2, 307-310, February 1963.

70. Hertig, A. T. and Sommers, S. C. *Genesis of endometrial carcinoma study of prior biopsies.* Cancer 2: #6, 946-956, November 1949.

71. Hieger, I. *Carcinogensis by cholesterol.* Brit. J. Cancer 13: #3, 439-451, September 1959.

72. Hieger, I. *Cholesterol as carcinogen. I. Sarcoma induction by cholesterol in a sensitive strain of mice. II. Croton oil a complete carcinogen.* Brit. J. Cancer 16: #4, 716-721, December 1962.

73. Hildreth, R. C. *Obesity - a complication in carcinoma cervix uteri.* J. Michigan State Med. Soc. 49: #10, 1175-1178, 1204, October 1950.

74. Hindhede, M. *Cancer statistics - cancer and diet.* Acta Med. Scand. 62: Fasc. V-VI, October 24, 1925.

75. Hirayama, T. *A study of epidemiology of stomach cancer with special reference to the effect of the diet factor.* Bull. Inst. Pub. Health 12: #2, 85-96, 1963.

76. Hoch-Ligeti, C. *Effect of fresh milk on the production of hepatic tumors in rats by dimethylaminoazobenzene.* Cancer Res. 6: #10, 563-573, October 1946.

77. Homburger, F., Bogdonoff, P. D. and Kelley, T. F. *Influence of diet on chronic oral toxicity of Safrole and butter yellow in rats.* Proc. Soc. Exp. Biol. Med. 119: #4, 1106-1110, August-September 1965.

78. Hower, G. *Observations on cystic moles and chorion-epitheliomas in Korea and South China.* Zschr. Geburtsch. Gynaek. 159: #3, 251-286, 1963.

79. Hueper, W. C. *Are sugars carcinogens? An experimental study.* Cancer Res. 25: #4, 440-443, May 1965.

80. Hueper, W. C. *Environmental carcinogenesis in man and animals.* Ann. New York Acad. Sc. 108, Art. 3, 963-1038, 4 November 1963.

81. Huseby, R. A., Ball, Z. B. and Visscher, M. B. *Further observations on the influence of simple caloric restriction on mammary cancer incidence and related phenomena in C3H mice.* Cancer Res. 5: #1, 40-46, January 1945.

82. Johnson, J. E., Ringsdorf, W. M. and Cheraskin, E. *Relationship of vitamin A and oral leukoplakia.* Arch. Dermatol. 88: #5, 607-612, November 1963.

83. Karnofsky, D. A. and Rawson, R. W. Foreword, *Symposium on medical advances in cancer.* Med. Clin. N. A. 50: #3, 611-612, May 1966.

84. Kensler, C. J., Sugiura, K., Young, N. F., Halter, C. R. and Rhoads, C. P. *Partial protection of rats by riboflavin with casein against liver cancer caused by dimethylaminoazobenzene.* Science 93: #2413, 308-310, 28 March 1941.

85. Kensler, C. J., Wadsworth, C., Sugiura, K., Rhoads, C. P., Dittmer, K. and DuVigneaud, V. *The influence of egg white and avidin feeding on tumor growth.* Cancer Res. 3: #12, 823-824, December 1943.

86. King, H. J., Spain, J. J. and Clayton, C. C. *Dietary copper salts*

and azo dye carcinogenesis. J. Nutrit. 63: #2, 301-309, 10 October 1957.

87. King, J. T., Casas, C. B. and Visscher, M. B. *The influence of estrogen on cancer incidence and adrenal changes in ovariectomized mice on calorie restriction.* Cancer Res. 9: #7, 436-437, July 1949.

88. Kirby, A. H. M. *Attempts to induce stomach tumors. I. The effect of cholesterol heated to 300° C.* Cancer Res. 3: #8, 519-525, August 1943.

89. Kirby, A. H. M. *Attempts to induce stomach tumors. III. The effects of (a) A residue of cholesterol heated to 300° C., and (b) 3,5-cholestadiene.* Cancer Res. 4: #1, 94-97, January 1944.

90. Kline, B. E. Miller, J. A. and Rusch, H. P. *Certain effects of egg white and biotin on the carcinogenicity of p-dimethylaminoazobenzene in rats fed a subprotective level of riboflavin.* Cancer Res. 5: #11, 641-643, November 1945.

91. Kocher, R. A. *The effect of a low lysine diet on the growth of spontaneous mammary tumors in mice and the N Balance in man.* Cancer Res. 4: #4, 251-256, April 1944.

92. Kraybill, H. F. and Shimkin, M. B. *Carcinogenesis related to foods contaminated by processing and fungal metabolites.* Advances in Cancer Res. 8: 191-248, 1964.

93. Kraybill, H. F. and Shimkin, M. B. *Liver tumors in rainbow trout.* Lancet 1: #7334, 654, 21 March 1964.

94. Krischke, W. and Graffi, A. *The transmission of the virus of myeloid leukaemia of mice by the milk.* Acta Unio. Int. Contra Cancrum 19: #1-2, 360-361, 1963.

95. Kroning, F. *Garlic as an inhibitor for spontaneous tumors in mice.* Acta Unio. Int. Contra Cancrum 20: #3, 855-856, 1964.

96. Lancaster, M. C., Jenkins, F. P. and Philip, J. M. *Toxicity associated with certain samples of ground nuts.* Nature 192: #4807, 1095-1096, 16 December 1961.

97. Larsen, C. D. and Heston, W. E. *Effects of cystine and caloric restriction on incidence of spontaneous pulmonary tumors in strain A mice.* J. Natl. Cancer Inst. 6: #1, 31-40, August 1945.

98. Larson, R. N., Saunders, A. L. and Cowen, R. D. *Breast cancer and heptaldehyde.* Canadian Med. Assoc. J. 75: #5, 486-588, 1 September 1956.

99. Lavik, P. S. and Baumann, C. A. *Dietary fat and tumor formation.* Cancer Res. 1: #3, 181-187, March 1941.

100. Lavik, P. S. and Baumann, C. A. *Further studies on the tumor-*

promoting action of fat. Cancer Res. 3: #11, 749-756, November 1943.

101. Lawson, R. N., Saunders, A. L. and Cowen, R. D. *Breast cancer and heptaldehyde.* Canad. M. A. J. 75: #5, 486-488, 1 September 1956.

102. Lemon, H. M. *Food-borne viruses and malignant hemopoietic diseases.* Bacteriological Rev. 28: #4, 490-492, December 1964.

103. LePage, G. A., Potter, V. R., Busch, H., Heidelberger, C. and Hurlbert, R. B. *Growth of carcinoma implants in fed and fasted rats.* Cancer Res. 12: #2, 153, February 1952.

104. Levenson, S. M. and Watkins, D. M. *Protein requirements in injury and certain acute and chronic diseases.* Federation Proc. 18: #4, 1155-1190, December 1959.

105. Li, M. C. *Choriocarcinoma of uterus and testis.* Med. Clin. N. A. 45: #3, 661-676, May 1961.

106. Marks, S. and Bustad, L. K. *Thyroid neoplasms in sheep fed radio-iodine.* J. Nat. Cancer Inst. 30: #4, 661-673, 1963.

107. McAlexander, R. A., Stevenson, J. K., Olch, P. D., Bogardus, G. M., Finley, J. W. and Harkins, H. N. *Accelerated mammary tumor development in C3H mice fed an iodine-deficient diet.* Surg. Forum 13, 105-106, 1962.

108. McCarrison, R. *Studies in deficiency diseases.* 1921. London, Frowder, H. Hadder & Stoughton.

109. McCay, C. M. *Chemical aspects of ageing and the effect of diet upon ageing.* Cowdrey's Problems of Ageing, 3rd Ed., Lansing, A. I., Ed. Chapter 6, 1952. Baltimore, Williams and Wilkins.

110. McCay, C. M. *Effect of restricted feeding upon aging and chronic diseases in rats and dogs.* Amer. J. Pub. Health 37: #5, 521-528, May 1947.

111. McCay, C. M., Crowell, M. F. and Maynard, L. A. *The effect of retarded growth upon the length of life span and upon the ultimate body size.* J. Nutrit. 10: #1, 63-79, July 1935.

112. McCay, C. M., Ellis, G. H., Barnes, L. L., Smith, C. A. H., and Sperling, G. *Chemical and pathological changes in aging and after retarded growth.* J. Nutrit. 18: #1, 15-25, July-December 1939.

113. McCay, C. M., Sperling, G. and Barnes, L. L. *Growth, ageing, chronic diseases, and life span in rats.* Arch. Biochem. 2: #3, 469-479, August 1943.

114. McCoy, T. A. *Neoplasia and nutrition.* In *World review of nutrition and dietetics.* Ed. Bourne, G. H., Vol. 1. 1959. Philadelphia, Lippincott.

115. Millar, F. K., White, J., Brooks, R. H. and Mider, G. B. *Walker carcinosarcoma 256 tissue as a dietary constituent. I. Stimulation of appetite and growth in tumor-bearing rat.* J. Natl. Cancer Inst. 19: #5, 957-967, November 1957.

116. Miller, E. C., Baumann, C. A. and Rusch, H. P. *Certain effects of dietary pyridoxine and casein on the carcinogenicity of p-dimethylaminoazobenzene.* Cancer Res. 5: #12, 713-715, December 1945.

117. Miller, J. A., Miner, D. L., Rusch, H. P. and Baumann, C. A. *Diet and hepatic tumor formation.* Cancer Res. 1: #9, 699-708, September 1941.

118. Miller, J. A., Miner, D. L., Rusch, H. P. and Baumann, C. A. *The carcinogenicity of p-dimethylaminoazobenzene in diets containing hydrogenated coconut oil.* Cancer Res. 4: #3, 153-158, March 1944.

119. Miner, D. L., Miller, J. A., Baumann, C. A. and Rusch, H. P. *The effect of pyridoxin and other B vitamins on the production of liver cancer with p-dimethylaminoazobenzene.* Cancer Res. 3: #5, 296-302, May 1943.

120. Moreschi, C. *Relation between nutrition and tumor growth.* Z. Immunforsch. 2: #6, 651-675, 6 July 1909.

121. Mori, K. *Effect of animal tissue feeding on experimental production of liver cancer especially in the inhibiting effect of kidney feeding.* Gann 35: #2, 86-105, April 1941.

122. Morigami, S. and Kasiwabara, N. *Inhibition of the experimental production of liver cancer by millet feeding.* Gann 35: #2, 65-70, April 1941.

123. Morris, H. P. and Voegtlin, C. *The effects of methionine on normal and tumor growth.* J. Biol. Chem. 133: #3, lxiv-lxx, May 1940.

124. Moss, W. T. *Common peculiarities of patients with adenocarcinoma of the endometrium, with special reference to obesity, body build, dietetics and hypertension.* Am. J. Roentgenol. 58: #2, 203-210, August 1947.

125. Nakahara, W., Mori, K. and Fujiwara, T. *Does Vitamin B1 inhibit the experimental production of liver cancer? (Second preliminary note on the effect of diet on the experimental production of liver cancer).* Gann 33: #1, 13-17, February 1939.

126. Nakahara, W., Mori, K. and Fujiwara, T. *Effect of liver feeding on experimental production of liver cancer (preliminary note).* Gann 32: #5, 465-469, October 1938.

127. Nakahara, W., Mori, K. and Fujiwara, T. *Inhibition of experimental production of liver cancer by liver feeding. A study of nutrition.* Gann 33: #5, 406-427, October 1939.

128. Opie, E. L. *The influence of diet on the production of tumors of the liver by butter yellow.* J. Exp. Med. 80: #3, 219-230, 1 September 1944.

129. Pareira, M. D., Conrad, E. J., Hicks, W. and Elamn, R. *Clinical response and changes in nitrogen balance, body weight, plasma proteins, and hemoglobin following tube feeding in cancer cachexia.* Cancer 8: #4, 803-808, July-August 1955.

130. Peller, S. 1930. Cited by McCoy, T. A. *Neoplasia and nutrition.* In *World review of nutrition and dietetics.* Vol. I. Ed. Bourne, G. H. 1959. Philadelphia, Lippincott.

131. Pelner, L. *Host-tumor antagonism. XXVII. Nutrition and cancer.* J. Am. Ger. Soc. 10: #8, 701-715, August 1962.

132. Poscharissky, T. 1930. Cited by McCoy, T. A. *Neoplasia and nutrition.* In *World review of nutrition and dietetics.* Vol. I. Ed. Bourne, G. H. 1959, Philadelphia, Lippincott.

133. Rigby, C. C. and Bodian, M. *Experimental study of the relationship between vitamin B12 and two animal tumor systems.* Brit. J. Cancer 17: #1, 90-99, March 1963.

134. Robertson, W., Yan, B., Dalton, A. J. and Heston, W. E. *Changes in a transplanted fibrosarcoma associated with ascorbic acid deficiency.* J. Nat. Cancer Inst. 10: #1, 53-60, August 1949.

135. Rous, P. *The rate of tumor growth in underfed hosts.* Proc. Soc. Biol. Med 8, 128-130, 1910.

136. Rous, P. *The influence of diet on transplanted and spontaneous mouse tumors.* J. Exp. Med. 20: #5, 433-451, 1 November 1914.

137. Rusch, H. P., Kline, B. E. and Baumann, C. A. *The influence of caloric restriction and of dietary fat on tumor formation with ultraviolet radiation.* Cancer Res. 5: #7, 431-435, July 1945a.

138. Rusch, H. P., Johnson, R. O. and Kline, B. E. *The relationship of caloric intake and of blood sugar to sarcogenesis in mice.* Cancer Res. 5: #12, 705-711, December 1945b.

139. Salmon, W. D. and Newberne, P. M. *Occurrence of hepatomas in rats fed diets containing peanut meal as a major source of protein.* Cancer Res. 24: #4, 471-575, May 1963.

140. Salmon, W. D., Newberne, P. M. and Prickett, C. O. *Hepatomas in rats fed diets containing commercial peanut meal.* Fed. Proc. 22: #2, 262, March-April 1963.

141. Saxton, J. A., Jr. An experimental study of nutrition and age as factors in the pathogenesis of common diseases of the rat. N. Y. State J. Med. Abstr. 41: #10, 1095-1096, 15 May 1941.

142. Saxton, J. A., Jr., Boon, M. C. and Furth, J. Observations on the inhibition and development of spontaneous leukemia in mice by underfeeding. Cancer Res. 4: #7, 401-409, July 1944.

143. Schottenfeld, D. and Houde, R. W. The changing pattern of cancer morbidity and mortality and its implications. Med. Clinics of N. A. 50: #3, 613-630, May 1966.

144. Schramm, T. Influence of fatty acids in carcinogenesis. Acta Unio. Int. Contra Cancrum 18: #1-2, 234-235, 1962.

145. Schweitzer, A. (personal communication) cited by Stefansson, V. Cancer: disease of civilization. 1960. New York, Hill & Wang.

146. Seelich, F. Recent findings in cancer research. Wien. Med. Wsch. 113: #2, 43-48, January 1963.

147. Shay, H., Gruenstein, M., Kessler, W. B. and Ashburn, L. L. Studies on cocarcinogens and cancer promoting agents in rats. Proc. Am. Assn. Cancer Res. 4: #1, 61, April 1963.

148. Shimkin, M. B. and Kraybill, H. F. Editorial: Moldy peanuts and liver cancer. J. A. M. A. 184: #1, 57, 6 April 1963.

149. Silverman, S., Jr., Renstrup, G. and Pindborg, J. J. Studies in oral leukoplakias. Acta Odont. Scand. 21: #3, 271-292, June 1963.

150. Silverman, S., Jr., Eisenberg, E. and Renstrup, G. A study of the effects of high doses of vitamin A on oral leukoplakia (hyperkeratosis) including toxicity, liver function and skeletal metabolism. J. Oral Thera. & Pharm. 2: #1, 9-23, July 1965.

151. Silvertone, H. The levels of carcinogenic azo dye in the livers of rats fed various diets containing p-dimethylaminoazobenzene. Relationship to the formation of hepatomas. Cancer Res. 8: #7, 301-308, July 1948.

152. Smith, J. F. Clinical evaluation of massive buccal vitamin A dosage in oral hyperkeratosis. O. Surg., O. Med., and O. Path. 15: #3, 282-292, March 1962.

153. Stefansson, V. Cancer: disease of civilization. 1960. New York, Hill and Wang.

154. Steyn, D. G. Food and beverages in relation to cancer. Acta Unio. Int. Cancrum XIII, #2, 342-355, 1957.

155. Strong, L. C. and Whitney, L. F. Treatment of spontaneous tumors in dogs by injection of heptylaldehyde. Science 88: #2274, 111-112, 29 July 1948.

156. Strong, L. C. The liquefaction of spontaneous tumors of the

mammary gland in mice by heptylaldehyde. Science 87: #2250, 144-145, 11 February 1938.

157. Sugiura, K. and Benedict, S. R. *The influence of insufficient diets upon tumor recurrence and growth in rats and mice.* J. Cancer Res. 10: #3, 309-318, October 1926.

158. Sugiura, K. and Rhoads, C. P. *The effect of yeast feeding upon experimentally produced liver cancer and cirrhosis.* Cancer Res. 2: #7, 453-459, July 1942.

159. Sugiura, K. *The relation of diet to the development of gastric lesions in the rat.* Cancer Res. 2: #11, 770-775, November 1942.

160. Sugiura, K. *Effect of feeding dried milk on production of liver cancer by p-dimethylaminobenzene.* Proc. Soc. Exp. Biol. Med. 57: #2, 231-234, November 1944.

161. Sugiura, K. *Effect of feeding dried milk on production of liver cancer by p-dimethylaminobenzene.* Proc. Soc. Exp. Biol. Med. 57: #2, 231-234, November 1944.

162. Sugiura, K., Kensler, C. J. and Rhoads, C. P. *Protection against the carcinogenic action of p-dimethylaminoazobenzene by liver and yeast fractions.* Cancer Res. 3: #2, 130, February 1943.

163. Szepsenwol, J. *Carcinogenic effect of egg white, egg yolk and lipids in mice.* Proc. Soc. Exp. Biol. Med. 112: #4, 1073-1076, April 1963.

164. Szepsenwol, J. *Carcinogenic effect of ether extract of whole egg, alcohol extract of egg yolk and powdered egg free of the ether extractable part in mice.* Proc. Soc. Exp. Biol. and Med. 116: #4, 1136-1139, August-September 1964.

165. Szepsenwol, J. *Carcinogenic effect of cholesterol in mice.* Proc. Soc. Exp. Biol. and Med. 121: #1, 168-171, January 1966.

166. Takahashi, E. *Coffee consumption and mortality for prostate cancer.* Tohohu J. Exp. Med. 82: #3, 218-223, April 1964.

167. Tannenbaum, A. *Dietary factors in carcinogenesis.* Acta Unio Int. Contra Cancrum 10: #3, 117-122, 1954.

168. Tannenbaum, A. *Nutrition and cancer.* In *Physiopathology in cancer.* Ed. Homburger, F. Second Edition. 1959. 517-562.

169. Tannenbaum, A. *Relationship of body weight to cancer incidence.* Arch. Path. 30: #2, 509-517, August 1940a.

170. Tannenbaum, A. *The dependence of the genesis of induced skin tumors on the caloric intake during different stages of carcinogenesis.* Cancer Res. 4: #11, 673-677, November 1944.

171. Tannenbaum, A. *The dependence of tumor formation on the*

degree of calorie restriction. Cancer Res. 5: #11, 609-615, November 1945a.

172. Tannenbaum, A. The dependence of tumor formation on the composition of the calorie-restricted diet as well as on the degree of restriction. Cancer Res. 5: #11, 616-625, November 1945b.

173. Tannenbaum, A. The genesis and growth of tumors. II. Effect of calorie restriction per se. Cancer Res. 2: #7, 460-475, July 1942.

174. Tannenbaum, A. The initiation and growth of tumors. Introduction. I. Effects of underfeeding. Am. J. Cancer 38. #3, 335-350, March 1940b.

175. Tannenbaum, A. The role of nutrition in the origin and growth of tumors. Approaches to tumor chemotherapy. 1947. Lancaster, Pa., Science Press.

176. Tannenbaum, A. and Silverstone, H. Dosage of carcinogen as a modifying factor in evaluation experimental procedures expected to influence formation of skin tumors. Cancer Res. 7: #9, 567-574, September 1947.

177. Tannenbaum, A. and Silverstone, H. Effect of low environmental temperature, Dinitrophenol, or sodium fluoride on the formation of tumors in mice. Cancer Res. 9: #7, 403-409, July 1949b.

178. Tannenbaum, A. and Silverstone, H. Failure to inhibit the formation of mammary carcinoma in mice by intermittent fasting. Cancer Res. 10: #9, 577-579, September 1950.

179. Tannenbaum, A. and Silverstone, H. The genesis and growth of tumors. IV. Effects of varying the proportion of protein (casein) in the diet. Cancer Res. 9: #3, 162-173, March 1949a.

180. Tannenbaum, A. and Silverstone, H. The genesis and growth of tumors. VI. The effects of varying the level of minerals in the diet. Cancer Res. 13: #6, 460-463, June 1953b.

181. Tannenbaum, A. and Silverstone, H. The influence of the degree of caloric restriction on the formation of skin tumors and hepatomas in mice. Cancer Res. 9: #12, 724-727, December 1949c.

182. Terepka, A. R. and Waterhouse, C. Metabolic observations during the forced feeding of patients with cancer. Am. J. Med. 20: #2, 225-238, February 1956.

183. Thedering, F. Tolerance of iron therapy with consideration of carcinogenic effect of the dextran-iron complex. Med. Welt 6: 277-282, 8 February 1964.

184. Torgersen, O., Oystese, B. and Refsum, S. *Some experimental aspects on precursors of gastric cancer.* Ed. Severi, L. *The morphological precursors of cancer,* 553-564, Perugia, Div. Cancer Res. 1962.

185. Tromp, S. W. and Diehl, J. C. *A statistical study of the possible relationships between cancer of the stomach and soil.* Brit. J. Cancer 9: #3, 349-357, September 1955.

186. Tschudy, D. P., Bacchus, H., Weissman, S., Watkins, D. M., Eubanks, M. and White, J. *Studies of the effect of dietary protein and caloric levels on the kinetics of nitrogen metabolism using N15 L-Aspartic Acid.* J. Clin. Invest. 38: #6, 892-901, June 1959.

187. Vialler, J. *Research on the in vivo carcinogenic activity of an iron-dextran complex in the rat.* C. R. Soc. Biol. (Paris) 156: #4, 691-693, July 1962.

188. Visscher, M. B., Ball, Z. B., Barnes, R. H. and Sivertsen, I. *The influence of caloric restriction upon the incidence of spontaneous mammary carcinoma in mice.* Surgery 11: #1, 48-55, January 1942.

189. Voegtlin, C., Johnson, J. M. and Thompson, J. W. *Glutathione and malignant growth.* Pub. Health Rep. 51: #49, 1689-1697, 4 December 1936.

190. Voegtlin, C. and Maver, M. E. *Lysine and malignant growth. II. The effect on malignant growth of a gliadin diet.* Pub. Health Rep. 51: #42, 1436-1444, 16 October 1936.

191. Voegtlin, C. and Thompson, J. W. *Differential growth of malignant and nonmalignant tissues in rats bearing hepatoma 31: Influence of dietary protein, riboflavin and biotin.* J. Nat. Cancer Inst. 10: #1, 29-52, August 1949.

192. Voegtlin, C. and Thompson, J. W. *Lysine and malignant growth. I. The amino acid lysine as a factor controlling the growth rate of a typical neoplasm.* Pub. Health Rep. 51: #42, 1429-1436, 16 October 1936.

193. Wahi, P. N., Bodkhe, R. R., Arora, S. and Srivastava, M. C. *Serum vitamin A studies in leukoplakia and carcinoma of the oral cavity.* Indian J. Path. Bact. 5: #1, 10-16, January 1962.

194. Walters, W. *Carcinoma of the stomach in this country and in the orient.* Am. Surg. 29: #6, 454-456, June 1963.

195. Walthard, B. *On precancerous and presarcomatous changes in the thyroid.* Editor, Severi, L. *The morphological Precursors of Cancer.* 745-749, Perugia, Div. Cancer Res. 1962.

196. Walthard, B. *Structural change of the struma maligna with respect to iodine prophylaxis of goiter.* Schweiz. Med. Wschr. 93: #23, 809-814, 8 June 1963.

197. Warren, H. *Trace elements and epidemiology.* J. Coll. Gen. Pract. 6: #4, 517-531, November 1963.

198. Watkins, D. M. *Nitrogen balance as affected by neoplastic disease and its therapy.* Am J. Clin. Nutrit. 9: #4, 446-460, July-August 1961.

199. Waxler, S. H. *The effect of weight reduction on the occurrence of spontaneous mammary tumors in mice.* J. Nat. Cancer Inst. 14: #6, 1253-1256, June 1954.

200. Waxler, S. H., Tabar, P. and Melcher, L. R. *Obesity and the time of appearance of spontaneous mammary carcinoma in C3H mice.* Cancer Res. 13: #3, 276-378, March 1953.

201. Wegelin, C. *Malignant disease of the thyroid gland and its relations to goitre in man and animals.* Cancer Rev. 3: #7, 297-313, July 1928.

202. White, F. R. and Belkin, M. *Effect of a low-nitrogen diet on the establishment and growth of a transplanted tumor.* J. Nat. Cancer Inst. 5: #4, 261-263, February 1945.

203. White, F. R. and White, J. *Effect of cystine per se on the formation of hepatomas in rats following the ingestion of p-dimethylazobenzene.* J. Nat. Cancer Inst. 7: #2, 99-101, October 1946.

204. White, F. R. and White, J. *Effect of diethylstilbestrol on mammary tumor formation in Strain C3H mice fed a low cystine diet.* J. Natl. Cancer Inst. 4: #4, 413-415, February 1944b.

205. White, F. R. and White, J. *Effect of a low lysine diet on mammary-tumor formation Strain C3H mice.* J. Nat. Cancer Inst. 5: #1, 41-42, August 1944a.

206. White, J., Andervont, H. B. *Effect of a diet relatively low in cystine on the production of spontaneous mammary gland tumors in Strain C3H female mice.* J. Nat. Cancer Inst. 3: #5, 449-451, June 1943.

207. White, J., Toal, J. N., Millar, F. and Brooks, R. *Walker carcinosarcoma 256 tissue as a dietary constituent. III. Sodium as a factor in stimulation of water and food intake and growth in tumor-bearing rats.* J. Nat. Cancer Inst. 24: #1, 197-209, January 1960.

208. White, J., Toal, J. N., Millar, F. K., Cool, H. T. and Mider, G. B. *Walker carcinosarcoma 256 tissue as a dietary constituent. II.*

Effect upon growth and nitrogen excretion in the normal rat. J. Nat. Cancer Inst. 19: #5, 969-975, November 1957.

209. White, J., White, F. R. and Mider, G. B. *Effect of diets deficient in certain amino acids on the induction of leukemia in DBA mice.* J. Nat. Cancer Inst. 7: #4, 199-202, February 1947.

210. White, P. R. *Preface of Cancer: Disease of civilization.* By Stefansson, V. 1960. New York, Hill & Wang.

211. Wissler, R. W., Frazer, L. F., Soules, K. H., Barker, P. and Bristow, E. C. *The acute effects of beta3 thienylalanine in the adult male albino rat.* AMA Arch. Path. 62: #1, 62-73, July 1956.

212. Wolf, H., Jackson, J. H. *Hepatomas in rainbow trout: Descriptive and experimental epidemiology.* Science 142: 3593, 676-678, 8 November 1963.

213. Wood, E. M. and Larson, C. P. *Hepatic carcinoma in rainbow trout.* Arch. Pathol. 71: #5, 471-479, May 1961.

214. Wynder, E. L. and Bross, I. J. *A study of etiological factors in cancer of the esophagus.* Cancer 14: #2, 389-413, March-April 1961.

215. Wynder, E. L., Escher, G. and Mantel, N. *An epidemiological investigation of cancer of the endometrium.* Cancer, 1966. (in press)

216. Wynder, E. L. and Hoffman, D. *Current concepts of environmental cancer research.* Med. Clin. N. A. 50: #3, 631-650, May 1966.

217. Wynder, E. L., Hultberg, S., Jacobsson, F. and Bross, I. J. *Environmental factors in cancer of the upper alimentary tract: A Swedish study with special reference to the Plummer-Vinson (Paterson-Kelly) syndrome.* Cancer 10: #3, 470-487, May-June 1957.

218. Zaki, F. G., Hoffbauer, F. W. and Grande, F. *Fatty cirrhosis in the rat. VIII. Effect of dietary fat.* Arch. Path. 80: #4, 323-331, October 1965.

219. Zollinger, H. U., Virchow's Arch. Path. Anat. 323: 694-710, 1953.

11. ISCHEMIC HEART DISEASE

THE UNITED STATES PUBLIC HEALTH SERVICE ESTIMATES RELATIVE to the incidence of cardiovascular disease, and ischemic heart disease in particular, are truly awesome. Of the 111,100,000 adults in the United States, 14,600,000 (13 per cent) have definite heart disease, and nearly the same number (13,200,000) are strongly suspected (81). Among American males between 20 and 25 years of age, close to 70 per cent have one or more coronary arteries significantly thickened by atherosclerosis, making them prime targets for a crippling coronary attack (84).

Figures from the Medical Research Council Atheroma Research Unit at the Western Infirmary in Glasgow, Scotland, indicate (17) that 55 to 59 year old males in the United States have the highest annual death rate from atherosclerotic heart disease, including coronary disease, in the world (Table 11.1). The age adjusted death rate for arteriosclerotic heart disease for the total United States population has progressively increased from 207 per 100,000 in 1940 to 238 per 100,000 in 1960. For white males alone, the comparable rates for the same period rose from 262 to 329 (82).

The cardiovascular diseases as a group (7) cause one-tenth of all deaths under age 35, one-third between ages 35 to 44, and approximately three-fourths of all deaths in individuals 75 years of age and older (Figure 11.1). Beyond age 25 coronary heart disease is the major cause of cardiovascular mortality. There is a steady increase in percentage of all deaths from cardiovascular disease with age. Additionally, the American Heart Association (7) reports a progressive rise in mortality since 1900 in the population as a whole (Figure 11.2).

Doctor William B. Kannel and associates (52), under the

Table 11.1
annual death rates from arteriosclerotic
heart disease including coronary
disease (1956-1959) for males
aged 55 to 59 in various countries

country	rate per 100,000 living persons
United States of America (whites)	737.5
South Africa (whites)	656.5
Canada	617.4
Scotland	581.1
Australia	574.1
Finland	549.1
Northern Ireland	530.2
New Zealand	497.3
England and Wales	443.6
Israel	434.2
Denmark	330.6
Norway	293.2
Austria	272.6
Netherlands	258.4
West Germany	256.8
Sweden	254.0
Czechoslovakia	235.4
Belgium	213.4
Venezuela	206.0
Switzerland	200.3
Italy	166.1
Hungary	152.2
France	127.2
Poland	113.6
Japan	61.9

sponsorship of the Heart Disease Epidemiology Study, Framingham, Massachusetts, and the National Heart Institute, have spoken quite pointedly as to the plan of attack upon coronary heart disease:

The need for a preventive approach in this disease is the chief lesson learned from study of the natural history of this disease. Prevention and not further innovations in treatment will be required if a significant reduction in the morbidity and mortality from this disease is to be achieved.

For prevention to be effective one must recognize the chronic nature of coronary heart disease. In a paper read

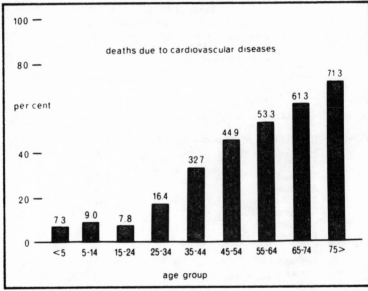

Figure 11.1. Per cent of deaths from all causes due to cardiovascular diseases (1962).

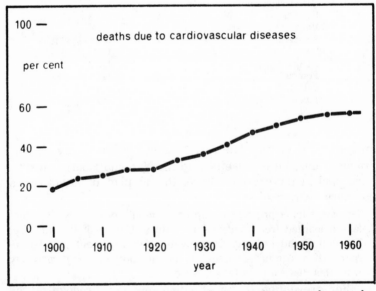

Figure 11.2. Per cent of deaths from all causes due to cardiovascular diseases (1900-1962).

before the Eighth International Congress of Internal Medicine at Buenos Aires, 23 November 1964, Captain George L. Calvy *(24)* (Director and Commanding Officer, Naval Medical Field Research Laboratory, Camp Lejeune, North Carolina) remarked:

> There is sufficient evidence available today to indicate that coronary heart disease has an incubation period just as do the well-known childhood infectious diseases, measles, mumps, etc.; however, in the case of coronary heart disease the incubation period may be 10 to 20 years. It has been shown further that coronary heart disease may be detected during the incubation period in nearly all such individuals. Once detection is made, the possibility of early and effective prevention becomes a reality.

Pathogenic alterations of the coronary arteries are occurring continuously during this quiescent period. In a Symposium on Myocardial Infarction presented in the Journal of the Florida Medical Association, Doctor Paul N. Unger *(118)* of Miami Beach outlined these changes:

> The developmental progress of atherosclerotic lesions as shown at post-mortem and by experimental production can be summarized briefly. Musculoelastic thickening is found in the first decade of life with differences noted between the sexes even at this early date. Fatty streaks occur in the second decade; fibrous plaques in the third; complicated lesions in the fourth; and clinically manifest disease in the fifth decade. Thus critical lesions occur in the coronary vessels 20 or more years before clinically manifest coronary artery disease.

Arterial pathosis has actually been noted quite early in the first decade. An examination of coronary arteries and aortas in 250 children (newborn to 15 years of age) revealed early atheromatous lesions as soon as three days after birth; they increased significantly in size and number with age, and by 15 years of age almost all were affected. Commenting on the preventive aspects of the very early evidence of atheroma, J. Van Belle, W. Stanley Hartroft, and W. L. Donahue *(119)* (Research Institute of the Hospital for Sick Children and the Department of Physiology, University of Toronto), in a presentation before the Canadian-United States Conference on Nutrition in Toronto (14-15 September 1964), asserted that:

> ...it should be realized that the disease is, in fact, a pediatric one in terms of initial onset....Reversal of these early lesions might be

more hopeful in the child than the adult.

Three staff members of New York University School of Medicine, Lee D. Cady, Jr., Menard M. Gertler, and Max A. Woodbury *(23)*, have effectively summarized a preventive philosophy for combatting coronary artery disease:

The problem resolves itself, therefore, in recognizing in the putatively normal population those individuals who are particularly prone to cardiovascular diseases during the incubation period and instituting preventive measures prior to overt symptomatology. It is emphasized at the onset that not all of the determining factors are present in each coronary patient; consequently it is not expected that all the determining factors will be found in each individual of the putatively normal group.

In agreement, Doctor Jeremiah J. Stamler *(113)* (Director, Division of Adult Health and Aging and the Heart Disease Control Program of the Chicago Health Research Foundation; and Assistant Professor, Department of Medicine, Northwestern University Medical School) has stated emphatically that:

It is now entirely feasible and realistic to strive for the prevention of first heart attacks....The key to the preventive effort lies in the new quantitative knowledge on coronary risk factors and their responsiveness to therapy.

An individual's susceptibility to ischemic heart disease has been characterized by the term *coronary proneness*. This predilection for coronary artery disease is the result of various combinations of both host and environmental variables. These risk factors may be collectively termed the *coronary profile*. Doctor Stamler *(113)*, in commenting on the profile of coronary proneness, has assured us:

...that medicine has the means to treat, correct and control the cardinal coronary risk factors....recognition of these abnormalities before clinical disease occurs, and effective treatment, creates the possibility of postponing and preventing clinical coronary heart disease.

A summary of many of the various risk factors which are correlated with an increase in coronary proneness may be observed in Table 11.2. Although not an exhaustive review of the literature, these components of the coronary proneness profile accentuate the fact that the etiology of ischemic heart disease is actually a *constellation* of host and environmental variables.

Table 11.2
host and environmental factors that
are known to be associated with an increased
risk of developing ischemic heart disease

	reference
psychologic	
aggressive personality	23,84,101,113
(exaggerated sense of time urgency)	
greater feelings of inner tension	88
more suspicions about motives of others	88
physiologic	
more rapid starch dextrinization by	117
salivary amylase	
minor electrocardiogram changes	68,113
(left heart strain, bundle branch	
block, minor T wave abnormalities)	
overweight–obesity	23,107,113,118
more rapid decrease in electromotive	42
force values in freshly collected saliva	
hypertension	23,24,68,77,107,113,118
low basal metabolic rate	42
sedentary living	23,113,118
increase in age	37
increased blood coagulability	69
sociologic	
urban American background	115
white collar workers	115
geographically mobile	115
occupationally mobile	115
more independent in social relationships	88
biochemical	
hypercholesterolemia	22-24,37,42,65,77,107,
	113,118
postprandial hyperlipemia	65,77,84,120
hyperuricemia	23,24,37,42,43,118
elevated serum phospholipids	23,37,43
decreased glucose tolerance	24,37-39,65,77,118
low serum 7S gamma-globulin	34
hypertriglyceridemia	22,65,118
elevated serum beta-lipoproteins	101
polycythemia	118
anthropometric	
short of stature	23,24,43
elevated mesomorphic index	23,24,43
nutritional	
cigarette smoking	23,107,113,118
high dietary lipid intake	65,77,84,120
dietary sugar intake	4,129,132
familial	
positive family history of coronary	23,24,37,43,118
heart disease	

Each of these factors exerts its effect, although not necessarily in every person. The strength of many factors is not only a function of their deviation from established physiologic standards *(38)* but also the length of time this has existed (Table 11.3). Thus, it may be noted that the per cent prevalence of coronary heart disease is significantly related to age and the percentile classification of the values for systolic blood pressure and one-hour blood glucose. For example, in the total group (irrespective of age) of 252 individuals comprising the 20 per cent with the lowest blood glucose values, 3.2 per cent demonstrated coronary heart disease. In contrast, in the upper 20 per cent (>80) with the highest blood glucose scores,

Table 11.3
per cent prevalence of coronary heart disease
in men by age and percentile class
for four physiologic variables
(Tecumseh, Michigan)

age (years)	percentile class	systolic blood pressure		cholesterol		1-hour blood glucose		relative weight	
		number	% coronary heart disease	number	% coronary heart disease	number	% coronary heart disease	number	% coronary heart disease
	<20	220	0.0	225	0.4	130	2.3	216	0.5
20-39	20-80	687	0.9	671	0.6	405	0.7	697	0.9
	>80	225	1.3	222	1.8	134	1.5	215	1.4
	<20	166	4.8	159	6.3	94	3.2	148	0.7
40-59	20-80	462	6.3	472	5.9	279	6.5	496	0.6
	>80	170	10.6 *	158	9.5	92	12.0 *	152	1.1
	<20	56	12.5	57	15.8	28	7.1	59	13.6
60+	20-80	190	17.9	179	17.3	92	17.4	180	16.7
	>80	57	24.6	59	22.0	29	34.5 **	61	26.2
	<20	442	3.4	441	4.5	252	3.2	423	4.5
total	20-80	1339	5.1	1322	4.8	776	4.8	1373	4.7
	>80	452	7.7 **	439	7.3	255	9.0 **	428	8.4

* P = 0.05
**P = 0.01

9.0 per cent showed coronary heart disease. Thus, there is an approximate threefold difference. In addition (Table 11.4), as these coronary proneness factors are compounded, the relative susceptibility to ischemic heart disease increases or the coronary profile worsens *(39)*. Thus, the group characterized by higher blood pressure, one-hour blood glucose, and serum cholesterol displays eleven times the coronary heart disease versus those with the lower values.

Table 11.4
relative prevalence of coronary heart disease
at two diagnostic levels by blood pressure,
blood glucose, and serum cholesterol range
(men aged 40 to 69 years)

blood pres- sure	1-hour blood glucose	serum choles- terol	rela- tive preva- lence
L	L	L	1.0
L	L	U	2.1
L	U	L	3.3
U	L	L	1.6
L	U	U	6.9
U	L	U	3.4
U	U	L	5.3
U	U	U	11.1

L is any value below age, sex-specific eightieth percentile (lower 80% range)
U is any value above age, sex-specific eightieth percentile (upper 20% range)

There is no known way of controlling many of the risks associated with coronary artery disease, such as family history, anthropometry, aggressive personality, or sociologic background. Therefore, the factors that are most readily amenable must be more thoroughly understood. Nutritional, endocrinologic, and metabolic status is, to a significant degree, a function of diet. Hence, diet as a manipulatable factor in the coronary proneness profile is deserving of serious attention.

The Council on Foods and Nutrition of the American Medical Association *(124)* is vitally interested in the dietary aspects of coronary artery disease and reflects its concern in the following statement:

> The Council believes that the development of coronary disease in young American men may be attributed to a combination of unfavorable genetic and environmental factors. One environmental factor of importance to the genetically predisposed person may be the American diet.

In fact, this American Medical Association Council (124) specifically encourages the practitioner to consider diet therapy for coronary disease prevention.

> After a thorough study, the Council reaffirms its previous position that physicians should advise persons with the hyperlipidemias to undertake diet therapy aimed at lowering the concentration of serum lipids and their associated macro-molecules. In addition, it recommends that physicians consider offering similar diet modifications to young men vulnerable to coronary disease in an attempt to prevent the rise in serum lipids which, in time, might put them into high-risk categories.

The dietary alterations suggested by the Council on Foods and Nutrition are primarily concerned with the regulation of dietary fat, especially the saturated fatty acids, with the ultimate purpose of preventing hyperlipemia and its consequence, coronary artery disease. This opinion has been repeatedly supported by noted medical authorities. Doctor Isadore Snapper (109), Director of Medicine and Medical Education at Beth-El Hospital in Brooklyn, reflected this consensus in a recent editorial:

> A diet with a high P/S ratio, i.e., one with a high proportion of polyunsaturated fatty acids, begun in early childhood as a life-long regimen will prevent the development of atherosclerosis, thrombosis and cholelithiasis.

On the other hand, there are strong objections to the exclusive emphasis on diet lipids. In the Chairmen's Address before the Section on Diseases of the Chest at the 111th Annual Meeting of the American Medical Association (Chicago, 25 June 1962) Doctor Arthur M. Master (67), Consultant Cardiologist for the Mount Sinai Hospital, voiced this viewpoint.

A prominent team of investigators from the Rockefeller Institute (32), Doctors Edward H. Ahrens, Jr., Jules Hirsch, William Insull, Jr., Theodore T. Tsaltas, Rolf Blomstrand, and

Malcolm L. Peterson *(32)*, have postulated that abnormal serum lipid levels may be the result of factors other than dietary fat. In a current review of diet and cardiovascular disease, Doctor Margaret J. Albrink *(4)* of the West Virginia University School of Medicine told the Symposium on Nutrition in Clinical Medicine (Chicago, 16 April 1964) that, from a historical review, two possible dietary hypotheses emerge: (1) that dietary fat causes atherosclerosis, and (2) that too many calories associated with too much carbohydrate or too highly purified carbohydrate cause atherosclerosis.

A review of the dietary habits of mankind and the changes in these habits suggests that an increase in total calories rather than of dietary fat coincides with the increase in atherosclerotic vascular disease in affluent countries. Serum triglycerides, unlike serum cholesterol, are associated with various measures of body fatness and may thus be used to test the importance of caloric excess in the pathogenesis of coronary artery disease. The fact that elevated triglyceride concentration is more closely associated with coronary artery disease than is serum cholesterol concentration, particularly after age fifty, supports the possibility that over-nutrition in general rather than an increased intake of dietary fat may be responsible for the increased incidence of coronary artery disease.

Doctor John Yudkin *(132)*, Professor of Nutrition and Dietetics at the University of London at Queen Elizabeth College, has also pointed out the importance of the simple carbohydrates in the etiology of ischemic heart disease (IHD):

My own view is that, in spite of the small amount of information we have so far accumulated regarding the role of dietary sugar in the etiology of IHD, it is already more convincing than the vastly greater body of information that has been adduced in the last 12 years or so in support of the hypothesis that dietary fat is a major culprit.

Two sources of information have provided evidence to substantiate the need for further investigation of the relationships between dietary carbohydrates and coronary heart disease: (1) that the only essential change in dietary intake during the twentieth century in economically advanced countries has been a dramatic increase in simple carbohydrates *(11,47,129)*, and (2) that international statistics show a closer relationship between ischemic heart disease mortality and sugar intake than with fat consumption *(14,116,132)*.

The diet of early man contained little carbohydrate until the discovery of agriculture. Increasing prosperity together with the cheapness of carbohydrates has resulted in the consumption of increasing quantities of sugar-containing manufactured goods. This occurs at the expense of nutritionally desirable foods, such as fruit or meat (129). According to a group of prominent investigators from the Department of Internal Medicine at the State University of Iowa (Mohamed A. Antar, Margaret A. Ohlson, and Robert E. Hodges) (11), the dietary changes related to the increased incidence of coronary heart disease have been in favor of carbohydrates rather than fats. From an analysis of retail market food supplies in the United States in the last 70 years they noted a decline in the intake of complex carbohydrates (starches) and a dramatic increase in simple sugars. This was cited in Chapter I, The American Diet (Figure 1.1). The slight increase in total fat consumption has been primarily in the unsaturated fatty acids. Referring to similar changes in the pattern of carbohydrate consumption in Britain, the Ministry of Agriculture, Fisheries and Food (47) reported that sugar in all its forms (excluding that used in brewing and distilling) now provides 18 per cent of the total calories consumed and 37 per cent of the total carbohydrate. This is twice that at the turn of the century and has resulted in a decrease in the starch:sucrose ratio from 4.5:1 to approximately 1.5:1.

This significant dietary change, together with the demonstration that international statistics show a relationship between ischemic heart disease mortality and sugar consumption, emphasize the need to examine more critically the dietary carbohydrates as they relate to coronary proneness. Doctor W. L. Ashton (14) of the Charing Cross Hospital Medical School, Department of Medicine, has shown with computed linear regressions that increased sugar consumption in Britain is significantly associated with an increased ischemic heart disease death rate. Similar results have also come from the Department of Hygiene in the Tohoku University School of Medicine, Sendai, Japan (116), when coefficients of correlation were calculated between the consumption of simple and complex carbohydrates (20 Western countries) and the corrected death rate for 30 to 69 year old people from arteriosclerotic heart disease (Table 11.5). Thus, the arteriosclerotic heart disease death rate correlates directly with the consumption of sugar and syrups and inversely with starch intake.

There is no question of the great strides made in food technology. However, Doctor John Yudkin has pointed out that these advances have not been without complications *(127)*.

> ...It used to be true that when we ate what we liked, we ate what our bodies needed both quantitatively and qualitatively. But today the ability of the food technologist to separate palatability from nutritional value means that taste is no longer a guide to good nutrition.

This chapter differs from the format of others in this section in two respects. First, evidence from lower animal investigation is not included since the volume of human data is truly overwhelming. Second, the design of this section has not considered, independently, the correlative and therapeutic studies. This manner of presentation was considered necessary because of the nature of the research data. In earlier chapters, for example (Congenital Defects, Chapter Seven), the therapeutic data revealed relatively clear-cut relationships between possible causes and end results (disease). The instance at hand, however, is that the great abundance of preventive and therapeutic data concerns itself with coronary proneness (risk) factors (Table 11.2) rather than cardiovascular disease per se. Hence, the nature of the evidence is principally correlative and necessitates this different approach.

Table 11.5
correlation between national average food
supplies and corrected death rate for
30-69 year old people from arteriosclerotic
heart disease (20 countries)

food	coefficient of correlation	
	female	male
potatoes and other starchy roots	−0.707***	−0.622**
sugar and syrups	0.472*	0.582**

* P < 0.05
** P < 0.01
***P < 0.001

In order to understand more effectively the published data relating diet to ischemic heart disease one should look, first, at the association in individuals with clinically evident disease; second, to the correlation in the coronary atherosclerotic; and, third, upon the relationships with predisposing factors for coronary artery disease.

CLINICAL CORONARY HEART DISEASE

Carbohydrate: National levels of consumption of fat and simple carbohydrates (dietary sugars) have been noted to be strikingly similar. This relationship is so close that statistics relating fat intake to ischemic heart disease or diabetes mellitus in different populations may, therefore, be only indirect, and the more direct association may be with sugar (Figure 11.3) *(131)*. Dietary surveys indicate that subjects with peripheral arterial disease or with a recent first myocardial infarction consume significantly more sugar than control subjects *(130)*. Doctor A. M. Cohen *(27)* from the Department of Medicine, Hadassah Medical School, Jerusalem, has made some very interesting observations concerning carbohydrate consumption and ischemic heart disease in immigrant Jews.

Thus neither the nature nor the amount of fat consumed by the Yemenite Jews in Yemen provides an obvious explanation of why they have less diabetes and ischemic heart disease than the Yemenites who have been long settled in Israel....There is no significant difference in the amount of protein consumed in the Yemen and in Israel....Whereas in the Yemen no sugar was eaten, about 20% of the carbohydrates taken by Yemenites in Israel is in the form of sucrose. No difference was apparent in the total amount of carbohydrates consumed or in the proportion of calories derived from carbohydrates.

In comparison with controls of the same age, a number of investigators have reported that, as a group, subjects with clinical coronary heart disease demonstrate a significant decrease in glucose tolerance *(29,40,58,78,89,98,110,111)*. The percentage of individuals with abnormally high oral glucose tolerance curves (Table 11.6) has been observed to range from 43 to 100 per cent *(29,40,58,78)*. Poor glucose tolerance was not only a significant finding in those with

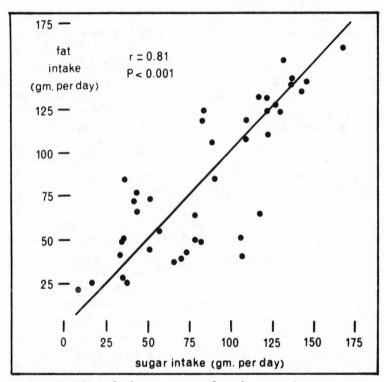

Figure 11.3. Relationship between average fat and sugar intake in 41 countries.

Table 11.6
carbohydrate metabolism in seven
patient groups with ischemic heart disease

group diagnosis	per cent with abnormal glucose tolerance	reference
myocardial infarction	100	110
myocardial infarction	77	29
myocardial infarction	73	111
angina pectoris & electro-cardiographic abnormalities	64	40
coronary heart disease	53-66	78
myocardial infarction	48	58
myocardial infarction	43	98

myocardial infarction but also in pre-infarction cases *(40)*. In the latter, with angina pectoris and electrocardiographic abnormalities, 25 per cent of those with elevated glucose tolerance curves had experienced a myocardial infarct within five years after the initial testing *(40)*.

Important electrocardiographic changes have been reported to follow the ingestion of 100 grams of glucose *(89,92)* in both normal subjects and patients with clinical heart disease. These changes, however, were more pronounced in the cardiac patients. The principal electrocardiographic alterations were an increase in heart rate, flattening and inversion of the T wave, and depression of the ST segment.

Data from the Tecumseh, Michigan, epidemiologic study have revealed a significant relationship between cardiovascular disease and hyperglycemia *(90)*. Of the individuals with coronary heart disease 40 years of age and older, 37.5 per cent of the men and 42.1 per cent of the women had hyperglycemia one hour after a 100 gram glucose challenge. The difference between these percentages and the expected ones of 22 and 24 per cent were significant at the one per cent level. Doctor Leon D. Ostrander, Jr. and co-workers *(90)* from the Department of Epidemiology in the University of Michigan School of Public Health also observed that the 87 known adult diabetics in the examined Tecumseh population had a higher prevalence of vascular disease than the nondiabetic persons of similar age and sex.

Hypoglycemia has also been noted to be related to coronary heart disease. Accordingly, a sudden lowering of the blood sugar which may occur in the hypoglycemic, normal, or hyperglycemic range was observed to precipitate objective signs of cardiac damage. Elimination of these episodes by employing a low-carbohydrate high-protein diet reportedly controlled the anginal attacks *(102)*.

In response to monoamine oxidase inhibition (iproniazid, nialamide, and mecamylamine), anginal symptoms have been reported to improve *(64)*. The clinical improvement correlated with a decrease in blood glucose and an increase in nonglucose sugars following a glucose (25 gm.)-galactose (25 gm.) tolerance test. No change in total blood sugar was observed.

Summarizing the relationship between dietary carbohydrates and ischemic heart disease, Doctor John Yudkin *(128)* places great significance upon the ingestion of simple carbohydrates.

...carbohydrate in general, with sugar in particular, is the likely dietary component amongst the complex of etiological factors of ischemic heart disease.

Fat: Patients suffering from coronary heart disease have been noted to be hyperlipemic. The hyperlipidemia is currently stated to be essentially composed of the triglycerides and beta-lipoproteins *(16,41)*. Others have indicated that survivors of a myocardial infarction demonstrate a decreased lipid tolerance and that this impairment in blood lipid clearance involves all lipids *(94)*. Thus, the role of dietary fat may be a prominent factor in ischemic heart disease.

To determine the effectiveness of a low dietary fat intake upon the recurrence of myocardial infarction, a research committee from four London hospitals initiated a controlled trial in 1957. In this study 264 male survivors of a first infarction were evaluated over a four-year period. Despite a lowering of blood cholesterol and a greater fall in body weight in the 40 gram low fat diet group, the relapse was not significantly different from the controls. At the end of four years the cumulative relapse rate (reinfarctions plus deaths) was 38 and 40 per cent for the low fat and control groups, respectively *(15)*.

However, in 814 male volunteers free of clinical coronary heart disease, the partial replacement of foods predominating in saturated fats by those rich in polyunsaturated fatty acids has been observed to lower the incidence of coronary heart disease. The Seven-Year Report *(25)* of the Anti-Coronary Club of New York revealed a significantly lower incidence rate for new coronary events in the experimental diet group, but not in the equally susceptible controls. In the 40-49 year old men the incidence rates were 196 and 642 per 100,000 person-years respectively. In the 50-59 year old group, the rates were 379 (experimentals) and 1,331 (controls).

In recent controlled studies of patients with myocardial infarction a disturbance in both carbohydrate and fat metabolism was noted *(29,110)*. In comparison with normal and diabetic subjects Doctor Louis A. Soloff *(110)*, Professor of

Medicine and Chief of the Division of Cardiology of Temple University Medical Center, found that myocardial infarction convalescents demonstrated two types of free fatty acid response to a 100 gram oral glucose supplement. One-third had an exaggerated normal response or decrease following the glucose load and a more precipitous postprandial rise. Two-thirds of the convalescents, however, showed a sluggish free fatty acid response (like diabetics) to glucose. Both groups of patients, nevertheless, had similar but abnormal glucose tolerance. Following a one gram per kilogram of body weight oral glucose load, an impaired glucose tolerance in 33 patients was accompanied in 21 by a prompt and prolonged decrease in serum free fatty acids. According to Doctors A. M. Cohen and E. Shafrir (29), this helps to confirm the association of diabetes or subdiabetes with myocardial infarction. A South African group of investigators reported that the abnormal carbohydrate and fat metabolism in coronary infarct cases were significantly improved following an 1800 calorie diet (starch 65 per cent, fat 25 per cent, protein 10 per cent) for eight to twelve months (36).

This dual flaw concept in coronary heart disease is also strengthened by the decrease in postprandial lipemia ($P < 0.001$) observed following an enhancement of glucose utilization in subjects with ischemic heart disease (61). The infusion of 50 grams of glucose and 10 units of crystalline insulin during a fat-containing meal produced a significant decrease in postprandial serum lipid levels without any change in the blood glucose level. Thus, the hyperlipemia and elevated serum triglycerides following a fat-containing meal apparently reflect (61), in part, abnormal carbohydrate metabolism (Figure 11.4).

The adhesive index of blood platelets has been compared in normal subjects and patients with coronary heart disease in the fasting state and following test meals of low or high fat content (80). Not only were the platelets more adhesive in the coronary patients but the increments in adhesiveness after high fat test meals were greater in those with heart disease.

Thus far it has been noted that hyperlipidemia, especially the serum triglycerides, is a prominent feature of individuals with coronary heart disease. The published evidence has revealed that dietary carbohydrate, in addition to dietary fats, is responsible for alterations in fat metabolism that result in decreased lipid tolerance.

Minerals: Doctor Henry A. Schroeder *(104-106)* from the Dartmouth Medical School in Hanover, New Hampshire, and the Brattleboro Memorial Hospital in Brattleboro, Vermont, has reported a very interesting relationship between municipal drinking water and cardiovascular death rates. According to his observations, softer water is associated with higher death rates. Thus, some factor either present in hard water or lacking in soft water appears to modify mortality rates from degenerative cardiovascular disease *(104)*. On the other hand, he has noted no correlation between hardness of water and noncardiovascular deaths.

Doctor Schroeder's original observations of a highly significant (statistically) negative correlation between the degree of water hardness and death rates from hypertensive and arteriosclerotic heart diseases (1949-1951 statistics) have persisted in his analyses of figures for 1960. Statistical study *(106)* of death rates from 88 cities of the United States with levels of bulk and trace elements in municipal water supplies showed negative correlations for 12 major and 4 trace constituents (Table 11.7). The purer the water in terms of dissolved elements, the higher was the cardiovascular death rate. According to Doctor Schroeder, the waters associated with the highest death rates were of a nature considered corrosive to metal pipes. The ability of water to dissolve metal from pipes depends directly upon the degree of softness and the concentrations of carbonic acid, alkaline bicarbonates, chlorides, and sulfates. Swedish investigators have also reported a highly significant negative correlation between the calcium ion concentration and deaths from arteriosclerotic heart disease *(20)*.

Further evidence that dietary trace elements may play a role in coronary heart disease has come from a comparison of the concentration of trace minerals in normal and infarcted heart tissue *(123)*. In injured tissue compared with uninjured there was a decrease in cobalt, cesium, potassium, molybdenum, phosphorus, rubidium, and zinc and an increase in

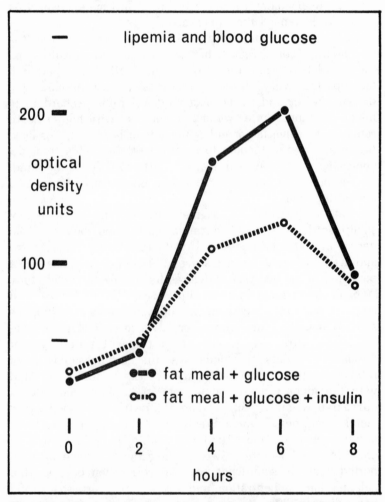

Figure 11.4. Effect of intravenous dextrose infusion with and without insulin upon postprandial lipemia (as measured in optical density units) in six ischemic heart disease patients for eight hours following a standard fat meal.

bromine, calcium, cerium, lanthanum, sodium, and samarium. A comparison of the concentration of trace elements in uninjured tissue from infarcted hearts with that in normal heart tissue revealed a decrease in copper and molybdenum and an increase in arsenic and cerium in the uninjured tissue *(123)*.

Protein: In a group of men with proven myocardial infarction, plasma albumin, an essential receptor of free fatty acid produced by the clearing system (lipoprotein lipase system), has been shown to be significantly deficient *(95)*. This cofactor defect of the fat clearing mechanisms was shown to be corrected, in vitro, by the addition of electrophoretically pure human albumin. These data may be quite significant when considered in the light of relationships between dietary and serum proteins and the current trends in the American diet.

Table 11.7
correlation of death rates from arteriosclerotic
heart disease and major and minor
constituents of municipal waters from 88 cities
(white males, aged 45 to 64 years)

major constituents	r	P
potassium	−0.475	< 0.0005
specific conductance	−0.434	< 0.0005
hardness	−0.411	< 0.0005
magnesium	−0.398	< 0.0005
silicon	−0.340	= 0.0005
bicarbonate	−0.337	< 0.0050
dissolved solids	−0.302	< 0.0050
chloride	−0.281	< 0.0050
sodium	−0.268	< 0.0100
sulfate	−0.254	< 0.0100
calcium	−0.231	< 0.0200
minor constituents		
vanadium	−0.344	= 0.0005
barium	−0.340	= 0.0005
copper	+0.294	< 0.0050
strontium	−0.287	< 0.0050
lithium	−0.280	< 0.0050
manganese	+0.262	< 0.0100
beta-radioactivity	−0.211	= 0.0250

Synopsis: From the discussions relating diet to clinical coronary heart disease, evidence has been presented from four aspects of metabolism: carbohydrate, lipid, mineral, and protein. In each of these areas, the significance of dietary constituents has been apparent. Therefore, diet must be considered as a prominent variable associated with both the morbidity and mortality of ischemic heart disease.

ATHEROSCLEROSIS

Atherosclerosis is described as a metabolic disease of dietary origin by three highly regarded investigators (Doctors Louis N. Katz, Jeremiah J. Stamler, and Ruth Pick) *(53)* in their book, *Nutrition and Atherosclerosis:*

Atherosclerosis is the chief pathologic lesion in coronary heart disease. It is a disease. Therefore, it is not inevitable, nor is it irreversible. Rather it is preventable and (at least up to a point) curable....Further, atherosclerosis is a metabolic disease, in which altered cholesterol-lipid-lipoprotein metabolism plays a critical and decisive (but not exclusive) role....Finally, and this is the decisive point in terms of the problem of the relationship between diet and atherosclerosis--the atherogenic alterations in cholesterol-lipid-lipoprotein metabolism are frequently brought about by the life-span pattern of diet. They are by-products of a habitually unbalanced diet excessive in total calories, empty calories, total fats, saturated fats, cholesterol, refined carbohydrates, salt, and inadequate (relatively and/or absolutely) in certain essential nutrients (vitamins, minerals, amino acids, and essential fatty acids) and in bulk. Empty calories are calories derived from processed, refined foods, high in energy value and low in essential nutrients (minerals, vitamins, essential amino acids and essential fatty acids) --foods such as sugar, white flour breads and pastries, solid cooking and table fats, and many others.

Discussing the role of nutrition in atherosclerosis, Doctor Robert E. Hodges and Doctor Willard A. Krehl *(49)* from the University of Iowa College of Medicine (Department of Medicine) summarized the currently available evidence in this fashion:

It may be assumed that diet plays an important role in the development of atherosclerosis....The bulk of epidemiologic evidence and much current investigation strongly suggest that elevated lipid levels associated with atherosclerosis are related to prolonged habitual consumption of excessive calories, saturated fats, cholesterol and refined carbohydrates....The publications which have been reviewed support the concept that hypercholesterolemia and atherosclerosis, as they relate to diet, are influenced by the type of carbohydrates as well as by fats and cholesterol.

In an address to the Seventh Inter-American Congress of Cardiology, Doctor Pierre Mandel *(76),* Professor of Biochemistry at Strasbourg Medical School, clarified the metabolic nature of atherosclerosis:

...if we are to conquer atherosclerosis we must never forget that it is a defect in energy metabolism, and the treatment of this condition must be our ultimate goal....In other words lipids by themselves do not create atherosclerosis. It is necessary to modify energy metabolism and the biosynthesis of proteins....We believe atherosclerosis is due to two phenomena inherent in aging-glycolysis increase and the decrease in biosynthesis of proteins and mucopolysaccharides.

It appears from this resume of current scientific opinion that even the nutritional influence upon atherosclerosis is multifactorial in nature *(44)* with many dietary substances playing a role. The following discussion will attempt to present the relationships between various aspects of tissue metabolism and coronary atherosclerosis.

Carbohydrate: Doctor Margaret J. Albrink *(5)* recently evaluated the association of impaired carbohydrate metabolism and atherosclerotic heart disease:

In recent years the pendulum of opinion regarding the etiology of atherosclerosis has swung away from the mechanistic view that ingested fat and cholesterol merely find their way through the blood stream to the arterial wall, toward the concept of an underlying metabolic abnormality. Growing evidence suggests that an important and perhaps basic defect is in the area of carbohydrate metabolism....The association between impaired carbohydrate metabolism and atherosclerosis--and between dietary carbohydrate and hyper-glyceridemia--are consistent with hypotheses that the common modern diseases of diabetes, atherosclerosis and obesity and associated hyperglyceridemia may be the present day manifestations of the effect of affluence on a once useful genetic trait, the ability to conserve carbohydrate.

A group of investigators *(6)* from the Second Clinic for

Internal Diseases, Medical Academy, in Warsaw, Poland, have reported that atherosclerotics show impaired tolerance to oral glucose. In response to a 50 gram oral glucose tolerance test, the atherosclerotic patients had significantly (statistically) higher blood glucose levels than healthy subjects at 30 minutes, one hour, and two hours. Symptoms of hypoglycemia were noted in the patients at the second through the fourth hour without any marked depression of blood glucose. Researchers from the Institute of Medical Pathology and Clinical Methodology, University of Pavia, Italy (35), reported that the significant decrease in plasma nonesterified fatty acids seen in diabetics occurred in 53 per cent of an arteriosclerotic sample. Thus, patients with atherosclerosis, in response to oral glucose loading, reveal abnormalities in both carbohydrate and fat metabolism.

Approaching this proposed relationship between impaired glucose tolerance and atherosclerosis from the opposite direction, Doctor H. Keen, Senior Lecturer in Medicine at Guy's Hospital in London, and associates (54) observed the prevalence of arterial disease in the general population according to the group level of blood sugar. Those designated diabetic had two hour (after 50 grams oral glucose) blood levels of 200 mg. per 100 ml. or greater; those with levels of 120 to 199 formed a borderline group; and the group with blood sugar levels less than 120 mg. per 100 ml. were classified as controls. In these groups the age-adjusted prevalence of both symptoms and electrocardiographic changes of arterial disease was lowest in the controls, intermediate in the borderline group, and highest in the diabetics. The authors concluded that:

...the association between these various manifestations of arterial disease and the level of glucose tolerance is real, and that this conclusion holds even at those levels of blood sugar at which a diagnosis of diabetes is considered doubtful.

It appears from their evidence that symptomless impairment of glucose tolerance may be one of the important accompaniments of atherosclerotic disease in the general population. Scientists from the Department of Epidemiology of the University of Michigan School of Public Health (90) recently reported data in agreement with this concept. The

87 known diabetics in the Tecumseh, Michigan epidemiologic study were noted to have a much higher prevalence of vascular disease than the nondiabetic persons of similar age and sex. Conversely, among participants with each of several manifestations of vascular disease, the proportion with elevated blood glucose levels was significantly greater than among others of the same age and sex in the total examined population (Table 11.8). According to recent controlled evaluations of oral glucose tolerance in coronary atherosclerotics (86, 121, 122), 35 to 95 per cent of the patients had a significantly decreased glucose tolerance. The latter figure was advanced by Doctor William R. Waddell and Doctor Richard A. Field from the Department of Medicine and Surgery of Harvard Medical School, the Surgical and Medical Services of Massachusetts General Hospital and the Department of Nutrition of the Harvard School of Public Health.

Table 11.8
prevalence of hyperglycemia among
persons with vascular disease
in three age groups

	16-39 years		40+ years		all ages	
	total persons	per cent hyperglycemic	total persons	per cent hyperglycemic	total persons	per cent hyperglycemic
males						
coronary heart disease	4	25.0	64	37.5**	68	36.8**
other vascular disease	2	50.0	62	32.3	64	32.8*
T wave inversion	6	50.0	48	37.5**	54	38.9**
systolic hypertension	261	26.1*	227	29.1**	448	27.5**
diastolic hypertension	261	26.4*	223	26.5	484	26.4*
females						
coronary heart disease	2	0.0	38	42.1**	40	40.0**
other vascular disease	2	50.0	60	41.7**	62	41.9**
T wave inversion	8	37.5	37	43.2**	45	42.2**
systolic hypertension	278	25.2	222	38.3**	500	31.0**
diastolic hypertension	261	23.8	224	35.3**	485	29.1**

* $P < 0.05$
**$P < 0.01$

Realizing the increasing incidence of atherosclerosis in affluent societies and its association with a decreased oral glucose tolerance, Doctor A. M. Cohen *(28)* asserted that the ingestion of sucrose might be an important factor. This knowledge, together with his nutritional studies on the Yemenite migrants to Israel, prompted the following remarks:

> If a nutrient is an etiological factor underlying the increased incidence of atherosclerosis and diabetes in Yemenites who have lived in Isreal for many years, it seems that suspicion must fall on the ingestion of sucrose. The increased consumption of sucrose might, therefore, also be responsible for the increased prevalence of these diseases in the general population.

Further implication of the role of dietary sucrose as an atherogenic factor has been advanced from controlled studies of dietary sugar supplementation in atherosclerotic patients. As a result of daily sucrose supplementation, significant elevations of serum cholesterol *(63,97)* and the serum triglycerides *(63)* have been observed. Alternating diet periods of high sugar and high starch content, Doctor Peter T. Kuo and Doctor David R. Bassett *(63)*, from the Edward B. Robinette Foundation of Cardiovascular Research in the University of Pennsylvania Hospital, succeeded in producing wide fluctuations in plasma total cholesterol, triglycerides, and phospholipids *(63)*. The plasma triglycerides were exceedingly responsive to these dietary alterations (Figure 11.5). This study revealed that sugar significantly elevated triglyceride levels, regardless of the initial value, and starch lowered the levels. Thus, sugar induced an endogenous lipogenesis and may well be the most important factor in the production of the commonly encountered type of hyperglyceridemia. The demonstration that high sugar intake can produce hyperglyceridemia even in normolipemic subjects indicates that the dietary habits of the individual and his inherent sugar tolerance are both important in the production of hyperglyceridemia *(63)*.

Fat: Reports concerning the relationships between dietary and serum fats and their effect upon the production of coronary atherosclerosis have produced, in the opinion of some researchers, what appears to be conflicting data. A group of investigators *(93)* from the Clinical Research Unit

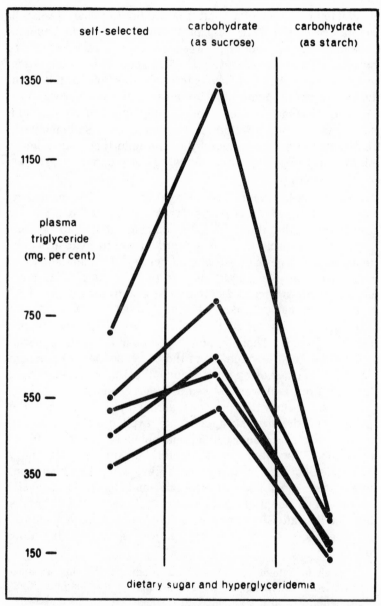

Figure 11.5. Comparison of plasma triglyceride levels in isocaloric self-selected, high sugar and high starch diets in five atherosclerotic hyperglyceridemic adults.

of Westminster Hospital and the Collip Medical Research Laboratory of the University of Western Ontario in London, Canada, reported recently on serum lipid levels and postmortem atherosclerosis. Correlations between antemortem serum cholesterol and cholesterol-phospholipid ratios and the severity of coronary atherosclerosis after death were evaluated in presumably adequately nourished 60 to 69 year old males. As a result of finding no significant relationship or trends, the authors concluded that the lipid theory of atherosclerosis remains unproved, as far as the coronary arteries are concerned.

On the other hand, however, a Veterans Administration research team (50) from Battle Creek, Michigan has clinically demonstrated the ability of a 10 per cent fat diet to prevent coronary atherosclerosis. In a ward of neuropsychiatric patients, two diet regimes (10 and 40 per cent fat calories) were evaluated from November 1958 until July 1961. The postmortem findings revealed coronary artery disease in 34 of 87 patients who had consumed the 40 per cent fat diet but no atherosclerotic lesions in the 13 autopsies of low fat (10 per cent) consumers. Though the 10 per cent fat diet appeared to have therapeutic value, 53 of the 87 consuming 40 per cent fat calories also showed no evidence of coronary disease even though all but two were 50 years of age or older.

Thus, neither the previous serum lipid levels nor the quantity of dietary fat appears to explain completely the development of coronary atheroma noted in postmortem examinations. Recently, the possibility of an essential fatty acid deficiency has been proposed. Reviewing the experimental evidence, Doctor Maurice Sandler and Doctor Geoffrey H. Bourne (Department of Anatomy, Emory University and Yerkes Regional Primate Center of Emory University, Atlanta, Georgia) have been convinced that these nutrients play an initiating role (103).

> Although to date no data has been produced showing a cause and effect relationship of arachidonic acid and a metabolic cellular alteration in the vessel wall, we feel that we have shown... that there is an essential fatty acid deficiency present in most instances in which atherosclerosis develops. In those instances in which it has been studied this deficiency in essential fatty

acids either primarily or in some as yet unknown secondary manner produces a metabolic defect in the arterial wall prior to the development of atherosclerosis. This defect may in fact be the initiating biochemical lesion.

Investigators (91) from the Institute of Thrombosis Research, University Hospital, in Oslo, Norway, have proposed that linolenic acid may prevent coronary thrombosis in patients with atherosclerosis or diabetes mellitus. The increased thrombotic tendency in these disorders has been demonstrated as a marked platelet adhesiveness. Linseed oil or purified linolenic acid dietary supplements were effective in reducing this factor to normal proportions (Figure 11.6). Linoleic acid and the pentaenoic and hexaenoic unsaturated fatty acids, however, were without effect. A South African team, investigating the effects of an 1800 calorie diet (starch 65 per cent, fat 25 per cent, and protein 10 per cent) upon the altered fat and carbohydrate metabolism in coronary thrombosis cases, noted a marked decrease in total fatty acids, an increase in serum linoleic and arachidonic acid to normal levels, and an improvement in glucose tolerance. This occurred during an eight to twelve month period (36).

Thus, the creation of deficiencies of one or more essential fatty acids through dietary and/or metabolic flaws, as a function of both fats and carbohydrates, is very likely promoting the development of coronary atheroma (59).

Vitamins: The utilization of dietary vitamin supplements as a therapeutic agent in atherosclerotics has only been very superficially investigated. It has been reported that intramuscular injections of B complex, ascorbic acid, and folic acid produced clinical improvement in patients with advanced arteriosclerosis (60). According to the author, weekly injections to patients with affected lower extremities reversed the signs and symptoms of arterial insufficiency by acting as a superior, long-lasting vasodilator.

Oral supplements of vitamin A and vitamin E have been observed to act as serum cholesterol reducing agents in patients with coronary atherosclerosis. Fifty to ninety mg. of E daily for 7 to 35 days was noted to produce a mean fall in serum cholesterol of 32 mg. per cent, with the maximal effect within eight days (85). The combination of vitamin A (100,000

I. U. daily) and vitamin E (60 mg. daily), intramuscularly for 7 to 20 days, has been effective in reducing serum cholesterol in cases of coronary atherosclerosis. Reportedly, a mean reduction of 70 mg. per cent was achieved and was accompanied by clinical improvement (112).

From these brief observations in individuals with advanced atherosclerotic heart disease, it appears that vitamins may play a preventive role if supplemented early in life.

Protein: A recent literature review cites evidence which may possibly indict the heating of animal protein as a factor in the etiology of atherosclerosis and subsequently, coronary thrombosis (9). Experimental studies are noted to show that

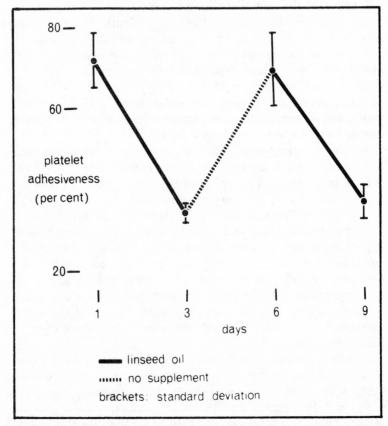

Figure 11.6. Effect of twenty milliliters of linseed oil daily upon mean per cent platelet adhesiveness in five atherosclerotic patients.

both heated animal protein and cyanocobalamin, freed during the heating process, enhance membrane permeability. The reviewer concluded that any factor enhancing this physical characteristic (membrane permeability) would tend to increase the deposition of lipids.

Synopsis: This review of nutrients and their assimilation substantiates the concept that the metabolic flaw in atherosclerosis is actually "a defect in energy metabolism" *(76)*. Thus, the problem is not just in carbohydrate, or lipid, or vitamin, or protein metabolism. The complexity of dietary nutrient interrelationships in the atheromatous process is consistent with the concept of nutrient interdependency (Chapter Four, Dietary Interrelationships).

CORONARY PRONENESS FACTORS

The first two sections of this chapter explored the relationships between dietary intake and nutrient metabolism and coronary artery disease. It is now appropriate to examine whether these associations are present *before* coronary artery disease becomes evident in the "presumably healthy" population. Thus, the effect of diet and assimilation upon various coronary proneness indicators will be summarized.

Carbohydrate: Investigators of apparently healthy subjects *(3)*, those with a defect in carbohydrate metabolism *(62)*, and patients with hyperglyceridemia *(51)* have noted that a decreased glucose tolerance was associated with an elevation of serum lipids. Actually, it is suggested that the primary event in the development of diabetes could be an abnormality of glyceride metabolism *(48)*. The fact that fasting blood sugar levels, even within the "normal range," are associated positively with serum triglycerides *(3)* suggests the existence of a common metabolic error. Facilitation of postprandial fat clearance, by enhancing glucose utilization (with insulin) in subjects with defective carbohydrate metabolism, also strengthens this concept *(62)*.

An evaluation of glucose tolerance in 14 hyperglyceridemic individuals resulted in the classification of nine glucose tolerance curves as abnormal and two as borderline *(51)*. Control curves were significantly lower at every point (Figure 11.7). Doctor John P. Kane and co-authors *(51)* from the

Department of Medicine of the University of California School of Medicine and the United States Public Health Service also noted other evidence of abnormal carbohydrate metabolism in the hyperglyceridemics, namely, (1) a reduced insulin sensitivity, (2) higher fasting free fatty acids with less decrease in response to a glucose load, intravenous insulin or glucagon, and (3) abnormal glucose and fatty acid responses to intravenous tolbutamide.

Doctor Edward H. Ahrens, Jr. and co-investigators (1) from the Rockefeller Institute, realizing the atherogenic effect of hyperlipemia, have emphasized the importance of knowing how the serum triglyceride levels are controlled.

Clearly there are two kinds of lipemia—one induced by dietary fat, the other by dietary carbohydrate, and it is not apparent on clinical grounds alone how to distinguish one from the other. We propose that carbohydrate induced lipemia is a common

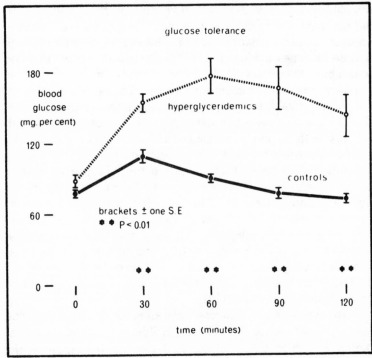

Figure 11.7. Glucose tolerance curves for twelve normal and fourteen hyperglyceridemic individuals.

phenomenon, especially in areas of the world distinguished by caloric abundance and obesity, where fat induced lipemia is probably a rare familial disorder encountered in all age groups. If the proper diagnostic procedures are carried out, clinical management becomes rational and effective.

In response to varying the quantity of dietary carbohydrate, a positive correlation has been observed with plasma triglycerides, serum cholesterol, and total serum lipids (19,114).

Even more important is the recent interest in carbohydrate quality as a determinant of serum lipid levels. Using data collected by the Interdepartmental Committee on Nutrition for National Development, scientists from the Department of Internal Medicine at the University of Iowa College of Medicine (66) have obtained significant correlations between simple (positive correlation) or complex (negative correlation) carbohydrates and serum cholesterol levels for 16 countries (Figure 11.8). Thus, the increased ingestion of simple sugars (carbohydrates) is associated with an increase in serum cholesterol and an increased intake of complex sugars (carbohydrates) with a depression of the serum cholesterol. The lipemic effect of dietary sucrose upon serum lipids is verified both by dietary supplementation (8) and elimination (99). The consensus, from controlled human experimentation, is that the concentration of atherogenic serum lipids can be altered by interchanging complex carbohydrate and sugar in the diet. It is generally agreed that, in the presumably healthy American male, sugar or sucrose exerts a hyperlipemic effect while the complex carbohydrates (starches) are principally hypolipemic in nature (10, 12, 46, 49). Alteration of serum lipid levels, with isocaloric exchanges of starch and sucrose, has actually been achieved in five days (74).

Doctor I. Macdonald (73) from the Department of Physiology in Guy's Hospital Medical School, London, has demonstrated a marked difference in the lipemic effect of dietary sucrose upon young men and women (Figure 11.9). In women 21 to 25 years of age, sucrose, which was hyperlipemic in men, produced a dramatic decrease in total serum lipids, serum cholesterol, and serum glyceride. A starch enriched diet, for both sexes, exerted no effect upon the serum glycer-

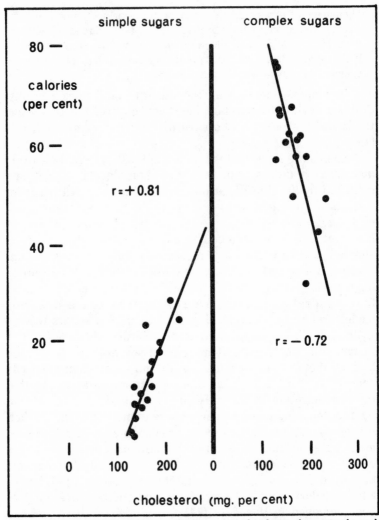

Figure 11.8. Correlation between the per cent of calories from simple and complex carbohydrates and serum cholesterol in sixteen countries.

ide and free sterols. However, it produced a reduction of the total serum lipids and serum cholesterol in men and women. According to Doctor Macdonald:

> These findings are compatible with the view that dietary sucrose in men leads to a serum lipid picture similar to that seen in ischemic heart disease.

This metabolic sexual difference remains until menopause. The lipemic effect of dietary sucrose in postmenopausal women and in men is very similar *(75)*. An increased susceptibility, at this time of life, to many of the chronic degenerative diseases (hypertension, ischemic heart disease, diabetes mellitus, and others) has been adequately demonstrated.

Further investigation into the effects of dietary carbohydrate quality upon serum lipid levels has revealed a difference in the metabolism of glucose and sucrose *(74,125)*. It appears that glucose activity is essentially hypolipemic in isocaloric substitution studies while sucrose is generally hyperlipemic

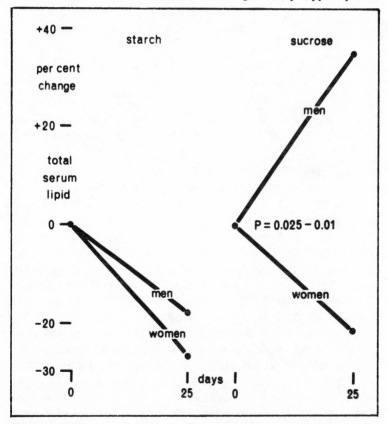

Figure 11.9. Per cent change in total serum lipids in men and women on isocaloric starch-enriched and sucrose-enriched diets.

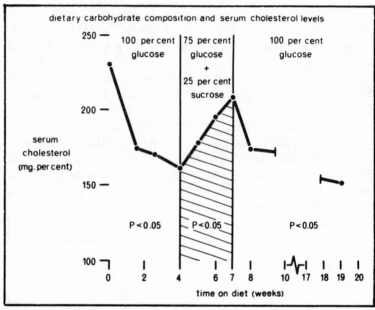

dietary carbohydrate composition and serum cholesterol levels

Figure 11.10. Variation of total serum cholesterol levels with synthetic diets differing only in the quality of the carbohydrate composition (healthy adult males).

(74,125). Since complete synthetic diets have been shown to support normal growth, lifespan, and reproduction in rats and positive nitrogen balance in man, a NASA-funded clinical study was initiated to determine their long term adequacy for man in space. Investigators *(125)* from the Life Sciences Laboratory, United Technology Center, Sunnyvale, California, observed a hypocholesterolemic action of such a synthetic diet in healthy adult males during 19 weeks of observation. The carbohydrate composition was, by weight, 100 per cent glucose. Although the findings indicated *(125)* that suitably formulated chemical diets will sustain man, it was observed that the hypocholesterolemic activity of glucose was reversed by a 25 per cent weight substitution of sucrose (Figure 11.10).

An increase in dietary carbohydrate (bread, potatoes, and sugar) *(59)*, especially sucrose *(70)*, has been reported to result in a significant lowering of the linoleic content of plasma fatty acids in normal subjects. Different metabolic effects of complex and simple carbohydrates have also been noted in regard to the coagulability of blood *(10, 21)*. In vitro, thrombus time and stypven time were, reportedly, longer after ingestion of complex carbohydrates than after isocaloric substitution of sugars in young men and women *(10)*. Another estimate of the coagulable state of blood, platelet-stickiness, was found to be markedly increased *(21)* following a 50 gram oral glucose supplement in normal subjects (Figure 11.11). Thus, a reduction in the number of free platelets indicates a greater platelet-stickiness, a situation regarded as a precursor of thrombosis. Addition of glucose to blood, in vitro, also caused an increase in platelet-stickiness. Intravenous glucose admin-istration and saline controls provided more evidence that, during periods of hyperglycemia, blood is hypercoagulable *(21)*. Parenthetic mention should be made that diabetics and those with ischemic heart disease, in comparison with normal subjects, have been observed to exhibit an increased platelet-stickiness *(21)*.

The effect of glucose ingestion upon the electrocardio-

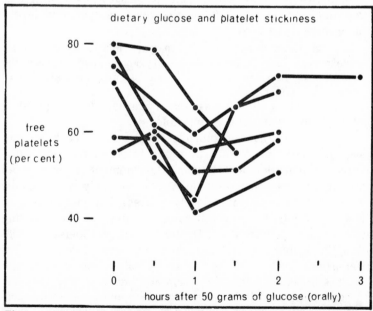

Figure 11.11. Per cent free platelets in relation to the initial count following rotation against a glass bulb for 20 minutes (platelet stickiness) following a 50 gram oral glucose supplement.

gram provides further evidence about the relationships of carbohydrate metabolism and coronary proneness (57, 89, 92). An increase in heart rate, flattening and inversion of the T wave, and depression of the ST segment have been noted in normal subjects following a 100 gram oral glucose supplement (89, 92). Significant ST segment and T wave changes were observed in 10 per cent of a group of normal adult males 22 to 66 years of age (89). Electrocardiographic changes typical of coronary insufficiency are reported in diabetics to occur during periods of both hyper- and hypoglycemia (57).

Relationships between dietary carbohydrate, carbohydrate metabolism, and various parameters equated with coronary proneness have been reviewed. From the published literature it appears that simple carbohydrates, especially sucrose, can produce in presumably healthy males and postmenopausal females a metabolic profile consistent with that observed in patients with ischemic heart disease.

Fat: Doctor T. B. Begg (17) of the Medical Research Council Atheroma Research Unit in Glasgow, Scotland, has proposed caution in ascribing changes in serum lipid levels solely to changes in dietary fat.

Although there is so much information which links a high fat intake with high blood lipids and ischemic heart disease, the relationship between the three is one of association and not of cause and effect.

He adds that alterations in dietary carbohydrate or physical activity may be equally responsible.

Actually, the average intake of fat and simple carbohydrate (sugar), according to data from the Interdepartmental Committee on Nutrition for National Development, is associated in a significantly positive fashion (66). Not only is the intake of fat and carbohydrate closely related, but metabolism of these nutrients is also intricately related. In commenting upon the interrelationships, Doctor Marvin D. Siperstein (108) from the University of Texas Southwestern Medical School (Department of Internal Medicine) in Dallas said in summary:

...it is becoming increasingly more apparent that fatty acid synthesis and oxidation, cholesterol synthesis and ketone body accumulation are all in part controlled by the rate at which glucose is broken down within the cell....In particular, it has been emphasized that glucose, in addition to serving the vital function of supplying substrate for the operation of Krebs cycle, acts as a generating system for the reduced pyridine nucleotides and it is through these coenzymes, and in particular triphosphopyridine nucleotide, that glycolysis may be able to exert its regulatory influence on lipid metabolism.

Doctor Margaret Albrink (3) has noted that overloading of adipose cells may contribute to the impairment of carbohydrate and lipid metabolism.

Adipose tissue is intimately associated with carbohydrate as well as triglyceride metabolism. The overloaded adipose cell may fail in its normal function, which is to regulate carbohydrate and fat metabolism with the result that hyperglyceridemia and impaired carbohydrate tolerance become manifest.

Great emphasis has been placed upon the serum cholesterol level as a predictor of coronary proneness. Although cholesterol intake may be positively correlated with the serum level (31), Doctor Ancel Keys (55) and associates from the Laboratory of Physiological Hygiene at the University of Minnesota, Minneapolis, pointed out the futility of considering it alone.

For the purpose of controlling the serum level, dietary cholesterol should not be completely ignored but attention to this factor alone accomplishes little.

These investigators (56) additionally suggest that the cholesterol-promoting-agents are saturated fatty acids, particularly palmitic acid. They note that, because of its abundance in most diets, palmitic acid may be primarily responsible for the contribution of dietary fat to the serum cholesterol level in man.

There are many reports which have demonstrated that increasing the dietary content of polyunsaturated fatty acids significantly lowers the serum cholesterol level (25,33,79). It has also been apparent that serum and adipose tissue levels of linoleic acid are significantly increased by such a dietary change (25,33). Determining the effect of a partial replacement of food predominating in saturated fats by those rich in polyunsaturated fatty acids upon the incidence of coronary heart disease has been an aim of the Anti-Coronary Club of New York. Starting with equally susceptible men, the Seven Year Report (25) revealed a significantly lower incidence of coronary heart disease in the experimental group. In 40-49 year old men the incidence rates for new coronary events in the experimentals was 196 per 100,000 person-years and 642 per 100,000 person-years for the controls. In the 50-59 year old group, the values were 379 and 1,331, respectively. The initial control rates were similar to those from other surveys, and the reported experimental incidence is much less than has been found in other epidemiologic studies of large populations (25).

Although serum cholesterol levels may provide evidence of a predisposition for coronary artery disease, Doctor Margaret J. Albrink (4) insists that the triglycerides are an even more prognostic factor.

As the serum triglycerides increase, the amount of cholesterol in the particulate lipids thought to be atherogenic also increases.... The triglycerides, then, not the cholesterol, determine the presence or absence of such particulate lipid as well as the type of particle in which cholesterol will be transported.

Experimental results suggest that the nature and proportion of fat in the diet may influence the rate of clearance of triglycerides from the blood stream, thereby affecting fasting serum triglyceride levels (13). A recent report indicated that the triglycerides were significantly higher after the consumption of emulsions of unsaturated fat than following saturated fat preparations rich in stearic acid (96). Delayed or poor absorption of this solid fat was advanced as the cause for the differences in postprandial triglyceride levels.

The current consensus is that hyperglyceridemia frequently may represent increased synthesis of lipid from carbohydrate (2,83). In a review of this concept, Doctor Margaret J. Albrink (2) succinctly summarizes the cholesterol-triglyceride controversy.

The low-density lipoproteins which have been implicated in coronary artery disease may be classified into two chief types or combinations thereof. In one, cholesterol is the predominant lipid component; in the other, the very low-density category, triglycerides are the major constituent. The first type, reflected in whole serum by an increase in the concentration of cholesterol but not of triglyceride, probably represents a deranged cholesterol metabolism. Although this disorder is associated with increased risk of coronary artery disease, it is found in only a small number of all patients with coronary artery disease, and rarely over age

50. The second type, characterized by increased triglyceride concentration with either normal or elevated cholesterol and slight to marked turbidity of serum, is the commonest lipid abnormality in coronary artery disease. Such hypertriglyceridemia in the post absorptive state indicates a defect in triglyceride metabolism resulting in the delayed removal of either endogenously or exogenously derived fat. The prolonged alimentary lipemia characteristic of this disease is further indication of such a defect. Not only are serum triglycerides and cholesterol relatively independent variables, but they respond differently to diet. The concentration of cholesterol and the cholesterol-dominated low-density lipoproteins is raised by feeding excessive animal fat and lowered by replacing the fat with vegetable oils. Postabsorptive concentration of serum triglycerides and very low-density lipoproteins is raised by increasing dietary carbohydrate, and reduced by caloric restriction and by substitution of fat for carbohydrate in the diet. The over-all influence of diet on serum lipids can usually be explained by the differing effect on serum cholesterol and triglycerides of dietary fat, type of fat, carbohydrate and total calories.

The metabolism of lipids, therefore, is not only affected by dietary fat but also by carbohydrate consumption. Reduced lipid tolerance frequently manifested as a postprandial or fasting hyperlipemia is often a result of defective carbohydrate metabolism. Thus, a reduced tolerance to dietary sugars, especially glucose and sucrose, may be expressed biochemically, through flaws in blood lipid clearing mechanisms, in the form of a hypertriglyceridemia.

Vitamins: Very little clinical research has been conducted to demonstrate the relationships between vitamin intake and various parameters of coronary proneness. No controlled evidence was noted except that favoring niacin as a hypolipemic agent *(26,45,100)*. With daily doses of 1 to 6 grams, significant reductions in serum cholesterol *(26,100)*, triglycerides *(45)*, and phospholipids *(45)* have been maintained for periods of three to seven years. These results have been observed in 80 per cent of those able to tolerate such a dosage. The incidence of side effects, however, has reduced the effectiveness of this form of therapy.

Minerals: Data relating the dietary mineral content to changes in any of the coronary risk factors is very incomplete. Since a reduction in glucose tolerance has been observed to play a prominent role in the development of coronary artery disease, the relationships between dietary potassium and carbohydrate metabolism are of importance. The impairment of carbohydrate tolerance associated with primary aldosteronism, which essentially is an inability of the beta cells to release insulin quickly in response to a rising blood sugar, has been shown to be correctable by potassium repletion *(30)*. On the other hand, potassium depletion to 200-500 milliequivalents per day for five days has been noted to decrease glucose tolerance by about 45 per cent even when serum potassium values had not changed *(30)*.

Calcium supplementation has been observed to cause a significant decrease in serum cholesterol (P<0.01) and in serum triglycerides (P<0.02). The hypolipemic mechanisms are not clear at the present *(126)*.

Protein: Evidence has been cited that heated animal protein may be a factor in coronary thrombosis since it, reportedly, causes a shortening of both the blood clotting time and platelet clumping time *(9)*.

In a controlled study of male students at Queen's University in Kingston, Ontario *(18)*, low protein diets (5 per cent of calories) for eight days caused a significant decrease (P= 0.02 − 0.05) in serum cholesterol, both with and without a 500 mg. cholesterol supplement. A high protein intake (25 per cent of calories) did not appreciably alter serum cholesterol. In female students, however, the high protein intake produced a significant decrease (P=0.01 − 0.02) in serum cholesterol levels.

Synopsis: The complexity of nutrient metabolic interrelationships indicates that the dietary influence upon various coronary proneness indicators is a multifactorial problem. The present picture has now been broadened to include, in addition to fats, the effects of carbohydrates, vitamins, minerals, and protein.

SUMMARY

The major nutrient groups have been considered separately as they relate to (1) clinical coronary heart disease, (2) atherosclerosis, and (3) coronary risk factors. Specifically, the metabolic effects of carbohydrate, fat, minerals, vitamins, and protein were noted.

Metabolism, however, cannot be dissected or compartmentalized. The interrelated activity of nutrients is quite complex. Emphasizing this fact before the Symposium on Nutrition at the 109th Annual Meeting of the American Medical Association (Miami Beach, Florida, 13 June 1960), Doctor Robert E. Olson *(87)* (Graduate School of Public Health, University of Pittsburgh) used as an example the two-carbon chain in metabolism.

Fat, carbohydrate and protein are broken down to acetyl coenzyme A prior to their terminal oxidation for energy production....The 2-carbon chain "active acetate" or acetyl coenzyme A is a highly reactive and important intermediary metabolite. It represents the point of fusion between many processes of catabolism and anabolism. It is the gateway to the terminal oxidation cycle of Krebs and a critical metabolite in the synthesis of ketone bodies, fatty acids and cholesterol. The effect of nutritional status upon the metabolism of acetyl CoA may be mediated via the control of cofactor concentrations which are functions of vitamin intake. Nutritional control of cellular metabolism, including that of acetyl CoA, may also be exercised by changing the substrates presented to the organism such as occurs when the amount and quality of dietary fat is altered. Nutrition and cellular physiology are inextricably associated. Only by referring to such fundamental considerations may one fully appreciate the pathologic physiology of nutritional disease and the effects of nutrition therapy.

The American diet has been recognized in many individuals as actively contributing to metabolic imbalances which ultimately terminate in the development of atherosclerosis and ischemic heart disease.

REFERENCES

1. Ahrens, E. H., Jr., Hirsch, J., Oette, K., Farquhar, J. W., and Stein, Y. *Carbohydrate-induced and fat-induced lipemia.* Trans. Assn. Amer. Phy. 74: 134-146, 1961.

2. Albrink, M. J. *Triglycerides, lipoproteins and coronary artery disease.* Arch. Int. Med. 109: #3, 345-359, March 1962.

3. Albrink, M. J. and Meigs, J. W. *Interrelationships between skinfold thickness, serum lipids and blood sugar in normal men.* Amer. J. Clin. Nutrit. 15: #5, 255-261, November 1964.

4. Albrink, M. J. *Diet and cardiovascular disease.* J. Amer. Dietet. Assn. 46: #1, 26-29, January 1965.

5. Albrink, M. J. *Carbohydrate metabolism in cardiovascular disease.* Ann. Int. Med. 62: #6, 1330-1333, June 1965.

6. Aleksandrow, D., Ciswicka-Sznajderman, M., Ignatowska, H., and Wocial, B. *Studies on disturbances of carbohydrate metabolism in atherosclerosis.* J. Atheroscler. Res. 2: #2, 171-180, March-April 1962.

7. American Heart Association. *Cardiovascular diseases in the U.S.; facts and figures.* February 1965. 44 East 23rd Street, New York, New York 10010.

8. Anderson, J. T., Grande, F., Matsumoto, Y. and Keys, A. *Glucose, sucrose and lactose in the diet and blood lipids in man.* J. Nutrit. 79: #3, 349-359, March 1963.

9. Annand, J. C. *The case against heated animal protein.* J. Atheroscler. Res. 3: #2, 153-156, March-April 1963.

10. Antar, M. A. and Ohlson, M. A. *Effect of simple and complex carbohydrates on thrombus formation, stypven time and serum lipids in young men and women.* Fed. Proc. 22: #2, Part I, 327, March-April 1963.

11. Antar, M. A., Ohlson, M. A., and Hodges, R. E. *Changes in retail market food supplies in the United States in the last seventy years in relation to the incidence of coronary heart disease, with special reference to dietary carbohydrates and essential fatty acids.* Amer. J. Clin. Nutrit. 14: #3, 169-178, March 1964.

12. Antar, M. A. and Ohlson, M. A. *Effect of simple and complex carbohydrates upon total lipids, nonphospholipids, and different fractions of phospholipids of serum in young men and women.* J. Nutrit. 85: #4, 329-337, April 1965.

13. Antonis, A. and Bersohn, I. *The influence of diet on serum*

triglycerides in South African white and Bantu prisoners. Lancet 1: #7167, 3-9, January 7, 1961.

14. Ashton, W. L. *Dietary fat and dietary sugar.* Lancet 1: #7386, 653-654, March 20, 1965.

15. Ball, K. P., Hanington, E., McAllen, P. M., Pilkington, T. R. E., Richards, J. M., Sharland, D. E., Sowry, G. S. C., Wilkinson, P., Clarke, J. A. C., Murland, C., and Wood, J. *Low-fat diet in myocardial infarction; a controlled trial.* Lancet 2: #7411, 501-504, September 11, 1965.

16. Bandyopadhyay, A. and Banerjee, S. *Plasma lipids in cardiovascular disorders.* Amer. J. Med. Sc. 248: #2, 203-205, August 1964.

17. Begg, T. B. *Dietary factors in ischemic heart disease.* Abs. World Med. 36: #4, 225-241, October 1964.

18. Beveridge, J. M. R., Connell, F., and Robinson, C. *Effect of the level of dietary protein with and without added cholesterol on plasma cholesterol in man.* J. Nutrit. 79: #3, 289-295, March 1963.

19. Bierman, E. L. and Hamlin, J. T. *The hyperlipemic effect of a low-fat, high-carbohydrate diet in diabetic subjects.* Diabetes 10: #6, 432-437, November-December 1961.

20. Biorch, G., Bostrom, H., and Widstrom, A. *On the relationship between water hardness and death rate in cardiovascular diseases.* Acta Med. Scandinav. 178: #2, 239-252, August 1965.

21. Bridges, J. M., Dalby, A. M., Millar, J. H. D., and Weaver, J. A. *An effect of D-glucose on platelet stickiness.* Lancet 1: #7376, 75-77, January 9, 1965.

22. Brown, D. F., Kinch, S. H., and Doyle, J. T. *Serum triglycerides in health and in ischemic heart disease.* New England J. Med. 273: #18, 947-952, October 28, 1965.

23. Cady, L. D., Jr., Gertler, M. M., and Woodbury, M. A. *Clues to the development of coronary heart disease.* Geriatrics 16: #2, 69-73, February 1961.

24. Calvy, G. L. *The prediction of disease.* Military Med. 129: #10, 929-932, October 1964.

25. Christakis, G., Rinzler, S. H., Archer, M., Winslow, G., Jampel, S., Stephenson, J., Friedman, G., Fein, H., Kraus, A., and James, G. *The anti-coronary club; a dietary approach to the prevention of coronary heart disease - a seven year report.* Amer. J. Pub. Health 56: #2, 299-314, February 1966.

26. Christensen, H. A., Achor, R. W. P., Berge, K. G., and Mason, H. L. *Hypercholesteremia; effects of treatment with nicotinic acid for three to seven years.* Dis. of Chest 46: #4, 411-416, October 1964.

27. Cohen, A. M., Barby, S., and Poznanski, R. *Change of diet of Yemenite Jews in relation to diabetes and ischemic heart disease.* Lancet 2: #7217, 1399-1401, December 23, 1961.

28. Cohen, A. M. *Fats and carbohydrates as factors in atherosclerosis and diabetes in Yemenite Jews.* Amer. Heart J. 65: #3, 291-293, March 1963.

29. Cohen, A. M. and Shafrir, E. *Carbohydrate metabolism in myocardial infarction; behavior of blood glucose and free fatty acid after glucose loading.* Diabetes 14: #2, 84-86, February 1965.

30. Conn, J. W. *Hypertension, the potassium ion and impaired carbohydrate tolerance.* New England J. Med. 273: #21, 1135-1143, November 18, 1965.

31. Conner, W. E., Hodges, R. E., and Bleiler, R. E. *The serum lipids in men receiving high cholesterol and cholesterol-free diets.* J. Clin. Invest. 40: #5, 894-901, May 1961.

32. Council on Foods and Nutrition, American Medical Association. Symposium III, *Fats in human nutrition with particular attention to fats, cholesterol and atherosclerosis.* 1957. Chicago 10, Illinois.

33. Dayton, S., Pearch, M. L., and Hiscock, E. *Can changes in the American diet prevent coronary heart disease?* J. Amer. Dietet. Assn. 46: #1, 20-25, January 1965.

34. Davies, D. F. *A serum protein deficiency related to coronary artery disease.* Lancet 1: #7375, 29-30, January 2, 1965.

35. DeCaro, L. G., Fattorini, A., and Gorini, M. *Plasma NEFA response to a glucose load in patients with diabetes, arteriosclerosis and obesity.* Metabolism 19: #1, 65-69, January 1966.

36. DeLange, D. J., Mey, H. S., and Vivier, F. S. *The effect of dietary therapy on abnormal carbohydrate and fat metabolism.* So. Afr. Med. J. 39: #16, 354-356, May 1, 1965.

37. Editorial. *Who are the coronary heart disease prone?* Rhode Island Med. J. 48: #5, 257, May 1965.

38. Epstein, F. H., Francis, T., Jr., Hayner, N. S., Johnson, B. C., Kjelsberg, M. O., Napier, J. H., Ostrander, L. D., Jr., Payne, M. W. and Dodge, H. J. *Prevalence of chronic diseases and distribution of selected physiologic variables in a total community, Tecumseh, Michigan.* Amer. J. Epidemiol. 81: #3, 307-322, May 1965.

39. Epstein, F. H., Ostrander, L. D., Jr., Johnson, B. C., Payne, M. W., Hayner, N. S., Keller, J. B., and Francis, T., Jr. *Epidemiological studies of cardiovascular disease in a total community, Tecumseh, Michigan.* Ann. Int. Med. 62: #6, 1170-1187, June 1965.

40. Fabrykant, M. and Gelfand, M. L. *Symptom-free diabetes in angina pectoris.* Amer. J. Med. Sc. 247: #6, 665-668, June 1964.

41. Fleischman, A. I. and Bierenbaum, M. L. *Dietary relationships of serum lipids in the young coronary male.* Fed. Proc. 23: #4, 876, Part I, July-August 1964.

42. Gertler, M. M., Garn, S. M., and White, P. D. *Young candidates for coronary heart disease.* J. A. M. A. 147: #7, 621-625, October 13, 1951.

43. Gertler, M. M., Woodbury, M. A., Gottsch, L. G., and White, P. D. *The candidate for coronary heart disease.* J. A. M. A. 170: #2, 149-152, May 9, 1959.

44. Goldsmith, G. A. *Highlights on the cholesterol fats, diets and atherosclerosis problem.* J. A. M. A. 176: #9, 783-790, June 3, 1961.

45. Goldsmith, G. *Niacin: antipellagra factor, Hypocholesterolemic agent.* J. A. M. A. 194: #2, 167-173, October 11, 1965.

46. Grande, F., Anderson, J. T., and Keys, A. *Effect of carbohydrates of leguminous seeds, wheat and potatoes on serum cholesterol concentrations in man.* J. Nutrit. 86: #3, 313-317, July 1965.

47. Greaves, J. P. and Hollingsworth, D. F. *Changes in the pattern of carbohydrate consumption in Britain.* Proc. Nutrit. Soc. 23: #2, 136-143, 1964.

48. Hales, C. N. and Randle, P. J. *Effects of a low-carbohydrate diet and diabetes mellitus on plasma concentrations of glucose, nonesterified fatty acid, and insulin during oral glucose tolerance tests.* Lancet 1: #7285, 790-794, April 13, 1963.

49. Hodges, R. E. and Krehl, W. A. *The role of carbohydrates in lipid metabolism.* Amer. J. Clin. Nutrit. 17: #5, 334-346, November 1965.

50. Kamp, H. V., Shipp, L. P., and Humphrey, A. A. *Prevention of coronary heart disease.* J. Michigan State Med. Soc. 61: #11, 1393-1394, November 1962.

51. Kane, J. P., Longcope, C., Pavlatos, F. C., and Grodsky, G. M. *Studies of carbohydrate metabolism in idiopathic hyperglyceridemia.* Metabolism 14: #4, 471-486, April 1965.

52. Kannel, W. B., Dawber, T. R., Thomas, H. E., Jr., and McNamara, P. M. *Comparison of serum lipids in the prediction of coronary heart disease.* Rhode Island Med. J. 48: #5, 243-250, May 1965.

53. Katz, L. N., Stamler, J., and Pick, R. *Nutrition and atherosclerosis.* 1948. Philadelphia, Lea and Febiger. pp. 15-16.

54. Keen, H., Rose, G., Pyke, D. A., Boyns, D., Chlouverakis, C., and Mistry, S. *Blood-sugar and arterial disease.* Lancet 2: #7411, 505-508, September 1965.

55. Keys, A., Anderson, J. T., and Grande, F. *Serum cholesterol response to changes in the diet. II. The effect of cholesterol in the diet.* Metabolism 14: #7, 759-765, July 1965.

56. Keys, A., Anderson, J. T., and Grande, F. *Serum cholesterol response to changes in the diet. IV. Particular saturated fatty acids in the diet.* Metabolism 14: #7, 776-787, July 1965.

57. Kilinskii, E. L. and Egart, F. M. *Coronary circulation in patients with diabetes mellitus (diurnal variations in ECG patterns).* Fed. Proc. (Trans. Supp.) 23: #2, Part II, T301-T303, March-April 1964.

58. Kimber, R. J. and Phear, D. N. *Glucose tolerance after myocardial infarction.* Med. J. Australia 1: #19, 686-687, May 8, 1965.

59. Kingsbury, K. J. *The essential fatty acids and human atheroma.* Geriatrics 20: #7, 554-562, July 1965.

60. Kopjas, T. L. *Treatment of chronic diffuse peripheral arteriosclerotic vascular disease with folic acid and vitamins B and C.* J. Amer. Geriat. Soc. 13: #10, 935-937, October 1965.

61. Krut, L. H. and Barsky, R. F. *Effect of enhanced glucose utilization on postprandial lipemia in ischemic heart disease.* Lancet 2: #7370, 1136-1138, November 28, 1964.

62. Krut, L. H. and Barsky, R. F. *Glucose and postprandial lipemia in ischemic heart disease.* Lancet 1: #7387, 707-708, March 27, 1965.

63. Kuo, P. T. and Bassett, D. R. *Dietary sugar in the production of hyperglyceridemia.* Ann. Int. Med. 62: #6, 1199-1212, June 1965.

64. Leak, D. and Dormandy, T. L. *Possible relations of hypoglycemia indicated by mono-amine oxidase inhibition and angina pectoris.* Proc. Soc. Exper. Biol. & Med. 108: #3, 597-600, December 1961.

65. Lees, R. S., Canellos, G. P., Rosenberg, I. H., and Hatch, F. T. *Myocardial infarction in one pair of twenty-seven year old identical male twins.* Amer. J. Med. 34: #5, 741-746, April 1963.

66. Lopez, A., Hodges, R. E., and Krehl, W. A. *Some interesting*

relationships between dietary carbohydrates and serum cholesterol. Amer. J. Clin. Nutrit. 18: #2, 149-153, February 1966.

67. Master, A. M. and Jaffe, H. L. Fads, public opinion and heart disease. J. A. M. A. 183: #2, 102-107, January 12, 1963.

68. Mathewson, F. A. L., Brereton, D. C., Keltie, W. A., and Paul, G. I. The University of Manitoba follow-up study: a prospective investigation of cardiovascular disease. Part II. Build, blood pressure and electrocardiographic factors possibly associated with the development of coronary heart disease. Canad. Med. Assn. J. 92: #19, 1002-1006, May 8, 1965.

69. McDonald, L. Studies on blood coagulation and thrombosis and on the action of heparin in ischemic heart disease. Amer. J. Cardiol. 9: #3, 365-371, March 1962.

70. Macdonald, I. Liver and depot lipids in children on normal and high carbohydrate diets. Amer. J. Clin. Nutrit. 12: #6, 431-436, June 1963.

71. Macdonald, I. Dietary carbohydrates and lipid metabolism. Proc. Nutrit. Soc. 23: #2, 119-123, 1964.

72. Macdonald, I. and Braithwhite, D. M. The influence of dietary carbohydrates on the lipid pattern in serum and adipose tissue. Clin. Sc. 27: #1, 23-30, August 1964.

73. Macdonald, I. The lipid response of young women to dietary carbohydrates. Amer. J. Clin. Nutrit. 16: #6, 458-463, July 1965.

74. Macdonald, I. The effects of various dietary carbohydrates on the serum lipids during a five-day regimen. Clin. Sc. 29: #1, 193-197, August 1965.

75. Macdonald, I. The lipid response of postmenopausal women to dietary carbohydrates. Amer. J. Clin. Nutrit. 18: #2, 86-90, February 1966.

76. Medical Tribune-World Wide Report. Catabolism in arterial wall held key to atherosclerosis. Med. Trib. 5: #79, 1, 23, August 3, 1964.

77. Medical Tribune-World Wide Report. Another risk factor cited in coronary heart disease. Med. Trib. 6: #77, June 28, 1965.

78. McKechnie, J. K. and Davidson, F. J. Coronary artery disease in Natal Indians. South African Med. J. 38: #11, 208-211, March 28, 1964.

79. McOsker, D. E., Mattson, F. H., Sweringen, H. B., and Kligman, A. M. The influence of partially hydrogenated dietary fats on

serum cholesterol levels. J. A. M. A. 180: #5, 380-385, May 5, 1962.

80. Moolten, S. E., Jennings, P. B., and Solden, A. *Dietary fat and platelet adhesiveness in arteriosclerosis and diabetes.* Amer. J. Cardiol. 11: #3, 290-300, March 1963.

81. National Center for Health Statistics. *Heart disease in adults; United States 1960-1962.* Series 11: #6, September 1964. Washington, D. C., Superintendent of Documents, Government Printing Office.

82. National Dairy Council. *Diet patterns and coronary heart disease.* Dairy Council Sig. 35: #6, November-December 1964.

83. Nestel, P. J. *Metabolism of linoleate and palmitate in patients with hypertriglyceridemia and heart disease.* Metabolism 14: #1, 1-9, January 1965.

84. *New hope in fights on heart disease.* Business Week, December 12, 1964.

85. Nikitin, J. P. *Effect of vitamin E on blood lipids and coagulability in patients with atherosclerosis.* Vop. Pitan. 21: #6, 22-27, 1962. Abstract in Nutrit. Abs. & Rev. 33: #2, 519, April 1963.

86. Nye, E. R. *Glucose tolerance test in hypertensive patients.* Brit. Med. J. 2: #5411, 727-730, September 19, 1964.

87. Olson, R. E. *The two-carbon chain in metabolism.* J. A. M. A. 183: #6, 471-474, February 9, 1963.

88. Ostfeld, A. M., Lebovits, B. Z., Shekelle, R. B., and Paul, O. *A prospective study of the relationship between personality and coronary heart disease.* J. Chron. Dis. 17: #3, 265-276, March 1964.

89. Ostrander, L. D., Jr. and Weinstein, B. J. *Electrocardiographic changes after glucose ingestion.* Circulation 30: #1, 67-76, July 1964.

90. Ostrander, L. D., Jr., Francis, T., Jr., Hayner, N. S., Kjelsberg, M. O., and Epstein, F. H. *The relationship of cardiovascular disease to hyperglycemia.* Ann. Int. Med. 62: #6, 1188-1198, June 1965.

91. Owren, P. A., Hellem, A. J. and Odegaard, A. *Linolenic acid for the prevention of thrombosis and myocardial infarction.* Lancet 2: #7367, 975-979, November 7, 1964.

92. Palma-Garcia, S. and Aspe-Rosas, J. *Postprandial electrocardiographic modifications.* Angiology 15: #4, 174-183, April 1964.

93. Paterson, J. C., Armstrong, R., and Armstrong, E. C. *Serum lipid levels and the severity of coronary and cerebral atherosclerosis in adequately nourished men, 60 to 69 years of age.* Circulation 27: #2, 229-236, February 1963.

94. Pelkonen, R. *Plasma vitamin A and E in the study of lipid and lipoprotein metabolism in coronary heart disease.* Acta Med. Scandinav. 174: Suppl. 399, 1963.

95. Pilgeram, L. D., Bandi, Z., and Thelander, P. F. *Albumin correction of the clearing factor defect in ageing, arteriosclerotic subjects.* J. Atheroscl. Res. 4: #3, 244-253, May-June 1964.

96. Pinter, K. G. and Karle, I. P. *Effect of ingestion of various mono- and triglycerides on serum triglyceride concentration.* Amer. J. Clin. Nutrit. 18: #3, 165-168, March 1966.

97. Pleshkov, A. M. *Effect of long-term intake of easily absorbed carbohydrates (sugars) on blood lipid level in patients with atherosclerosis.* Fed. Proc. Trans. Suppl. 23: #2, Part II, 334-336, March-April 1964.

98. Reaven, G., Calciano, A., Cody, R., Lucas, C., and Miller, R. *Carbohydrate intolerance and hyperlipemia in patients with myocardial infarction.* J. Clin. Endocrinol. & Metab. 23: #10, 1013-1023, October 1963.

99. Ringsdorf, W. M., Jr. and Cheraskin, E. *Effect of a relatively high-protein low-refined-carbohydrate diet upon serum cholesterol concentration.* J. Amer. Geriat. Soc. 11: #2, 156-165, February 1963.

100. Rivin, A. U. *Hypercholesterolemia; use of niacin and niacin combinations in therapy.* California Med. 96: #4, 267-269, April 1962.

101. Rosenman, R. H., Friedman, M., Straus, R., Wurm, M., Kositchek, R., Hahn, W., and Werthessen, N. T. *A predictive study of coronary heart disease; the western collaborative group study.* J. A. M. A. 189: #1, 15-22, July 6, 1964.

102. Sandler, B. P. *The control of the anginal syndrome with a low carbohydrate diet.* Med. Ann. D. C. 10: #10, 371-380, October 1941.

103. Sandler, M. and Bourne, G. H. *Dietary effects on the arterial wall.* Angiology 16: #7, 375-378, July 1965.

104. Schroeder, H. A. *Relation between mortality from cardiovascular disease and treated water supplies.* J. A. M. A. 172: #17, 1902-1908, April 23, 1960.

105. Schroeder, H. A. *Relations between hardness of water and death rates from certain chronic and degenerative diseases in the United States.* J. Chron. Dis. 12: #6, 586-591, December 1960.

106. Schroeder, H. A. *Municipal drinking water and cardiovascular death rates.* J. A. M. A. 195: #2, 125-129, January 10, 1966.

107. Schwartz, D., Lellouch, J., Anguera, G., Beaumont, J. L., and Lenegre, J. *Tobacco and other factors in the etiology of ischemic heart disease. Results of a retrospective survey.* J. Chron. Dis. 19: #1, 35-55, January 1966.

108. Siperstein, M. D. *Inter-relationships of glucose and lipid metabolism.* Amer. J. Med. 26: #5, 685-702, May 1959.

109. Snapper, I. *Diet and atherosclerosis: truth and fiction.* Amer. J. Cardiol. 11: #3, 283-289, March 1963.

110. Soloff, L. A. and Schwartz, H. *Relationship between glucose and fatty acid in myocardial infarction.* Lancet 1: #7285, 449-452, February 26, 1966.

111. Sowton, E. *Cardiac infarction and the glucose tolerance test.* Brit. Med. J. 1: #5271, 84-86, January 13, 1962.

112. Spirt, J. J., Davidenkowa, I. M., and Sewrjugina, A. T. *Use of vitamins A and E in different forms of atherosclerosis.* Ztschr. Ges. Inn. Med. 17: 431-436, 1962. Abstract in Nutrit. Abs. & Rev. 33: #2, 516, April 1963.

113. Stamler, J. J., Berkson, D. M., Lindberg, H. H., Hall, Y., Miller, W. A., Mojounier, L., Cohen, D. B., Levinson, M., and Young, Q. D. *Coronary risk factors - their impact and their therapy in the effort to achieve primary prevention of clinical coronary heart disease.* Chicago Med. 68: #11, 467-469, May 29, 1965.

114. Straus, R., Kositchek, R. J., Wurm, M., Toto, A. J., and Olsberg, A. E. *Changes in serum lipoproteins, lipids and body weight induced by an ad libitum low-fat, low-calorie diet.* J. Amer. Geriat. Soc. 10: #11, 954-968, November 1962.

115. Syme, S. L., Hyman, M. M., and Enterline, P. E. *Some social and cultural factors associated with the occurrence of coronary heart disease.* J. Chron. Dis. 17: #3, 277-289, March 1964.

116. Takahashi, E. *An epidemiological approach to the relation between diet and cerebrovascular lesions and arteriosclerotic heart disease.* Tohoku J. Exp. Med. 77: #3, 239-257, August 25, 1962.

117. Turner, N. C., Gertler, M. M., and Cady, L. D., Jr. *Some aspects of carbohydrate metabolism and coronary heart disease.* Geriatrics 17: #1, 20-25, January 1962.

118. Unger, P. N. Coronary proneness; can it be identified? J. Florida Med. Assn. 51: #9, 579-581, September 1964.

119. Van Belle, J., Hartroft, W. S., and Donohue, W. L. Early atheromatous lesions in aortas and coronary arteries of infants and children. Fed. Proc. 23: #4, Part I, 880, July-August 1964.

120. Van Itallie, T. B. and Hashim, S. A. Diet and heart disease - facts and unanswered questions. J. Amer. Dietet. Assn. 38: #6, 531-535, June 1961.

121. Waddell, W. R. and Field, R. A. Carbohydrate metabolism in atherosclerosis. Metabolism 9: #9, 801-806, September 1960.

122. Wahlberg, F. The intravenous glucose tolerance test in atherosclerotic disease with special reference to obesity, hypertension, diabetic heredity and cholesterol values. Acta Med. Scand. 171: #1, 1-7, January 1962.

123. Wester, P. O. Trace elements in human myocardial infarction determined by neutron activation analysis. Acta Med. Scand. 178: #6, 765-788, December 1965.

124. White, P. L. Diet and the possible prevention of coronary atheroma; a council on foods and nutrition statement. J. A. M. A. 194: #10, 1149-1150, December 6, 1965.

125. Winitz, M., Graff, J., and Seedman, D. A. Effect of dietary carbohydrate on serum cholesterol levels. Arch. Biochem. & Biophy. 108: #3, 576-579, December 1964.

126. Yacowitz, H., Fleischman, A. I., and Bierenbaum, M. L. Effects of oral calcium upon serum lipids in man. Brit. Med. J. 1: #5446, 1352-1354, May 22, 1965.

127. Yudkin, J. Nutrition and palatability with special reference to obesity, myocardial infarction, and other diseases of civilization. Lancet 1: #7295, 1335-1338, June 22, 1963.

128. Yudkin, J. Dietary carbohydrates and ischemic heart disease. Amer. Heart J. 66: #6, 835-836, December 1963.

129. Yudkin, J. Patterns and trends in carbohydrate consumption and their relation to disease. Proc. Nutrit. Soc. 23: #2, 149-162, 1964.

130. Yudkin, J. and Roddy, J. Levels of dietary sucrose in patients with occlusive atherosclerotic disease. Lancet 2: #7349, 6-8, July 4, 1964.

131. Yudkin, J. Dietary fat and dietary sugar in relation to ischemic heart disease and diabetes. Lancet 2: #7349, 45, July 4, 1964.

132. Yudkin, J. Dietetic aspects of atherosclerosis. Angiology 17: #2, 127-133, February 1966.

PART THREE

EPILOGUE

MAN'S QUEST FOR CATEGORIZATION HAS PRODUCED AN ELABORATE system of distinct disease entities. Once a set of symptoms and signs is christened, the pattern is deemed to be unique and the syndrome regarded as separate and distinct from other such entities. Hence, diabetes mellitus becomes a problem apart from ischemic heart disease and cancer. To a degree, this is a useful approach for the understanding and management of these disorders. For example, in Part Two (Disease States), this conventional classification has proved helpful in communicating the relationship of diet to such syndromes.

The conventional classification, however, is not without limitations. This was brought into focus by Sir Thomas Lewis:

> The continued separation of disease into types can be pressed too far, and a subdivision which may perhaps have some immediate practical use can help to conceal underlying mechanisms held in common and thus to hinder progress in studying disease.

In other words, diseases appear to cluster both clinically and metabolically. The interrelationships of many of these chronic disorders will be the concern of Chapter Twelve in this section.

If there is any validity to the theme of this book, namely a relationship between diet and disease, it must become evident, at least by implication, that there is also a relationship between diet and health. It is reasonable to expect that there ought to be generalizations which permit the development of an optimal diet. Perhaps assistance in the construction of such a regime can be gained by examining the diets of individuals with obvious illness. Possibly, additional information could be derived from a study of the food consumption among persons with marginal sickness. Lastly, it may be informative to analyze the dietary habits of healthy subjects. Conceivably, from such a three-pronged analysis, it would be possible to create the optimal diet. The final chapter (Thirteen) thus faces up to this admittedly difficult task.

Man's myopia frequently is reflected in his inability to note the obvious. This nearsightedness prevails in the thesis that Americans eat well. Unfortunately, this has served to dampen investigation and has muted interest in the correlation of diet and disease. Of the many who have called attention to the hazards which stem from ignoring the obvious, perhaps none has expressed it more penetratingly than Francis Bacon (Novum Organum, First Book, page 119) when he said:

> Nothing has been so injurious to philosophy as this circumstance, namely, that familiar and frequent objects do not arrest and detain men's contemplation, but are carelessly admitted, and their causes never inquired after.

12. DISEASE STATE INTERRELATIONSHIPS

IN THE BOOK, TRANSITIONS IN MEDICINE, DOCTOR IAGO GALDSTON, one of the foremost medical philosophers, emphasizes that nutrition was not only "the foundation of Hippocratic medicine" but is, today, "the foundation of physiological medicine" (15).

The science of nutrition is without doubt one of the greatest, most significant, and most permeative attainments of modern medicine. It impinges upon and affects every phase and aspect of life and being. It is basic to human well-being and to medicine. Unfortunately, what is known about nutrition is as yet not fully utilized in the practice of medicine, or in the maintenance of health.

Thus, it is quite possible that the proper application of dietary and nutritional knowledge could appreciably improve health and increase life expectancy in the United States. Doctor James M. Hundley, Chief of the Laboratory of Biochemistry and Nutrition at the National Institutes of Health, has called attention to medicine's poor progress in conquering the diseases which afflict older people. The national scope of these "chronic degenerative disorders" has been summarized in Chapter Two. It is apparent (Figure 12.1) that, at 50 years of age, little increase in life expectancy has occurred since 1900 (18).

OVERNUTRITION

According to the late Doctor Thomas D. Spies (Professor of Nutrition and Metabolism, Northwestern University Medical School and Director of the Nutrition Clinic, Hillman Hospital, Birmingham, Alabama) "germs are not our principal enemy" (39).

Our chief medical adversary is what I consider a disturbance of the inner balance of the constituents of our tissues, which are

built from and maintained by necessary chemicals in the air we breathe, the water we drink and the food we eat.
In an analysis of what we eat, Doctors Louis N. Katz (Director, Cardiovascular Department, Medical Research Institute, Michael Reese Hospital), Jeremiah Stamler (Director, Heart Disease Control Program, Chicago Board of Health), and Ruth Pick (Assistant Director, Cardiovascular Department, Medical Research Institute, Michael Reese Hospital) have emphasized in their text, *Nutrition and Atherosclerosis*, that malnutrition is actually prevalent in this country (22).
In the economically developed countries a marked change in nutritional patterns has occurred during the last century. In conjunction with industrialization, urbanization, and increase in per capita national income, "richer" diets have become commonplace— diets containing sizeable quantities of the more expensive high-lipid foods of animal origin plus "elegant" white bread and refined sugar. These foods are now consumed en masse in countries like the United States. As a result, intake en masse of total cal-

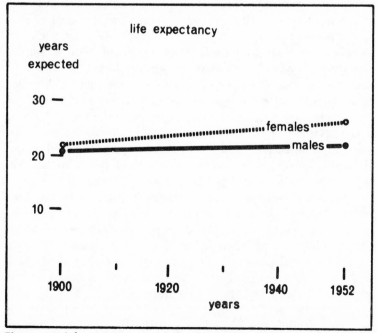

Figure 12.1. Life expectancy trends for 50 year old white males and females in the United States (1900 - 1952).

ories, empty calories, total fats, cholesterol, saturated fats has tended to increase significantly in these economically developed countries.... In fact, the calorie intake is frequently in excess of the total required to balance energy expenditure, with consequent widespread obesity.... Thus, malnutrition of a different type is actually widespread in the economically developed countries—malnutrition in the literal meaning of the word, bad nutrition.

Doctor Rene Dubos *(12)* of the Rockefeller Institute recently warned of the consequences of this dietary pattern:

Thus, history repeats itself. Like the prosperous Romans of 2,000 years ago, many prosperous citizens of the Western world today dig their own graves through overeating.

The clinical effect of so-called overnutrition upon energy metabolism in the United States is evident in the alarming prevalence of obesity. An excess of 20 pounds above the ideal weight is frequently taken as evidence of overweight. By this standard, 25 per cent of men over 30 years and 40 per cent of women over the age of 40 are obese. Similar figures are quoted for adolescents *(35)*. Excess weight also makes a significant contribution to morbidity (Table 12.1) *(11)* and mortality (Table 12.2) *(30)*. From Table 12.1 many chronic diseases occur in pairs much more frequently than expected. For example, hypertensive vascular disease and arthritis are observed 1.47 more times than anticipated. However, the relationship between hypertensive vascular disease and arthritis occurs even more frequently than expected (2.28 times) in the obese patient. It is also apparent that excessive weight (Table 12.2) is significantly related to mortality. In Chapter Two (National Scope of Health and Disease) it was emphasized that chronic disorders are the principal public health concern.

Diabetes mellitus is also, in part, a product of the prevailing dietary habits of the economically developed countries *(7,8,28)*. The close ties between these two disorders of metabolism (obesity and diabetes mellitus) are evident not only from the morbidity and mortality data presented in Table 12.1 and Table 12.2, respectively, but also from observations of increased insulin *(20,21,43)* and adrenocortical activity *(38)* in apparently healthy obese subjects. Actually, at least 80 per cent of adult diabetics living in the United States are or were obese *(3)*. The exaggerated serum insulin levels observed after administration of glucose (orally or intravenously) in maturity onset diabetic patients correlate with the degree of obesity and do not differ qualitatively from the hyperresponse of insulin to glucose in obesity *(21)*. Following weight reduction *(25)*, in some patients, there is a normalization of both blood sugar and serum insulin levels as clearly shown in an 18 year old patient (Figure 12.2 *(21)*. In the diabetic American male an increase in weight above the accepted normal is associated with a considerable increase in the risk of dying (Figure 12.3). For example, an individual with 20 per cent above average weight has a 350 per cent greater mortality risk.

Table 12.1
significant chronic disease interrelationships in the
same person and their association with overweight

related chronic conditions	per cent actual (observed) of expected occurrences together*
hypertensive vascular disease--gall bladder disease	223
hypertensive vascular disease--gall bladder disease in overweight subjects	345
hypertensive vascular disease--arthritis	147
hypertensive vascular disease--arthritis in overweight subjects	228
heart disease--gall bladder disease in overweight subjects	415
heart disease--diabetes in overweight subjects	452
arthritis--gall bladder disease	167
psychoneurosis--gall bladder	279
overweight--heart disease	134
overweight--hypertensive vascular disease	134
overweight--arthritis	137
overweight--diabetes mellitus	148
overweight--gall bladder disease	146

$$\frac{\text{*actual (observed) occurrence together}}{\text{expected occurrence together}} \times 100$$

Table 12.2
principal causes of death among men
and women significantly related
with overweight

cause of death	per cent actual of expected deaths	
	men	women
principal cardiovascular-renal diseases	149	177
diabetes mellitus	383	372
cirrhosis of the liver	249	—
appendicitis	223	195
biliary calculi	206	284
tuberculosis (all forms)	21	35
gastric and duodenal ulcers	67	—
suicide	78	—
accidents (total)	—	135

According to figures from the Nutrition Research Laboratories, Department of Preventive Medicine, Washington University School of Medicine, the prevalence of diabetes is increasing in the United States at a more rapid rate than the total population (28). From current death rates by the World Health Organization (13), the United States is one of the leaders in diabetic deaths (Table 12.3) among the economically developed countries. It is interesting to note, also, that most of these nations have demonstrated a significant increase in the diabetic rate during the last decade.

From an observation of the diseases that accompany diabetes mellitus (Table 12.4) (37) and of the principal causes of death in diabetics (Table 12.5) (11), it is evident that frank diabetes is closely associated with the chronic degenerative diseases which are presently of national concern. In each chapter of Part Two (Disease States) a relationship was noted between a disturbance in carbohydrate metabolism and the disease state under consideration.

DISEASE CLUSTERS

The American Diet (Chapter One), therefore, does not just contribute to specific diseases but may foster deranged energy metabolism which appears to play a role in many of the prevalent chronic disorders. Disease state interrelationships have been observed as "disease clusters" and multiple diagnoses are commonly made in patients *(6)*. For example, in a study of 170 stroke patients at Wayne State University Center for Cerebrovascular Research, Doctor John Sterling Meyer *(33)* (Chairman, Department of Neurology) noted significantly high frequencies of accompanying disease states (Table 12.6).

Considerable interest is being shown concerning the interrelationships between hyperuricemia, gout, diabetes mellitus, atherosclerotic vascular disease, obesity, hypercholesterolemia, coronary disease, hypertension, and neoplasia

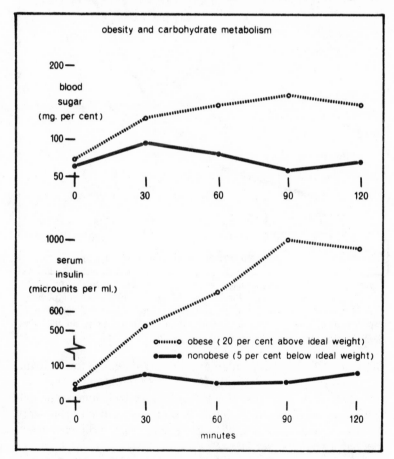

Figure 12.2. The effect of weight reduction upon blood sugar and serum insulin levels following a 100 gram oral glucose load in an 18 year old girl.

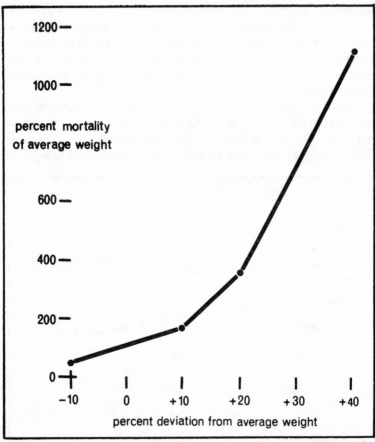

Figure 12.3. Risk of dying from diabetes mellitus relative to degree of departure from average weight for height and age group at time of physical examination for life insurance (white males, low risk group, medium to upper income, midwest, east and south of United States, between 1887 and 1908, aged 45 years and over at time of death).

(5,17,19,26,27,31,34,40). In an excellent review, Doctor William K. Ishmael *(19)*, Associate Professor of Medicine and Director of the Arthritis Clinic at the University of Oklahoma Medical Center, pointed out that gout, diabetes, atherosclerosis, and obesity are causally related to dietary sucrose induced hypertriglyceridemia.

The association between impaired carbohydrate metabolism and atherosclerosis, and between dietary carbohydrate (sucrose)

Table 12.3
death rates from diabetes mellitus in
selected countries in 1950-1952 and 1960-1962

country	death rates per 100,000		per cent change
	1950-1952	1960-1962	
Australia	12.8	12.1	− 5
New Zealand	12.6	12.1**	− 4
England and Wales	8.2	8.1	− 1
United States	16.3	16.7	+ 2
Canada	11.2	11.8	+ 5
South Africa (whites)	10.0	10.6***	+ 6
Switzerland	13.4	14.7**	+10
Ireland	7.4	8.7	+18
Netherlands	11.4*	14.4	+26
France	10.1	12.9	+28
Germany (West)	10.2	13.6**	+33
Denmark	6.1*	8.3**	+36
Sweden	10.2	14.1**	+38
Belgium	15.6	23.2**	+49
Italy	8.6	12.9**	+50
Spain	6.1	9.3**	+52
Japan	2.4	3.7	+54

*   1951-1952
** 1960-1961
***1960

Table 12.4
associated diseases among 225 cases of
diabetes mellitus admitted to the Mary
Johnston Hospital from January 1
through December 31, 1964

disease	per cent cases with disease
arteriosclerotic heart disease	31
pulmonary tuberculosis	18
pyelonephritis-urolithiasis group	14
hypertension	11
myocardial infarction	8
cerebrovascular accident	8
deranged hepatic function	8
gall bladder disease	6
azotemic-uremic group	4

and hypertriglyceridemia, and the increased triglyceride concentration accompanying hyperuricemia, are consistent with the hypothesis that the genetically associated diseases of gout, diabetes, atherosclerosis and obesity are causally related to carbohydrate (sucrose) induced or aggravated hypertriglyceridemia.

An increasing consumption of "empty calories" was noted in an earlier discussion in this section and in Chapter One (The American Diet). Thus, more simple sugars and less complex carbohydrates appear to be the principal dietary changes in this country during the last century.

Table 12.5
principal causes of death among diabetic
patients at the Joslin Clinic in
Boston, Massachusetts (1960-1964)

causes of death	per cent of all causes
vascular diseases	77.9
cancer	9.5
infections	5.8
accidents	1.7
diabetic coma	1.1
cirrhosis of the liver	1.0
number of deaths	2,634

Table 12.6
per cent of 170 stroke patients
with accompanying disease states

disease	per cent of patients with disease
hypertension	75.8
arteriosclerotic heart disease	51.7
hypercholesterolemia	44.7
hypothyroidism	38.0
gout or hyperuricemia	33.0
diabetes mellitus	31.0
postural hypotension	16.0
anemia	13.1
myocardial infarct	10.0
peripheral arteriosclerotic ischemia	5.0
syphilis	5.0
rheumatic heart disease	4.5
polycythemia	1.5

Doctor Ishmael *(19)* has also noted that coronary artery disease, obesity, diabetes, and hyperglyceridemia may be different manifestations of the same genetic trait, which possibly exists in as much as 40 per cent of the population. The common association together of coronary artery disease, obesity, diabetes and hyperglyceridemia and their frequent familial occurrence suggests that all these conditions may be different manifestations of the same genetic trait. This genetic tendency may exist with more frequency than the usually quoted incidence of clinical diabetes of one to two per cent. Mildly impaired glucose tolerance, prevalent in many, could not be diagnosed as unequivocal clinical diabetes, yet could play a vital role in atherogenesis. If clinical diabetes mellitus represents the homogeneous state of a single recessive gene and if a "degree" of clinical diabetes is present in as much as four per cent of the population, the heterogeneous state might be expected to be present in thirty to forty per cent of the population.

Dental caries is intimately associated with the geographic incidence of these "diseases of civilization." Doctor Fred L. Losee *(29)*, Dental Research Facility, United States Naval Training Center, has observed a strong geographic correlation between digestive tract cancer and dental decay. As was noted for coronary artery disease, obesity, diabetes, and gout, the ingestion of large quantities of refined carbohydrates is causally related to the carious lesion. It has been emphasized throughout this book that this type of overnutrition may be a potentiating factor in a variety of chronic conditions.

A pathologic oral finding which has been observed to occur in relation to coronary artery disease is dental calculus (tartar). From Table 12.7 it appears that the rate of deposition is positively correlated with the personal and family history of coronary heart disease *(42)*.

Doctor Sidney Cobb and Doctor William Hall *(6)* from the Survey Research Center of the University of Michigan recently reported what they termed a "newly identified cluster of diseases." In a study of 244 employed men they found that rheumatoid arthritis is significantly associated with tuberculosis and peptic ulcer. According to these investigators, this disease cluster is negatively associated with the occurrence of myocardial infarction, obesity, and hypertension. Also associated with rheumatoid arthritis is the problem of subfertility. The Chelsea and Kensington Group Rheumatism Units at St. Stephen's Hospital in London (24) have found fertility to be lowered before and after the onset of the disease (Table 12.8).

There is considerably more information concerning "disease clusters" or disease state interrelationships. A sufficient number of examples, however, have been presented to illustrate the complex associations. In many of the prevalent chronic disorders, "bad nutrition" appears to be a possible responsible denominator for the clustering effect.

Table 12.7
rate of deposition of dental calculus
(tartar) versus cardiovascular findings

	low (n=27)	low medium (n=36)	high medium (n=42)	high (n=??
percentage of subjects with prior history of coronary heart disease	11.1	13.8	28.5	34.5
number of family members with coronary heart disease per subject	1.23	1.28	1.28	1.75

Table 12.8
fertility in 54 pairs in which both
patient and control were married before
onset of rheumatoid arthritis in the patient

series	patients	controls	difference
total live births	91.00	142.00	51.00
total mean size of family	1.68	2.62	0.94
live births before onset	76.00	124.00	48.00
mean size of family before onset	1.40	2.29	.89

METABOLIC INTERRELATIONS

In Chapter Four (Diet and the Nature of Health and Disease) it was observed that one of the characteristics of disease and especially chronic disease, is its progressive nature. Thus, before the disease is clinically apparent, there are biochemical aberrations. Therefore, the cause of disease clustering may be (1) that a metabolic flaw, in different people,

Table 12.9
Interrelationships between dietary
carbohydrate, biochemical parameters of
energy metabolism, and disease states

diet	metabolism	disease state
a high carbohydrate intake	increases serum tri- glycerides, circulat- ing insulin and in- sulin resistance	enhancing athero- sclerosis and the de- velopment of diabetes mellitus
a high refined carbohydrate in- take	results in a defi- ciency of specific carbohydrate enzymes and a decrease in glucose tolerance	giving rise to diabetes mellitus and athero- sclerosis
most of dietary carbohydrate as sucrose or glucose	causes an increase in serum triglycerides	which is a feature of: obesity diabetes mellitus gout atherosclerosis
most of dietary carbohydrate as starch	produces a reduction in serum triglycer- ides	
a 100 gram glucose tolerance supple- ment or 60 grams intravenously	produces an exces- sive serum insulin response	in obesity in hyperglyceridemia
a 100 gram oral or a 25 gram intra- venous glucose tolerance supple- ment	yielded evidence of a close association between impaired glu- cose tolerance and increased serum tri- glycerides	and support to the possibility that ele- vation of plasma tri- glycerides is a manifestation of in- sulin resistance and represents a stage in the development of maturity onset diabetes

can produce different disorders, and (2) that faulty metabolism is initiated and/or enhanced by faulty nutrition.

Tables 12.9 and 12.10 *(1,2,4,10,14,16,19,21,23,32,36,41)* provide some examples of the complex associations between dietary carbohydrate, biochemical parameters of energy metabolism, and disease states. The positive associations of hypertriglyceridemia, hyperuricemia, and impaired glucose tolerance make it evident that energy metabolism cannot be dissected into fat, protein, and carbohydrate compartments. It is, therefore, quite understandable that disease state clusters are common. It is also apparent from Table 12.9 and other evidence cited in this chapter that an excessive refined carbohydrate (simple sugar) intake may be causally related to a greater extent than has been previously suspected in obesity, diabetes mellitus, atherosclerosis, coronary heart disease, gout, and hypertension.

Table 12.10
Interrelationships between biochemical
parameters of energy metabolism
and disease states

metabolism	disease state
a positive association exists between hypertriglyceridemia. hyperuricemia, and impaired glucose tolerance	
a primary association between hypertriglyceridemia and impaired glucose tolerance	helps explain the increased frequency of diabetes in diseases such as coronary atherosclerosis. hypertension. hyperlipemia and gout (which have elevated triglyceride levels as a common feature)
decreased carbohydrate tolerance, abnormal lipid patterns. excessive insulin response to glucose, and excessive synalbumin insulin antagonism	exist in diabetes mellitus, atherosclerosis, and ischemic heart disease
correction of elevated serum triglyceride levels occurred	in maturity onset diabetes that responded to tolbutamide
impaired carbohydrate metabolism or an impaired glucose tolerance	is evident in: pregnancy women taking ovulatory suppressants

SUMMARY

In the world of traditional diagnosis, there is the implication that each disease is a separate and distinct entity. On the basis of this hypothesis, it becomes comprehensible for an individual to suffer with, for example, ischemic heart disease and be otherwise "healthy." In contrast, the data contained in this chapter are representative of the emerging viewpoint that an individual with one chronic problem very likely is afflicted with other degenerative syndromes. In other words, some diseases appear in clusters. Furthermore, evidence of common etiologic threads of a dietary nature interlacing these clusters of degenerative disorders has been presented.

It has been pointed out that man's ability to survive is a function of homeostasis. This capacity to live with the many ever-present environmental challenges is a product of numerous defense mechanisms implicating, for example, phagocytosis, immune bodies, and the enzymes. Though the understanding of such systems is incomplete, the fact remains that they depend, to a degree, upon an adequate diet.

The link between diet and aberrations in energy metabolism has been documented. It should be underscored that noncarbohydrate nutrients, for example, vitamin fractions (Chapter Four), influence energy metabolism. Furthermore, carbohydrate foodstuffs alter noncarbohydrate parameters of metabolism. The effect of dietary sucrose upon serum lipids is typical of this relationship (Chapter Eleven, Ischemic Heart Disease). Finally, the interrelationships between all nutrients have been described (Chapter Four). For the reasons just offered, it should be clear that there must be other nutritional threads in the fabric of disease.

The Council on Foods and Nutrition of the American Medical Association has expressed its awareness of these nutritional strands and their applicability to the health sciences *(9)*.

The concepts of nutrition integral to the practice of medicine are applicable in diagnosis of disease, treatment of disease, in rehabilitation from chronic illness, in disease prevention, and in health promotion.

Not only does the nutritional status of the patient influence the development and regression of many diseases, but many disorders, whether infectious, metabolic, degenerative, or neoplastic, influence the nutritional status of the patient.... Undergraduate teaching of nutrition is centered around nutritional deficiency diseases. This is too limited a focus for present-day problems. It is necessary to think more in terms of disturbances of the metabolic and biochemical reactions of the body. Nutritional diagnosis implies evaluation of biochemical changes within and outside the cell, as well as abnormalities of function and structure of the organs and tissues of the body.

REFERENCES

1. Albrink, M. J. *Diet, diabetes and serum lipids.* Diabetes 13: #4, 425-429, July-August 1964.

2. Albrink, M. J. and Davidson, P. C. *Impaired glucose tolerance in patients with hypertriglyceridemia.* J. Lab. & Clin. Med. 67: #4, 573-584, April 1966.

3. Aldersberg, D. *Obesity, fat metabolism and diabetes.* Diabetes 7: #8, 236-243, May-June 1958.

4. Ashton, W. L. *Atheroma, glucose, lipid, and insulin.* Lancet 2: #7704, 347-348, August 14, 1965.

5. Bradley, R. F. and Partamian, J. O. *Coronary heart disease in the diabetic patient.* Med. Clin. N. A. 49: #4, 1093-1104, July 1965.

6. Cobb, S. and Hall, W. *Newly identified cluster of diseases.* J. A. M. A. 193: #13, 1077-1079, September 27, 1965.

7. Cohen A. M. *Fats and carbohydrates as factors in atherosclerosis and diabetes in Yemenite Jews.* Am. Heart J. 65: #3, 291-293, March 1963.

8. Cohen, A. M. and Teitelbaum, A. *Effect of dietary sucrose and starch on oral glucose tolerance and insulin-like activity.* Am. J. Physiol. 206: #1, 105-108, January 1964.

9. Council on Foods and Nutrition, American Medical Association, *Nutrition teaching to medical schools.* J. A. M. A. 183: #11, 955-957, March 16, 1963.

10. Davidson, P. and Albrink, M. J. *Excessive plasma insulin in non-obese, non-diabetic hyperglyceridemic persons.* Clin. Res. 13: #3, 417, October 1965.

11. Downes, J. *Association of the chronic diseases in the same person and their association with overweight.* Milbank Mem. Fund Quart. 31: #2, 125-140, April 1953.

12. Dubos, R. *Man adapting.* 1965. New Haven, Yale University Press. p. 77.

13. Entmacher, P. S. and Marks, H. H. *Diabetes in 1964, a world survey.* Diabetes 14: #4, 212-223, April 1965.

14. Erlander, S. R. *Common enzyme deficiencies may cause athero-sclerosis and diabetes mellitus.* Enzymologia 28: #3, 139-151, 1965.

15. Galdston, I. *Medicine in transition.* 1965. Chicago, The University of Chicago Press.

16. Gershberg, H., Javier, Z. and Hulse, M. *Glucose tolerance in women receiving an ovulatory suppressant.* Diabetes 13: #4, 378-382, July-August 1964.

17. Hall, A. P. *Correlations among hyperuricemia, hypercholesterolemia, coronary disease and hypertension.* Arth. & Rheumat 8: #5, Part I, 846-852, October 1965.

18. Hundley, J. M. *Diabetes—overweight: U. S. problems.* J. Am Dietet. Assn. 32: #5, 417-422, May 1956.

19. Ishmael, W. K. *Atherosclerotic vascular disease in familial gout, diabetes and obesity.* Med. Times 94: #2, 157-162, February 1966.

20. Karam, J. H., Grodsky, G. M. and Forsham, P. H. *Excessive insulin response to glucose in obese subjects as measured by immunochemical assay.* Diabetes 12: #3, 197-204, May-June 1963.

21. Karam, J. H., Grodsky, G. M. and Forsham, P. H. *The relationship of obesity and growth hormone to serum insulin levels.* Ann. New York Acad. Sc. 131: #1, 374-387, October 8, 1965.

22. Katz, L. N., Stamler, J. and Pick, R. *Nutrition and atherosclerosis.* 1958. Philadelphia, Lea and Febiger. pp. 16-20.

23. Kaufmann, N. A., Poznanski, R., Blondheim, S. H. and Stein, Y. *Changes in serum lipid levels of hyperlipemic patients following the feeding of starch, sucrose and glucose.* Am. J. Clin. Nutrit. 18: #4, 261-269, April 1966.

24. Kay, A. and Bach, F. *Subfertility before and after the development of rheumatoid arthritis in women.* Ann. Rheumat. Dis. 24: #2, 169-173, March 1965.

25. Klimt, C. R. and Goldner, M. G. *Epidemiologic associations of environmental factors with diabetes mellitus.* J. Kentucky Med. Assn. 62: #7, July 1964.

26. Kolbel, F., Gregorova, I., and Sonka, J. *Hyperuricemia in hypertension.* Lancet 1: #7384, 519-520, March 6, 1965.

27. Lea, A. J. *Diabetes and neoplasia.* Lancet 1: #7441, 821-822, April 9, 1966.

28. Levin, M. E. and Recant, L. *Diabetes and the environment.* Arch. Environ. Health 12: #5, 621-630, May 1966.

29. Losee, F. L. *Geographic isolation: its value in epidemiologic research.* J. Dent. Res. 42: #1, Part 2, 202-208, January-February 1963.

30. Marks, H. H. *Influence of obesity on morbidity and mortality.* Bull. New York Acad. Med. 36: #5, 296-312, May 1960.

31. Marks, H. H. *Diabetes, overweight and elevated blood pressure.* Diabetes 11: #6, 544-545, November-December 1962.

32. Medical Tribune. *Elevated triglyceride levels: a role in gout and diabetes?* 6: #91, 14, July 31-August 1, 1965.

33. Medical News. *Stroke patients show various disease states.* J. A. M. A. 194: #9, 30, November 29, 1965.

34. Mikkelsen, W. M. *The possible association of hyperuricemia and/or gout with diabetes mellitus.* Arth. & Rheumat. 8: #5, Part I, 853-859, October 1965.

35. National Dairy Council. *Obesity and its management.* Dairy Council Dig. 36: #3, May-June 1965.

36. Peel, J. *Diabetes and the gynecologist.* Canad. Med. Assn. J. 92: #23, 1195-1202, June 5, 1965.

37. Reyes, E. and Fernando, R. E. *Diseases accompanying diabetes mellitus among diabetics admitted at Mary Johnston Hospital.* J. Fed. Priv. Med. Practit. 13: #11, 741-743, November 1964.

38. Schteingart, D. E. and Conn, J. W. *Characteristics of the increased adrenocortical function observed in many obese patiets.* Ann. New York Acad. Sc. 131: #1, 388-403, October 8, 1965.

39. Spies, T. D. *Some recent advances in nutrition.* J. A. M. A. 167: #6, 675-690, June 7, 1958.

40. Stare, F. J. *Coronary disease and preclinical diabetes.* Nutrit. Rev. 23: #11, 323-326, November 1965.

41. Sullivan, J. F., Lankford, H. G., and Grinnell, E. H. *Serum lipid abnormalities in diabetes mellitus.* Current Therap. Res. 7: #1, 28-34, January 1965.

42. Wiener, S. P., Ward, H. L., and Archer, M. *The rate of deposit of supragingival calculus as an indicator of individuals prone to coronary heart disease: a preliminary study.* J. Chron. Dis. 17: #2, 191-198, February 1964.

43. Yalow, R. S., Glick, S. M., Roth, J., and Berson, S. A. *Plasma insulin and growth hormone levels in obesity and diabetes.* Ann. New York Acad. Sc. 131: #1, 357-373, October 8, 1965.

13. THE OPTIMAL DIET

FROM THE STORY THAT HAS UNFOLDED, SEVERAL CONCLUSIONS ARE evident. First, while widespread starvation or classical malnutrition syndromes are unlikely findings in the United States, trends in food purchases and consumption strongly suggest that the eating patterns of many individuals leave much to be desired. Second, the increase in chronic disease is both real and relative. Third, many of these disease states occur in clusters and are characterized by common, dietary etiologic threads. Finally, the determination of precise dietary requirements is clouded by the subtle and myriad interrelationships of the many nutrients.

An insight into the ingredients of an optimal diet may be derived from observations in three health-disease categories made at three points in the health-disease spectrum. First, it would be informative to analyze the dietary patterns associated with gross illness. Second, it should be equally helpful to study the dietary regimes of those with incipient illness (the incubation period of disease). Lastly, it may prove rewarding to ferret out possible relationships between diet and performance in the relatively healthy subject.

DIETARY PATTERNS AND GROSS ILLNESS

Examination of Table 13.1 reveals the areas of major investigative emphasis concerning diet and the disorders mentioned in Part Two as determined by the volume of reported literature. It will be noted that the principal concern is concentrated in lower animal therapeutic research. The general statement can be made that much is now known about the optimal diet for many lower animal species. From an examination of Table 13.2, it is clear that inanition, suboptimal protein intake, increased sugar consumption, massive vitamin overdose, and vitamin and mineral deficiencies are not conducive to good health in lower animals as measured in terms of the disease states enumerated in Part Two. Conversely, it appears within the limits of these observations that vitamin supplementation particularly promotes optimal health. Obviously, such generalizations, while possibly useful as guidelines, can be misleading and must be interpreted with caution.

In the history of medicine, lower animal investigation has generally been the prelude to human research and, in many instances, to fruitful application. It is noteworthy, from Table 13.3 which summarizes the human findings in Part Two, that the results are quite consistent with observations in lower animals (Table 13.2). For example, good quality diets, relatively high protein regimes, and vitamin supplements seem quite in harmony with optimal health. On the other hand, the converse parallels an increased incidence and severity of disease. Surely, the quantity and quality of the data and the consistency of the findings in lower animals and humans are sufficient to warrant their consideration in the development of an optimal diet.

Table 13.1
relative number of reported observations

disease state	correlative findings lower animal	human	therapeutic findings lower animal	human
infertility			*	
obstetrical complications		*	*	*
congenital defects		*	*	
mental retardation		*	*	*
psychologic disorders			*	*
cancer			*	
ischemic heart disease		*	*	

*major emphasis as determined by volume of reported literature

Table 13.2
summary of findings relating diet and disease states
(lower animal correlative and therapeutic observations)

variable	infertility	obstetrical complications	congenital defects	mental retardation	psychologic disorders	cancer
inanition	+	+	+		+	−
reduced obesity	−					−
induced overeating or obesity	+					+
excessive protein or amino acids	+		+			
low protein	+	+		+	+	
moderate underfeeding						
high fat	+					+
low fat						−
increased sugar	+	+	+			
alcohol supplement	+					
vitamin overdose	+	+	+			
vitamin supplements	−	−	−	−		
vitamin deficiencies	+	+	+	+	+	
vitamin antimetabolites			+		+	
adequate or high protein or amino acid supplement	−			−		
mineral excesses						+
mineral supplements	−					−
mineral deficiencies	+	+		+		+
food contaminants					+	

+ = increased incidence or severity
− = decreased incidence or severity

DIETARY PATTERNS AND THE INCUBATION OF DISEASE

A legitimate complaint which could be registered is that such conclusions regarding the optimal diet are based upon observations made in gross disease states characterized by relatively *specific* symptoms and signs. More often, the so-called healthy citizen is beset with *nonspecific* complaints. In reality, these vague findings may precede by years the full-blown picture of chronic disease. The question which may be reasonably posed is whether the same dietary principles which prove successful in the *treatment* of classical disease are equally effective in the *prevention* of gross disease.

Dietary denominators in diverse disease states have been identified earlier in this chapter. There is general agreement that the *specific* symptoms and signs of most chronic diseases are antedated by *nonspecific* findings (e.g. fatigability, insomnia, headache). Hence, it is in order to scrutinize the diets of persons during this incubation phase of disease for these same dietary denominators.

One technique for detecting these nonspecific findings is a health questionnaire. An attempt has been made to correlate the number of symptoms and signs as measured by the Cornell Medical Index Health Questionnaire *(6)* with the ingestion of several major nutrients (refined carbohydrates, animal protein, nicotinic acid). These foodstuffs, from earlier descriptions, appear to correlate with health and disease. Parenthetic mention should be made that this questionnaire has been studied extensively and the results correlate with absenteeism in industry and performance in the military *(1-5, 14-16)*. Perhaps, for want of a better phrase, one could regard the discussion to follow as an analysis of the diets of *complainers* versus *noncomplainers*.

One phase of this study, the correlation of refined carbohydrate consumption (principally sugar) and cardiovascular findings, has been reported *(9)*. For purposes of this study, 74 dental practitioners and their wives recorded their diets for seven days. Figure 13.1 shows, on the abscissa, the daily refined (processed) carbohydrate consumption. It will be noted that the intake ranged from 6 to 195 grams per day. Near-equal groups were established as shown on the x-axis with 25 individuals consuming the least amount (6-46 grams),

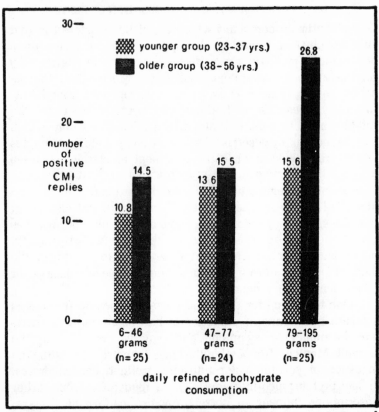

Figure 13.1. The relationship of daily refined carbohydrate consumption and positive responses on the Cornell Medical Index Health Questionnaire.

24 in the middle (47-77 grams), and 25 ingesting the largest quantity (79-195 grams) of refined carbohydrate foodstuffs per day. Each of the subjects also completed the Cornell Medical Index Health Questionnaire. Described on the ordinate are the number of affirmative replies.

Since an important ingredient in chronic disease is its duration, each of the subgroups in terms of carbohydrate consumption has been further subdivided by age. The youngest subject was 23 and the oldest 56. Near-equal subgroups could be derived by dividing the entire sample into a younger group (23-37 years) portrayed by the hatched columns and an older group (38-56 years) pictured by the black bars. Figure 13.1

describes the mean number of positive responses on the Cornell Medical Index for the two age groups. It is clear that, with increasing refined carbohydrate consumption, the mean number of positive replies increases from 10.8 to 13.6 to 15.6 for the relatively younger subjects. In the older age groups the pattern is similar but even more sharply defined (14.5, 15.5, and 26.8).

It would appear, within the limits of these very simple observations, that there are correlations between nonspecific complaints and the daily refined carbohydrate consumption. Furthermore, they are consistent with the findings described throughout this text and earlier in this chapter.

Evidence has been presented in Tables 13.2 and 13.3 to suggest the possibility of a relationship between the daily protein consumption and various disease syndromes. In another phase of this investigation an attempt was made to relate the daily animal protein intake to the number of positive replies on the Cornell Medical Index Health Questionnaire (CMI). A portion of this survey has been released *(10)*. Daily animal protein consumption is the basis for dividing these same subjects into three near-equal subgroups. Overall, the animal protein consumption per day ranged from 9 to 160 grams (Figure 13.2). Twenty-four of the subjects consumed the least amount (9-66 grams); 25 of the individuals ate 67 to 85 grams; 25 subjects consumed 86 to 160 grams. Also, as in the case of carbohydrate intake, the CMI scores are analyzed in terms of age with hatched and black bars for the younger and older groups, respectively. Once again, regardless of food intake, the younger groups demonstrate fewer complaints. However, the greatest score (24.2 per person) is observed in older subjects consuming the least amount of animal protein. In fact, this group reports twice as many affirmative answers as older subjects consuming the greatest amount of animal protein (24.2 versus 12.3). It would appear, from these limited observations, that there are parallelisms between diet and the disease incubation period.

Because so much of the concern about diet and disease centers about vitamin deficiencies and supplementations, the relationship between the Cornell Medical Index Health Questionnaire and one of the common vitamin B fractions was

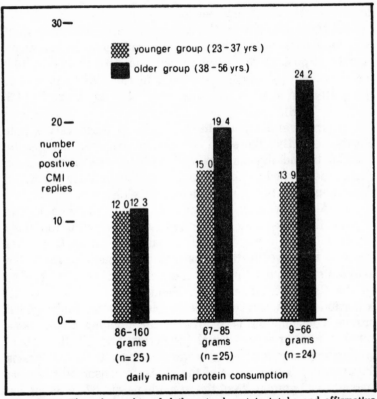

Figure 13.2. The relationship of daily animal protein intake and affirmative responses to the Cornell Medical Index Health Questionnaire.

analyzed. The format is essentially that previously described in connection with refined carbohydrate and protein intake. Figure 13.3 shows the relationship of daily nicotinic acid consumption on the abscissa versus the number of positive replies on the Cornell Medical Index Health Questionnaire on the ordinate. It will be noted that, in the younger age group, the relationship is not sharply defined. In contrast, in the older age bracket, as the intake of nicotinic acid decreases, the number of positive responses rises.

Three points are worthy of special mention. First, the three illustrations given only emphasize relationships and not necessarily cause-and-effect. Second, the three examples cited are designed to underline the correlation of nonspecific

Table 13.3
summary of findings relating diet and disease states
(human correlative and therapeutic observations)

	infertility	obstetrical complications	congenital defects	mental retardation	psychologic disorders	cancer	ischemic heart disease
undernutrition	+				+	−	
caloric excess or obesity		+				+	+
poor quality diet		+	+	+	+	+	
good quality diet	−	−		−		−	
high protein diet	−			−	−		
low protein diet		+	+		+	+	+
low carbohydrate diet			+		−		
sugar increased					−	+	+
sugar decreased	−						−
alcoholism	+					+	
wartime diets	+	+ −	+ −				
vitamin supplements	−	−	−	−	−	−	−
vitamin deficiency	+	+	+	+	+	+	
vitamin decrease or anti-metabolites		+	+	+	+	−	
altered amino acid intake					−		
mineral deficiencies		+	+	+	+	+	+
mineral excesses (especially salt)		+			+	+	
mineral supplements	−					−	−

+ =increased incidence or severity
− =decreased incidence or severity

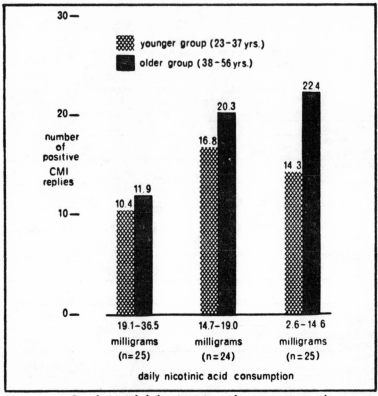

Figure 13.3. Correlation of daily nicotinic acid consumption and response pattern on the Cornell Medical Index Health Questionnaire.

symptoms and signs and common nutrients Lastly, parenthetic mention should be made that an analysis of many other nutrients in this same group of complainers versus noncomplainers provides very similar answers.

PATTERNS IN HEALTH

Weight change is probably one of the most sensitive reflections of metabolic status in the relatively healthy person. Fluctuations in body weight are indicative of changes in metabolic homeostasis. It has been pointed out that obesity enhances the morbidity and mortality from many chronic disorders (Chapter 12, Disease State Interrelationships). The experiment now to be demonstrated has been selected for three reasons. First, it is designed to show the effects of the addition and deprivation of a common nutrient (sugar) upon the health status of presumably healthy dental students. Second, the study is relevant because it deals with a very common metabolic barometer of health and disease, namely weight. Parenthetic mention should be made that a literature search reveals a paucity of evidence concerning the effect of sugars upon weight. Finally, the experiment permits insight into a possible relationship of diet to the incipient states (electrocardiographic) of a major killing and crippling problem, the cardiovascular diseases.

One hundred and twenty-one dental students participated in this experiment. On Monday of a week, at 10:00 A.M. (two hours after breakfast), weight was recorded to the nearest pound. The group was then subdivided into five categories (Table 13.4). Group I (n = 23) was given 50 grams of sucrose (C.P.) in solution twice daily under supervision. Group II (n = 16) received nothing. Group III (n = 21) was supplied three times per day with 75 grams of glucose in solution. Group IV (n = 21) received thrice daily a low calorie artificially sweetened drink indistinguishable in volume or color from the glucose preparation. Finally, Group V (n = 40) was instructed to eliminate refined carbohydrate foods from the diet. On Friday of the same week at precisely the same hour, weight was remeasured by the same examiner with the same scale with no knowledge by the examiner or the student of the earlier scores, the type of supplement, or the nature or purpose of the experiment.

Table 13.4 summarizes the mean weight changes. It will be observed that statistically significant changes occurred with sucrose or glucose supplementation and refined carbohydrate deprivation (11).

It is, of course, true that the statistically significant changes in weight are admittedly very small. However, it must be remembered that these findings occurred within a four-day period in relatively healthy young people. The practical implications are suggested by simple extrapolation. Figure 13.4 pictorially portrays the observed data during the one-week experimental period (the continuous lines) and the projections for one month (assuming, of course, that the re-

Table 13.4
weight response to one-week change in
consumption of refined carbohydrate foodstuffs

group	sample size	supplement	daily dosage	mean weight change (pounds)
I	23	sucrose	100 grams	+0.5*
II	16	none	—	−0.4
III	21	glucose	225 grams	+0.8*
IV	21	low-calorie	—	+0.1
V	40	dietary restriction of refined carbohydrate foodstuffs	—	−1.2*

*statistically significant difference

lationship is linear). It will be observed that a weight gain of 0.8 pounds in one week with a daily 225 gram glucose supplement may mean a 3.2 pound weight rise in approximately one month. In contrast, a 0.5 pound one-week increment with 100 grams of sucrose daily suggests a 2.0 pound weight gain in the four-week period. Finally, the elimination of refined carbohydrate foods from the diet yielded a 1.2 pound weight loss in one week which, extrapolated to 28 days, indicates a projected decrease of 4.8 pounds. This experiment communicates quickly (within one week) and simply (via gross dietary change) a possible relationship of diet (in this case sugar) to a common metabolic barometer of health and disease (weight).

A relatively complete review of the correlation between refined carbohydrate food consumption and ischemic heart disease was presented (Chapter Eleven). Limited studies are available (19,22-24,26) which indicate the effect of these same foodstuffs upon the electrocardiographic picture in relatively healthy individuals.

Like all other diagnostic tools, the significance of the electrocardiographic waves, segments, and intervals can be questioned. However, it is agreed that depression or inversion of the T-wave in Lead I should arouse a suspicion of myocardial pathosis (8,20,21,28,29).

Mention should be made that electrocardiograms were recorded in the student groups (I-IV) at the same time that weight was measured. Table 13.5 summarizes the effects of sucrose and glucose versus placebo supplementation upon T-wave height (Lead I). A significant (P < 0.025) mean decrease of 0.32 mm. occurred in one week in the student group supplied with the glucose supplement *(12)*. Thus, the ingestion of glucose, under these conditions, is not incompatible with developing risk of myocardial pathosis.

The two very simple cause-and-effect studies cited are examples of the physiologic changes which follow the addition and elimination of a common nutrient. Other illustrations could be cited. The cardinal point is to emphasize that the parallelisms enumerated earlier in this chapter do have cause-and-effect implications.

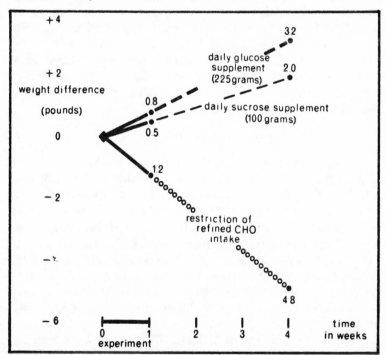

Figure 13.4. Time is pictured on the abscissa showing the one-week experimental period and extrapolation to one month. Weight change is described on the ordinate. The observed findings during one week are shown by the continuous lines; the projected findings by discontinuous lines.

Evidence concerning the influence of dietary patterns in the relatively healthy have also been provided by many other investigators. Performance statistics provide an additional estimate, in the relatively healthy, of the importance of diet and nutrition in the maintenance of optimal health. Table 13.6 clearly shows the significantly improved performance in the vitamin-supplemented group of young military volunteers. The test involved both running a course and carrying out specific coordinated activity *(18)*.

Mention has been made that the ecologic formula for disease recognizes the importance of environmental trauma as it relates to host resistance and susceptibility (Chapter 3, Diet and the Nature of Health and Disease). Hence, one way to view the effect of diet in a healthy man is to observe how well certain dietary foodstuffs change him in the face of environmental challenges. For example, football players at Louisiana State University were randomly divided into two groups on a matched player basis. Water-soluble citrus bioflavonoid and placebo supplements were administered in a double-blind fashion. Not only were the number of injuries reduced in the bioflavonoid group but the days of disability were dramatically decreased (Table 13.7)*(7)*.

PRACTICAL DIETARY GUIDELINES

There are three prime specifications in the formulation of an optimal diet. The regime should avoid those foodstuffs which seem to correlate with disease and should stress those which have been reported to enhance health. Second, it must be economically realistic. Finally, it should be couched in terms readily grasped and understood by the general public. Few people will remember, much less consume, prescribed portions (e.g. ounces, grams) of the various food groups. Probably the best that can be realistically achieved is that certain foods are to be eaten liberally and others sparingly or even avoided.

Findings cited (Tables 13.2 and 13.3) in this book indicate that some nutrients seem to increase susceptibility to disease while others enhance the body's resistance to it. Obviously, the former should be minimized and the latter encouraged. The major flaw in the American diet (Chapter One) appears

Table 13.5
T wave height (Lead I) changes

group	supplement	mean change	P
I (n = 23)	sucrose (100 gms. daily)	−0.02	> 0.500
II (n = 16)	none	+0.01	> 0.500
III (n = 21)	glucose (225 gms. daily)	−0.32	< 0.025*
IV (n = 21)	low-calorie	−0.11	> 0.100

*statistically significant difference

Table 13.6
effect of vitamin and placebo supplementation
for six days on coordinated muscular effort
in healthy young military volunteers

	initial time (seconds)	final time (seconds)	difference (seconds)
group A (ascorbic acid, 100 mg.; riboflavin, 5 mg. and nicotinamide, 50 mg.)	111.3	107.6	−3.7*
group B (riboflavin, 5 mg.; and nicotinamide, 50 mg.)	115.8	113.2	−2.6*
group C (placebo)	121.0	120.5	−0.5

*statistically significant

Table 13.7
effect of citrus bioflavonoid (900 mg. per
day) and placebo supplementation on contact
injuries in Louisiana State University football
players* during the 1962 season

	placebo group (n = 24)	bioflavonoid group (n = 24)
bruises and contusions		
total injuries	27	23
disability days	113	87
sprains		
total injuries	28	14
disability days	164	69

*randomly arranged into two groups on a matched player basis.

to be an excessive consumption of nutrient-poor products. Moreover, their metabolism requires considerable quantities of the vitamins and minerals. They also frequently displace protein, vitamin and mineral-rich foods in the diet and may create a caloric intake in excess of body requirements. Sugar is a cardinal case in point. Table 13.8 (25) emphasizes three facts regarding the sugar (in addition to that which might be naturally present) in foods. First, some foods are almost exclusively pure sugar (e.g. four ounces of hard candy contain 20 teaspoonsful). Second, sugar is frequently hidden in other foods (e.g. sweetened gelatin). Third, while certain products admittedly contain only small quantities of sugar, the nature of their use (e.g. chewing gums and gum drops) makes for overall large sugar intake.

Such foods should be restricted. In their stead, tissue-building foods rich in protein, minerals, and vitamins should be substituted. In other words, while counting calories may be indicated in many instances, making every calorie count in terms of its protein, vitamin, and mineral content may be equally important.

Breakfast, lunch, and dinner menus which make every calorie count, nutrientwise, are compared with inadequate meals in Tables 13.9-13.11. It becomes quite evident that the caloric yield in terms of tissue building nutrients can be markedly increased through wise food selection. The recommended dietary allowances proposed by the National Academy of Sciences (National Research Council) for most Americans *(17)* leaves little room for the intake of nutrient-poor foods. Thus, the prime need in dietary guidance is to make the American public aware of the relative nutrient value of foods. These have been extensively reviewed and published by the United States Department of Agriculture *(13)*.

The selection of a diet is, in part, economically determined. Table 13.12 *(27)* portrays the marked variation in nutrients furnished per ten cents' worth for soft drinks and fruit juices. It is evident that the soft drinks contain only carbohydrate calories. In contrast, the juices contain an array of vital nutrients. Table 13.13 similarly reveals comparative nutrient analysis furnished per dollar of representative foods frequently purchased for household consumption *(27)*. For the same dollar, it is possible to obtain foods rich or poor in nourishment (e.g. eggs versus doughnuts for breakfast).

Table 13.8
approximate amount of sugar added
to popular foods and expressed in
teaspoonsful of granulated sugar

food item	size portion	sugar content in teaspoonsful
hard candy	four ounces	20
chocolate cake (iced)	four ounce piece	10
cherry pie	one slice	10
sherbet	one-half cup	9
ice cream sundae	one	7
donut (glazed)	one	6
jelly	one tablespoon	4-6
rice pudding	one-half cup	5
fig newton	one	5
orangeade	eight ounces	5
jello	one-half cup	4 1/2
ice cream cone	one	3 1/2
fruit salad	one-half cup	3 1/2
chocolate sauce	one tablespoon	3 1/2
cola drink	six ounces	3 1/2
chocolate bar	one & one-half ounces	2 1/2
oatmeal cookie	one	2
gumdrop	one	2
whiskey sour	three ounces	1 1/2
chewing gum	one stick	1/2
lifesavers	one	1/3

Table 13.9
comparative nutritional value of
two isocaloric breakfasts

nutrients	adequate* breakfast (700 calories)	inadequate** breakfast (700 calories)	adequate: inadequate ratio
ascorbic acid (mg.)	50	0.0	50.0
nicotinic acid (mg.)	15	0.6	25.0
phosphorus (mg.)	760	100	7.6
calcium (mg.)	460	65	7.1
riboflavin (mg.)	1.07	0.18	5.9
protein (gram)	45	8	5.6
iodine (mcg.)	17	4	4.3
iron (mg.)	7	2	3.5
vitamin A (I. U.)	4200	1400	3.0
thiamine (mg.)	0.8	0.4	2.0
fat (gram)	40	30	1.3
carbohydrate (gram)	40	100	0.4

* 1/2 grapefruit, 2 eggs, 3 oz. ham, 1 slice whole grain bread
and butter, 1 glass of milk
**3 hot cakes with butter and syrup, 1 cup coffee with sugar
and cream

Table 13.10
comparative nutritional value of
two isocaloric lunches

nutrients	adequate* lunch (655 calories)	inadequate** lunch (655 calories)	adequate: inadequate ratio
riboflavin (mg.)	0.53	0.1	53.0
iodine (mcg.)	34	1.4	24.3
ascorbic acid (mg.)	10	1	10.0
iron (mg.)	4	0.6	6.7
calcium (mg.)	370	75	4.9
vitamin A (I. U.)	1930	420	4.6
phosphorus (mg.)	440	120	3.7
thiamine (mg.)	0.26	0.07	3.7
protein (gram)	28	11	2.5
fat (gram)	27	21	1.3
nicotinic acid (mg.)	3	2.5	1.2
carbohydrate (gram)	75	105	0.7

* 1 bowl vegetable soup, shrimp salad, 1 slice whole grain bread
and butter, 1 glass buttermilk, 1 apple
**1 ham sandwich, 1 soft drink, 1 piece of pie

The basic outline of a desirable diet embraces foods which should be consumed liberally, foodstuffs which must be taken sparingly, and those which should be avoided. Fortunately, the foods to be consumed in liberal amounts are well dispersed in nature. Generally speaking, the most nutritious protein foods are obtained from animal sources (meat, fish, fowl) and should be consumed in generous quantities at each meal. Other excellent sources of protein include eggs, hard cheeses and cottage cheese, and milk (including buttermilk and skim milk). When available, one should eat daily fresh seasonal fruits. Ideally, one should be of the citrus variety. Generally speaking, raw fruits are preferable. Fruit juices may be utilized in addition to fresh fruits and can serve as substitutes for soft drinks and other beverages. Any kind of fruit juice including the canned types, except those with added sugar, are acceptable. Canned fruits are useful when fresh seasonal fruits are not available. However, it is advisable in such instances to use canned fruits with no sugar added. The list of nutrient-rich vegetables is bountiful. Green and yellow vegetables are excellent examples and should be consumed daily both cooked and raw. The potato, properly prepared, is a valuable adjunct. It is evident, from the above description, that the preferred foods are many and varied.

On the other hand, especially by the overweight, there are foodstuffs which should be consumed sparingly. Breads and cereals fit this category. Within this group, the whole grain varieties are preferable. There is an almost universal tendency in the American diet to consume considerable quantities of fats. The reduction of saturated fats provides a more physiologic caloric intake. On the other hand, the fats to be consumed should be largely of the unsaturated type.

Finally, Table 13.8 lists foods illustrative of those to be avoided. Yet, these are the foods commonly consumed because of their reward and snack appeal. The avoidance of such foods in our present culture is extremely difficult. Fruits, fruit juices, nuts, cheeses, and raw vegetables serve as desirable snack or dessert substitutes. Adequate nutrient intake, especially protein, at mealtimes mutes the desire for between meal snacks.

Table 13.11
comparative nutritional value of
two isocaloric dinners

nutrients	adequate* dinner (890 calories)	inadequate** dinner (890 calories)	adequate: inadequate ratio
ascorbic acid (mg.)	90	10	9.0
riboflavin (mg.)	1.4	0.29	4.8
iodine (mcg.)	45	11	4.1
nicotinic acid (mg.)	16	4.5	3.6
calcium (mg.)	600	175	3.4
thiamine (mg.)	0.84	0.26	3.2
phosphorus (mg.)	860	320	2.7
vitamin A (I.U.)	4900	1900	2.6
protein (gram)	70	28	2.5
iron (mg.)	10	4	2.5
fat (gram)	30	40	0.8
carbohydrate (gram)	85	105	0.8

* 4 oz. tomato juice, mixed green salad with vinegar dressing, 6 oz. roast beef, baked potato with 1 square butter, green peas, 1/2 cantaloupe with 1 oz. cheddar cheese, 1 glass buttermilk

** spaghetti and meat balls, mixed green salad with French dressing, French bread and 1 square butter, French pastry, coffee with sugar and cream.

Table 13.12
comparison of nutrients furnished per
ten cents' worth of soft drinks and fruit juices

nutrients	tomato juice (12 oz.)	orange juice (4 oz. frozen)	grapefruit juice (4 oz. frozen)	ginger ale (8 oz.)	cola drinks (8 oz.)
protein (gm.)	3.6	0.4	0.3	0	0
fat (gm.)	0.7	1.0	0.5	0	0
carbohydrate (gm.)	15.0	50.0	52.0	20	19
calories	75.0	200.0	200.0	86	78
calcium (mg.)	25.0	46.0	42.0	0	0
phosphorus (mg.)	54.0	80.0	68.0	0	0
iron (mg.)	1.5	1.4	1.6	0	0
vitamin A (I.U.)	3800.0	440.0	40.0	0	0
thiamine (mg.)	0.2	0.3	0.2	0	0
riboflavin (mg.)	0.1	0.1	0.1	0	0
nicotinic acid (mg.)	2.7	1.0	1.0	0	0
ascorbic acid (mg.)	60.0	180.0	180.0	0	0

Table 13.13
comparative quantities of nutrients furnished
per retail dollar of food frequently purchased

quantity	protein gms.	fat gms.	carbo hydrate gms.	calories	minerals					vitamins				
					calcium mgs.	phosphorus mgs.	Iron mgs.	Iodine mgs.	A I.U.	B1 thiamin mgs.	B2 riboflavin mgs.	nicotinic acid mgs.	ascorbic acid mgs.	D I.U.
6-1/2 lbs. oatmeal	425	220	2046	11700	1590	12150	135	40	-	18	4.2	30	-	-
3 lbs. corn flakes	118	11	1063	4930	5'	993	39	8	4030	6.0	3.2	48	-	-
1-3/4 lbs. leg of lamb	119	116	-	1550	60	1400	17	60	-	1.0	1.5	35	-	-
1-1/4 lbs. bacon	52	370	-	3570	75	610	5	40	-	2.7		11	-	-
1-1/4 quarts ice cream	30	90	150	1500	880	700	0.5	-	-	0.30	1.35	0.5	5	-
5 qts. whole milk	170	190	240	3330	5760	4540	3.5	100	7700	1.75	8.40	6	55	2000
18 eggs	1.0	99	5	1380	470	1820	19.4	30	9900	.72	1.94	1	-	-
30 oz. utility sirloin	142	164	-	2080	80	1270	26.0	96	-	0.70	1.50	34	-	-

In conclusion, the general statement can be made that there is an inverse relationship between the nutrient value of food and its preparation. In this regard, the chief offender is likely to be cooking (Chapter One, The American Diet). Finally, because of the difficulties in food selection and preparation inherent in the American culture, the utilization of nutritional supplements may play a role in approaching an optimal diet.

REFERENCES

1. Brodman, K., Deutschberger, J., Erdmann, A. J., Jr., Lorge, I., and Wolff, H. G. *Prediction of adequacy for military service.* U. S. Armed Forces Med. J. 5: #12, 1802-1808, December 1954.

2. Brodman, K., Erdmann, A. J., Jr., Lorge, I., Deutschberger, J., and Wolff, H. G. *The Cornell Medical Index Health Questionnaire: VII. The prediction of psychosomatic and psychiatric disabilities in army training.* Amer. J. Psychiat. 111: #1, 37-40, July 1954.

3. Brodman, K., Erdmann, A. J., Jr., Lorge, I., and Wolff, H. G. *The Cornell Medical Index: an adjunct to medical interview.* J. A. M. A. 140: #6, 530-534, 11 June 1949.

4. Brodman, K., Erdmann, A. J., Jr., Lorge, I., and Wolff, H. G. *The Cornell Medical Index Health Questionnaire: II. As a diagnostic instrument.* J. A. M. A. 145: #3, 152-157, 20 January 1951.

5. Brodman, K., Erdmann, A. J., Jr., Lorge, I., and Wolff, H. G. *The Cornell Medical Index Health Questionnaire: VI. The relation of patients' complaints to age, sex, race, and education.* J. Gerontol. 8: #3, 339-342, July 1953.

6. Brodman, K., Erdmann, A. J., Jr., and Wolff, H. G. *Cornell Medical Index Health Questionnaire: Manual.* 1949. New York, Cornell University Medical College.

7. Broussard, M. J. *Evaluation of citrus bioflavonoids in contact sports.* Citrus in Med. 2: #2, October 1963.

8. Burch, G. E. and Winsor, T. *A primer of electrocardiography.* Fifth edition. 1966. Philadelphia, Lea and Febiger.

9. Cheraskin, E., Ringsdorf, W. M., Jr., Setyaadmadja, A. T. S. H., and Barrett, R. A. *Carbohydrate consumption and cardiovascular complaints.* Angiology 18: #4, 224-230, April 1967.

10. Cheraskin, E., Ringsdorf, W. M., Jr., Setyaadmadja, A. T. S. H., and Barrett, R. A. *Protein consumption and cardiovascular complaints.* Brit. J. Clin. Pract. (in press)

11. Cheraskin, E., Ringsdorf, W. M., Jr., Setyaadmadja, A. T. S. H., and Barrett, R. A. *The teaching of nutrition to medical students: I. An experiment in weight and processed carbohydrate foodstuffs.* Ala. J. Med. Sc. 4: #3, 311-314, July 1967.

12. Cheraskin, E., Ringsdorf, W, M., Jr., Setyaadmadja, A. T. S. H., and Barrett, R. A. *Effect of carbohydrate foodstuffs upon the height of the T wave in Lead I.* Angiology (in press)

13. Consumer and Food Economics Research Division, Agricultural Research Service, United States Department of Agriculture. *Composition of foods, raw, processed, prepared.* Agriculture

Handbook No. 8. United States Government Printing Office, Washington, D. C., December 1963.

14. Erdmann, A. J., Jr. *Experiencès in use of self-administered health questionnaire.* Arch. Indust. Health 19: #3, 339-344, March 1959.

15. Erdmann, A. J., Jr., Brodman, K., Deutschberger, J., and Wolff, H. G. *Health questionnaire use in an industrial medical department.* Indust. Med. & Surg. 22: #8, 355-357, August 1953.

16. Erdmann, A. J., Jr. Brodman, K., Lorge, I., and Wolff, H. G. *The Cornell Medical Index Health Questionnaire: V. Outpatient admittance department of a general hospital.* J. A. M. A. 149: #6, 550-551, 7 June 1952.

17. Food and Nutrition Board, National Academy of Sciences, National Research Council. *Recommended dietary allowances.* Sixth revised edition. Publication 1146. Washington, D. C. 1964.

18. Frankau, I. M. *Acceleration of coordinated muscular effort by nicotinamide: preliminary report to the medical council.* Brit. Med. J. 2: #4323, 601-603, 13 November 1943.

19. Kilinskii, E. L. and Vysokii, F. F. *Production of electrocardiographic changes in sugar tests.* Fed. Proc. 25: #5, Part II, T794-796, September-October 1966.

20. Lamb, L. E. *Electrocardiography and vectorcardiography, instrumentation, fundamentals and clinical application.* 1965. Philadelphia, W. B. Saunders Company.

21. Massie, E. and Walsh, T. J. *Clinical vectorcardiography and electrocardiography.* 1960. Chicago, The Year Book Publishers.

22. Ostrander, L. D. *The effect of glucose ingestion upon electrocardiograms in an epidemiological study.* Amer. J. Med. Sc. 251: #4, 399-404, April 1966.

23. Ostrander, L. D. and Weinstein, B. J. *Electrocardiographic changes after glucose ingestion.* Circulation 30: #1, 67-76, July 1964.

24. Palma-Garcia, S. and Aspe-Rosas, J. *Postprandial electrocardiographic modifications.* Angiology 15: #4, 174-183, April 1964.

25. Roberts, S. E. *Ear, nose and throat dysfunctions due to deficiencies and imbalances.* 1957. Springfield, Illinois, Charles C. Thomas. p. 115.

26. Sotgin, F. and Tumioto, G. *Modification of the electrocardiogram after glucose administration.* Acta Cardiologica 14: #3, 284-293, 1959.

27. Walsh, M. J. *Nutrition by the calorie and by the dollar.* Beverly Hills, California. 1954.

28. Wolff, L. *Electrocardiography, fundamentals and clinical application.* 1962. Philadelphia, W. B. Saunders Company.

29. Zeisler, E. B. *Electrocardiography, principles and practice.* 1960. Chicago, Login Brothers.

Index